Market Reforms
in Health Care
Current Issues,
New Directions, Strategic Decisions

Edited by Jack A. Meyer

D0930984

American Enterprise Institute for Public Policy Research
Washington and London

Library of Congress Cataloging in Publication Data

Main entry under title:

Market reforms in health care.

    1. Medical care—United States—Cost control—
Congresses. 2. Medical policy—United States—Congresses.
3. Medical care, Cost of—United States—Congresses.
4. Insurance, Health—United States—Congresses.
I. Meyer, Jack, 1944–   . II. Series. [DNLM: 1. Marketing
of health services. 2. Cost control—Trends.
3. Public policy—United States. 4. Quality of health care—
Trends, United States. 5. Delivery of health care—Trends,
United States. W 74   M3456]
RA410.53.M37   1983   362.1'0973   82-22678
ISBN 0-8447-2242-1
ISBN 0-8447-2236-7 (pbk.)

AEI Symposia 82F

Contributors

William J. Baroody, Jr.
American Enterprise Institute

Rosemary Gibson
American Enterprise Institute

Paul B. Ginsburg
Congressional Budget Office

Warren Greenberg
George Washington University

Clark C. Havighurst
School of Law, Duke University

William G. Kopit
Epstein, Becker, Borsody & Green, P.C.

Jack A. Meyer
American Enterprise Institute

Lynn Paringer
School of Business and Economics
California State University

Charles E. Phelps
Rand Corporation

John B. Reiss
Baker & Hostetler

Patricia W. Samors
American Enterprise Institute

William B. Schwartz
Tufts University

Lynn E. Shapiro
Epstein, Becker, Borsody & Green, P.C.

Sean Sullivan
American Enterprise Institute

Amy K. Taylor
National Center for Health Services Research

Burton A. Weisbrod
J. F. Kennedy School of Government
Harvard University

Gail R. Wilensky
National Center for Health Services Research

Contents

Foreword

Since June 1981 AEI's Center for Health Policy Research has conducted a study analyzing the implications of market reform or "procompetitive" health care proposals. The study, funded by The John A. Hartford Foundation of New York City, was designed to explore some of the key decisions and barriers that must be confronted in implementing a system of incentives fostering cost-conscious choices in health care. In addition to assessing objectively the cost-saving and revenue-enhancing potential of market-oriented reforms in health care, the study sought to highlight possible pitfalls that could frustrate the achievement of the goals of the reforms, and to suggest and evaluate alternative means of avoiding these problems.

To guide our research and policy analysis, we established and coordinated five working groups, most of which met twice. The purpose of these meetings was to assemble a diverse group of experts—professors of economics, law, and medicine; government officials; and representatives of private sector groups including insurers, providers, employers, and unions—to identify the legal, economic, and social ramifications of reforming the existing incentive structure.

Each of the five working groups analyzed one aspect of the debate over reform of the health care market. The groups served as advisory panels that guided the study design. The sessions were characterized by open and candid discussion, and no attempt was made to forge a consensus on every issue. I would like to acknowledge each working group participant for his or her expert guidance and substantial effort in ensuring that we explored the relevant issues thoroughly.

This volume has grown out of the task forces' meetings, and the working papers prepared for each group form its core. In addition to revised versions of these working drafts, the volume includes a number of in-house and commissioned papers.

The difficult trade-offs between cost containment and medical efficacy or freedom of choice are examined in the chapters in part one. Conflict over such trade-offs is viewed by some health experts as the primary impediment to cost savings. This part also identifies some of the obstacles to cost-reducing innovations that result from insufficient flexibility in the private contract system covering new financing and delivery arrangements.

The chapters in part two provide the bridge between our interest in federal health policy reforms and the creative initiatives that state and local governments are taking in their own health care markets. The final two parts of this volume examine the tax, regulatory, administrative, and legal implications of implementing market-oriented changes in federal health care policy. Although it appears that there are no insurmountable or wholly intractable legal problems that would undermine market-oriented federal legislative proposals, there are a number of areas where legal or regulatory barriers might thwart or limit fulfillment of the intent of these reforms. The overriding issue raised when analyzing the administrative and tax implications is the trade-off between efficiency and equity.

As part of our work we also prepared an analytical review of private sector initiatives in health care. This effort forged an important link between our analysis of health care and our longstanding interest in the proper and possible role of the private sector in helping to meet a broad spectrum of human needs.

In the past year this interest received heightened attention at AEI as we prepared a comprehensive review of private sector initiatives through detailed case studies in areas such as education, housing, unemployment, child welfare, health care, and youth crime. This study culminated in a volume that also featured a thorough analysis of many government policies that relate to, and sometimes stifle, private efforts addressed to our toughest social problems.

The programs conducted by AEI's Center for Health Policy Research have always focused on issues in the forefront of public debate. In response to the heated discussions over National Health Insurance (NHI) proposals in the 1970s, we analyzed the impact of mandatory national health insurance plans and assessed their potential for solving the problems in health care. As the focus of interest moved to the issues of sharply rising health care costs and market versus regulatory reform, AEI followed the shift. Our publication *A New Approach to the Economics of Health Care,* edited by Mancur Olson, reviewed experiences with health care regulation in the United States and abroad and assessed the general merit of market-oriented changes in health policy. In our current volume we have carried the transition a step further by obtaining practical and detailed information on the consequences of implementing competitive policies and on the pitfalls lying between proposed changes in legislation and a world in which true competition is actualized.

This effort has encouraged us to take a step beyond our recent interest in market-oriented changes in health care policy at the federal level. We have come to realize the importance of efforts being developed by state and local governments that actually change the basic incentives associated with the delivery and financing systems of their Medicaid programs. Thus, our next major project will focus on incentives-based cost-containment initiatives undertaken by state and local governments.

WILLIAM J. BAROODY, JR.
President
American Enterprise Institute

Acknowledgments

The American Enterprise Institute would like to acknowledge the support of The John A. Hartford Foundation of New York City, which enabled us to conduct the program of seminars and research that culminated in this volume. The support of the Hartford Foundation enabled us to assemble on a regular, periodic basis a wide range of knowledgeable health care scholars and practitioners whose advice guided our research. I would like to thank all the participants in these seminars for their willingness to share their insights with us. Many of them also contributed articles to this volume, and I would like to express my appreciation to all the authors.

I am particularly indebted to the staff of AEI's Center for Health Policy Research for their countless hours of work and their continuous advice and assistance. Rosemary Gibson deserves special mention for her multi-faceted and crucial role in the project. She helped devise the initial work plan for the study, participated actively in planning the seminars that shaped the work, contributed a key chapter on new directions in Medicaid policy, and was coauthor of two other chapters. Sean Sullivan also provided invaluable assistance in preparing the seminars and this book, and is the coauthor of three chapters. Patricia Samors, coauthor of two chapters of this volume, provided a link between our studies of health care and private sector initiatives in a variety of social program areas.

I would also like to express my gratitude to Gretchen Erhardt and Melinda Schwenk for their professional typing and clerical assistance, as well as their office management skills, which kept both the seminar program and the book on schedule. Richard Epstein also provided helpful advice regarding the initial design of our seminar program.

JACK A. MEYER
American Enterprise Institute

Market Reforms
in Health Care

Introduction

Jack A. Meyer

The principal problem in health care today is the need for a workable mechanism to achieve a proper balance between acceptable cost and an ensured level of quality. At the core of the trade-off between cost and quality faced by consumers, employers, and state and federal governments is the question of how to pay the providers of health care enough to get them to supply services, but to do so in a way that is affordable for those paying the bill.

This book examines the potential of a new approach to controlling health care costs that features market reforms based on incentives. This approach stresses the need for fair, cost-conscious choices among alternative health plans for consumers and prudent buyer concepts for bill payers. By altering the system of incentives to which providers, insurers, and consumers respond, market-oriented proposals strive to reduce costs while maintaining or enhancing the quality of care and access to it. In place of government regulation of providers, these plans would induce providers to hold down costs because people who chose such providers would reap the savings, while those who chose inefficient providers would pay the extra cost.

Thus, arbitrary cost control is not the core challenge in health care today. The real challenge is to devise methods of cost management that are not inextricably tied to unacceptable service cutbacks or benefit restrictions. The answer lies in finding ways to isolate waste, deny payment for unnecessary care, induce providers to offer services in an efficient way, and induce beneficiaries (consumers) to seek cost-effective care. This book evaluates the potential of the incentives approach for achieving these objectives, isolates the problems facing this approach, and assesses the relative merits of alternative ways of overcoming these problems.

Cost increases associated with technological improvements, an aging population, changing consumer tastes and preferences, and general price inflation explain a considerable amount of the rising cost of care, and these factors are not major reasons for alarm about spending increases if the health care market is functioning well otherwise. There is substantial evidence, however, that this market is not functioning efficiently. Although sector-specific inflation appears to be negligible, rapid increases in the use of health services have contributed significantly to the escalation of health expenditures, and the increased use of the system cannot be fully explained by the rising incomes or relative price effects that have occurred over the last three decades.

A problem for consumers arises from the disparity between the definition of the health care problem offered here and the perspective on the problem typically characterizing public policy. Too often, the government defines the problem through the narrow prism of its own frantic search for ways to bring rising government outlays in line with a shrinking fiscal resource base. As government views it, we have a cost problem, and the objective is to get those costs down. The notion of a trade-off between cost and quality has often become lost in public policy making. The incentives approach to health policy promises to introduce this notion and make it the hallmark of both public and private decision making.

Ironically, while the federal government complains loudly about rising health care costs, its own policies set the tone for cost escalation. Moreover, the federal government's proposed "cures" for cost increases gloss over the fundamental source of inefficiency in the health care system; indeed, in recent years government's solutions have been a part of the problem. Government policy has centered on a "cost pass-through" approach in which the inefficient delivery of services has been rubber-stamped, if not rewarded, while open-ended federal tax breaks have encouraged the use of health care resources beyond the point at which benefits are commensurate with costs. Then, having contributed to cost increases through such policies, the federal government has vainly sought to contain the inevitable outcome of these policies through an elaborate network of cost controls ranging from certificate-of-need programs limiting capital investment projects by hospitals to formulas for allowable increases in hospital charges. These policies entrench inefficiency in the health care system and foster "cost control" at the expense of considerations of the quality and availability of services. By contrast, greater reliance on market-oriented incentives to economize on the use of health services would encourage health care providers to deliver services of acceptable quality at a lower cost.

Budgetary Backdrop

Public policy is now on a collision course. Our government is trying to achieve a major buildup in national defense spending while holding down the tax burden and leaving benefits under some of our most costly social programs untouched. The result is intense pressure on the remaining portion of the federal budget, pressure that will jeopardize the basic nutrition, health, and housing requirements of our most needy citizens.

The squeeze on federal outlays for health care arising from the tension among our national security, economic, and social objectives has led to pressure on state and local governments, private employers, and consumers. The cost of health care is being shifted from the federal government to states in the Medicaid program, to employers and the elderly in Medicare, and to all private-pay patients as government's insufficient reimbursement of providers is "compensated" by corresponding increases in charges to others.

State and local governments, companies, unions, and insurers are desperate for new ideas to contain costs without reneging on commitments to their beneficiaries or employees. Incentives-based reforms are spreading quietly around the country as those who are stuck with a rising portion of the health care tab hope to avert slashing coverage under health insurance policies. Meanwhile, the federal government is still sending out a mixed message. It feeds the escalation of costs and utilization of services through ever more expensive programs for beneficiaries, open-ended tax subsidies, and retrospective cost-based reimbursement with one hand while clamping on new controls with the other.

In this volume, the authors discuss and debate the merits of a federal health care policy that would reinforce and accelerate the market-based reforms cropping up in many local areas. Combining incentives for greater efficiency with deregulation, this approach would permit the federal government to send a consistent, rather than a mixed, message to lower levels of government and the private sector, and then remove itself from the process of experimentation and innovation that is best conducted locally.

The conflict between ongoing social needs and the diminished capacity of the federal government to address these needs necessitates the development of fundamental reforms in the benefit structure, the delivery, and the financing mechanisms of social programs. By delivering adequate social services at a lower cost, we can lessen the need to (1) restrict eligibility, (2) reduce benefits per eligible recipient, and (3) put price controls or new ceilings on service providers that lead to a reduction in services. None of these strategies is desirable.

Regrettably, structural reforms in social programs often fall victim to short-term budgetary concerns. Long-term budgetary reform is sacrificed because of the reluctance of any regime to forgo short-term savings or to incur a temporary upturn in outlays.

To the extent that these opportunities for reform are missed or postponed, efforts by the federal government to cap or to reduce involvement in these programs will only shift to lower levels of government the difficult choices between tax increases, benefit reductions, and price controls. Numerous programs could be redirected from costly delivery mechanisms to more effective strategies that are also more consistent with consumer choice and the dignity of program participants.

The Problem with Regulation

We seem always to be striving for marginal savings in federal health outlays, without sufficient regard for the impact of the regulatory devices used to effect such savings on the quality and accessibility of care. Also we often underestimate the likelihood of "regulatory failure" when we reach for formulas and caps designed to hold down spending. Government regulation of the health care industry has papered over the real problems and failed to arrest cost escalation.

That elaborate controls have not worked should come as no surprise. Government policy responses have typically overlooked the fundamental forces driving spending in health care: open-ended federal tax subsidies to purchase increasingly comprehensive insurance; retrospective cost-based reimbursement systems in both government programs and much of the private market that reward and entrench inefficiency; and, in some cases, ironically, regulation itself, which serves to protect profligate providers and to impede innovators.

The adverse effects of regulation may take years to develop, and they may be a price that today's citizens are willing to pay to release resources now to spend on other goods and services. Before the future of the health care system is mortgaged for yearly budgetary relief, however, new approaches deserve careful study. This book attempts to shed light on the feasibility of an incentives-based alternative to the command-and-control regulatory model that has governed health policy for so long.

Some Guiding Principles

The purpose of this book is to evaluate a set of principles and strategies that constitute an incentives-based approach to health care policy. These principles include: (1) a system of sharing costs that encourages people to economize on the use of routine health services, while offering greater protection from the costs of serious illness; (2) federal aid to low-income people that increases with increasing need, and vice versa; (3) fixed-dollar, instead of open-ended, federal subsidies to aid those unable to purchase adequate health insurance; and (4) fair competition among alternative health care plans.

4

Several legislative proposals introduced in the 97th Congress incorporate these principles: the National Health Care Reform Act, H.R. 850, sponsored by Congressman Richard A. Gephardt (Democrat, Missouri); the Catastrophic Health Expense and Cost Constraint Act, H.R. 7000, sponsored by Congressmen James Jones (Democrat, Oklahoma) and James G. Martin (Republican, North Carolina); the Health Incentives Reform Act, S. 433, sponsored by Senator David Durenberger (Republican, Minnesota); and the Comprehensive Health Care Reform Act, S. 139, sponsored by Senator Orrin G. Hatch (Republican, Utah). This book does not focus exclusively on any of these bills, although occasionally some of their features are compared. Rather, the book assesses a general strategy for implementing these principles of reform through the following measures: (1) a ceiling on the chief open-ended tax subsidy for health care—the tax-free status of employer contributions to employee health insurance; (2) protection against expenses associated with catastrophic illness under Medicare, combined with a greater measure of cost-sharing for routine services; (3) the conversion of Medicare to a program of premium subsidies to be used for Medicare coverage or any qualified alternative plan; (4) continued deregulation of health care in areas such as certificate-of-need and flexibility for states under Medicaid; (5) antitrust law to encourage fair competition among alternative health care plans and providers.

Important new findings by Gail Wilensky and Amy Taylor illustrate the need for a new approach to health cost containment. Some of these findings are presented for the first time in this volume. The work of Wilensky and Taylor and their colleagues at the National Center for Health Services Research provides detailed national estimates of the use of health services, health care expenditures, and health insurance coverage. This work has quantified with a reliable national data base what we have known on a selected regional or anecdotal basis: that most employees have little, if any, choice in health care plans. Where choice exists, the deck is typically stacked against the less expensive plans; nevertheless, many of those who have a choice—even a biased one—are opting for the less expensive coverage.

These conclusions can be linked with the authors' finding of a significant short-term relationship between the amount of insurance purchased and the effective price of insurance (as reflected in the purchaser's marginal tax rate), as well as the likelihood of an even more sizable response to price over the long run. The combination of these findings makes one rather sanguine about the ultimate cost-saving (and revenue-enhancing) potential of a cap on the tax-free nature of employer contributions. A likely scenario is that a tax cap would begin to stimulate multiple choice (even without a requirement for choice), and that, as

5

more individuals have an effective choice, the relationship between the amount of insurance coverage and the price of insurance will become stronger. Thus, a tax cap, in addition to its initial bite, could trigger a series of changes in the employer-based group insurance market that would ultimately enhance the cost savings.

Recent government actions have not significantly reformed Medicare and Medicaid. With a few exceptions, the numerous health care provisions of the Tax Equity and Fiscal Responsibility Act of 1982 (H.R. 4961) that were designed to improve Medicare and Medicaid are a classic example of the Band-Aid approach to the problems of escalating health costs. This act is a collection of measures that shift costs to employers and patients, extend the grip of federal regulation in a vain attempt to close loopholes, cut back provider reimbursement, reduce benefits, and provide small technical corrections.

The Organization of This Book

This volume contains four parts. Part one develops a conceptual framework for assessing the potential of incentives-based reforms in the financing and delivery of health care. The four authors all discuss the trade-offs between cost containment on one hand and the risks, quality, and availability of care on the other. Although the authors present different perspectives on these key issues, the chapters as a group convey the clear message that cost containment will not be "free." Changes in the practice patterns of providers and the purchasing patterns of employers, consumers, and government will not occur without some challenges, nor will these changes unfold overnight. In the first chapter, William Schwartz warns that "much of what is medically effective does not meet standards of economic efficiency," so that the decision to limit the amount of money spent on health care implies that treatment will not be provided to all who might benefit from it. Schwartz argues that the trade-off between cost control and medical efficacy does not mean that we should avoid moving ahead with market reforms. He stresses, however, that the magnitude of truly wasteful, duplicative, or unnecessary health care is not as great as many people believe; this means that achieving greater efficiency will at times entail loss of care that has some value.

In chapter 2, Clark Havighurst explores some of the difficulties in moving away from what is viewed as a uniform standard of care toward a pluralistic system in which differences in either risk or style of care are associated with different costs of care. Havighurst argues that the standards of care currently enforced by the courts reflect medical practices that do little to discourage inappropriate spending. He attempts to encourage the courts to tolerate departures from conventional standards and practices of medical care that could be incorporated in private contracts. For example, insurers, employers, and consumers could design policies that exclude desirable but nonessential services from insurance coverage. Havighurst suggests that, while the courts need to maintain the integrity of contracts and protect consumers against abuse, they need not impose obstacles to private initiation of changes that would make medical practice more efficient.

Warren Greenberg, writing about the effects of competition on health care costs, maintains that the conflict between medical efficacy and economic efficiency is the most important impediment to cost savings. Greenberg notes that removal of the tax-based distortions in the purchase of health insurance would substantially improve the efficiency in the purchase of health services by motivating consumers and providers to scrutinize medical procedures more closely for the benefits they would afford. Greater use of deductibles and copayments would help bring medical efficacy and economic efficiency considerations into line. Yet, according to Greenberg, there are considerable obstacles to making consumers, providers, and insurers more cost-conscious to the point where marginal benefits are commensurate with marginal costs.

Burton Weisbrod in chapter 4 plays the role of skeptic, questioning whether competition can be made to work as economists say it does for a "good" like health care. He suggests three reasons why it may not: (1) consumers lack sufficient information to make economic choices; (2) because of distortions caused by the dominant system of cost reimbursement, the subsidization of health insurance, and the prevalence of third-party payment for medical services, prices fail to reflect the real marginal costs of "production"—leading to overconsumption; (3) the importance of nonproprietary providers makes it uncertain that more competition would result in more efficiency and lower prices. The author does concede, however, that if consumers had better information and if prices could be made to reflect costs more truly, health care would more likely behave like other goods and respond to the forces of competition.

Part two traces new frontiers or battlegrounds in the effort to contain health costs. This section reveals that incentives approaches are now being tried out in Medicaid at the state government level, in Medicare by the federal government, and in the private sector by employers, unions, insurers, and providers. An increased public interest in the states' role in financing and regulating health care has resulted from both block grants and the new regulations that allow states more flexibility in designing their Medicaid programs. In chapter 5, Rosemary Gibson examines state Medicaid developments that test some of the key principles involved in market-oriented health policy. Gibson discusses innovations designed to allow states to be "prudent purchasers" of medical services by steering

7

patients toward more cost-conscious providers, eliminating profligate providers from program involvement, and substituting care at home for institutional care.

In chapter 6, Paul Ginsburg discusses options for changing incentives under the Medicare and Medicaid programs. Three kinds of options are analyzed for Medicare: (1) redesigning benefits to increase cost-sharing for routine outlays while improving catastrophic protection, coupled with policies to counter the existing incentives to buy supplemental coverage that could frustrate efforts to increase cost sharing; (2) paying hospitals on a prospective basis, and health maintenance organizations (HMOs) on a per capita basis for enrollees, to introduce incentives for cost saving in place of the existing reimbursement mechanism; (3) converting Medicare to a fixed-payment voucher system instead of an open-ended entitlement program.

Ginsburg discusses both the administrative issues and the implications for the problem of adverse risk selection associated with a Medicare voucher system. Adverse selection is the process by which consumers choose their health plan on the basis of their expected rate of use of services, so that a disproportionately large number of low-risk consumers choose low-premium plans and high-risk consumers choose high-premium plans. Most analysts agree that, under a voucher system, Medicare would have to establish a minimum set of benefits and supervise enrollment in qualified plans. Ginsburg points out that the adverse selection problem would be less serious under a mandatory voucher scheme than under a voluntary scheme, because a mandatory plan would avoid a situation in which better risks opt for vouchers while high-risk beneficiaries remain in the traditional cost-reimbursement system.

In chapter 7, Lynn Paringer analyzes the implications of applying an incentives approach to long-term care. Paringer explores the use of alternative delivery systems, the role of federal subsidies, and alternative sources of financing long-term care in the private sector. She discusses the special characteristics of the long-term care market that affect the way it functions—such as the lack of private insurance, heavy public sector financing of nursing homes, and the long time dimension of patient service use.

Patricia Samors and Sean Sullivan have studied the role of the private sector in moderating the increase in health costs. In chapter 8, they pinpoint various forms of private sector activities—those sponsored by individual employers, unions, insurers, and providers, as well as coalitions of interested parties in a given community. Some of these initiatives correspond closely with the current procompetitive proposals by trying to change consumer or provider incentives. Most, however, attempt to improve the existing system without altering the basic incentives.

The authors found that a prime example of the incentives approach is the "cafeteria plan" offered by several employers around the country. These plans offer flexible benefits, allowing employers to shape their benefit packages to meet individual needs while giving employees incentives to choose less expensive plans. Wellness programs, offered by companies to promote the health of their employees, and the provision of direct care by companies and unions are examples of approaches that work to lower costs within the framework of the existing health care system.

The final two parts of this volume examine specific issues in federal health policy. They include detailed analysis of the comprehensive market reform plans involving caps on tax subsidies, vouchers for federal health programs, and deregulation. Part three highlights fiscal and administrative issues. It begins with the chapter by Gail Wilensky and Amy Taylor, which presents detailed estimates of the effect on taxpayers and federal revenues of alternative ceilings on the tax-exempt status of employer contributions to health insurance.

In their chapter on tax-related issues in health care market reform, Sean Sullivan and Rosemary Gibson note that growing tax expenditures related to health care now amount to more than $25 billion annually—equaling a third of the government's direct spending on health and exceeding all federal health programs except Medicare. More than three-fourths of this total comes from the unlimited exclusion of employer contributions for health insurance from employee income, and the authors assert that limiting this subsidy would change incentives for consumers, insurers, and providers—reducing the demand for comprehensive health insurance and, thereby, for medical services.

The authors also discuss the arguments for and against offering consumers cash payments for choosing less expensive insurance plans. Some analysts believe that such "rebates" would be necessary to induce consumers to make cost-conscious choices, whereas others feel that the revenue loss and possible exacerbation of adverse selection more than offset any advantages.

Sullivan and Gibson also consider proposals for giving tax credits to all individuals who must purchase their own health insurance. They argue that such a credit would be more equitable than current law, subsidizing everyone instead of just those with generous employers, and that it would begin to effect a fundamental structural change in the marketplace by moving the locus of decision making from the employer to the individual consumer.

Charles Phelps in chapter 11 examines the interrelationships of tax policy, health insurance, and the demand for health care. He cites evidence suggesting that demand increases with insurance coverage, and notes that present tax policies subsidize the provision by employers of extensive coverage to their employees. Consumers often lack an incentive to balance costs against benefits under current market arrangements. Limits on the growth of utilization and the consequent rise of prices would require new market relationships between consumers and providers.

Phelps suggests that some mix of higher deductibles and more co-payments could help to create a more competitive marketplace of price-conscious consumers and cost-conscious providers. He considers the insurance marketplace to be the crucial forum for affecting consumer demand for health care. Evidence does not suggest that tightening the tax deduction for itemized medical expenses (a step taken by Congress in 1982) will have any favorable effect on health costs or prices. Such action could even raise prices by increasing the demand for health insurance. Phelps would rely instead on limiting the subsidy for insurance to reduce demand and, thereby, prices.

In chapter 12, Sean Sullivan and Patricia Samors examine practical questions raised by trying to implement sweeping changes in federal health policies. The core concept of leading reform plans would administer a cap or limit on the tax-free level of employer contributions for employee health insurance. One critical question the authors examine is how to set the limit, whether nationally at a uniform level or regionally to reflect differences in costs.

In addition, Sullivan and Samors examine the administrative process of "qualifying" health care plans, a procedure to be overseen by the Department of Health and Human Services (HHS). They conclude that the systems outlined in the various legislative proposals would impose a considerable administrative burden on both HHS and employers.

The comprehensive proposal by Congressman Gephardt is carefully examined. It would establish its own regulatory apparatus, even though it would dismantle most of the existing regulatory apparatus. The authors also note that the Gephardt plan is the only one that proposes fundamental reform of public programs (Medicare and Medicaid) as well as of the private marketplace.

Part four analyzes regulatory and legal issues relating to an incentives-based plan for federal health policy reform. Chapter 13, on regulatory issues, by Rosemary Gibson and John Reiss, explores a number of areas where regulatory barriers might thwart or limit fulfillment of the intent of these reforms. The authors address the following areas of regulation: state occupational and facility-licensing laws, certificate-of-need programs, hospital regulation, premium taxes on commercial insurers, reserve and other financial requirements, scope of practice limitations, and free-choice-of-doctor provisions. In addition, they cite a variety of federal regulations as possible barriers to market reforms, including federal regulations governing access to care for the indigent, federal forms pertaining to allowable hospital costs, regulatory requirements for the qualification of HMOs, and detailed federal requirements for the physical plant of hospitals.

In chapter 14, Lynn Shapiro provides a thorough review of possible legal impediments and conflicts that could block the implementation of market reforms. Although Shapiro found no insurmountable or wholly intractable legal problems that would undermine market-oriented federal legislative proposals, she did uncover a number of important areas where proposed health care reforms could conflict with other federal laws and trigger challenging litigation. Such challenges, if successful, could partially frustrate or delay fulfillment of the intent of procompetition legislation. In each of these areas, which include labor law, freedom of information, and health-related laws pertaining to certificates of need, Shapiro proposes ways in which the reform proposals could be modified or sharpened to remove the roadblocks.

This part also examines the question of whether existing antitrust doctrine—perhaps with more rigorous enforcement—would be adequate to reinforce and help achieve the basic thrust of the new competitive proposals. A chapter by Clark Havighurst argues that vigorous enforcement of existing antitrust rules would do the job, whereas a chapter by William Kopit suggests that some legal revisions would be necessary. Kopit argues that to encourage a broad choice of insurers for employees, insuring entities will require the right to enter into exclusive or preferential agreements with groups of providers, and that such agreements should be accorded explicit antitrust protections.

Part One

Incentives-Based Reforms:
Assessing the Trade-offs

1

The Competitive Strategy: Will It Affect Quality of Care?

William B. Schwartz

What will be the effect of a successful procompetition strategy on the provision of health services? In relying on market forces to squeeze "wasteful" activities out of the system, will we be significantly affecting the quality of care? Or will cost-consciousness simply rid the system of costly but "unnecessary" activities?

Procompetition legislation would encourage consumers to abandon first-dollar, fee-for-service coverage and to purchase health insurance that either provides membership in a health maintenance organization (HMO) or has a substantial coinsurance feature. Under these circumstances, both patients and providers would become aware of costs and could be expected to modify their behavior.[1] Undoubtedly, fewer medical services would be consumed and dollars would be saved.[2] But to appreciate what, if any, loss of medical benefits would ensue, we must define the kinds of services that might be eliminated. Critical to this analysis is a framework that allows us to examine the meaning of such vague terms as "wasteful" or "unnecessary" care. Only then can we determine whether substantial dollar savings can be achieved while the quality of care is maintained at present levels. Under a leaner, more cost-conscious system, can we have our cake and eat it too, or will fewer dollars mean fewer medical benefits?

"Wasteful" and "Unnecessary" Services

Zero-Benefit Analysis. In a competitive environment, there will be a powerful incentive to eliminate care that yields no perceptible medical benefits. When costs are of no concern, it is easier to request that a battery of blood tests be carried out daily than to decide, on a day-to-day

NOTE: The work of the author cited in this paper was supported in part by a grant from the Robert Wood Johnson Foundation, Princeton, New Jersey.

15

basis, whether additional laboratory studies will yield useful information. Other riskless, painless procedures, such as electrocardiograms and chest X-rays, are also often ordered on a routine basis with little thought to the possible benefits that may accrue. All this will change once the patient faces a coinsurance provision or the HMO physician faces the prospect of wasting the resources of his group practice. Patient and doctor will become sensitive to such expenditures and to the question of whether useful information is being purchased by their dollar investment. Under such circumstances, tests and treatments not expected to yield any benefits will largely disappear from the medical scene. This change in behavior achieves a desirable economic goal without posing any conflict in values. Economic efficiency is achieved without any sacrifice of medical efficacy. Indeed, to the extent that the patient is spared the slight discomfort of a venipuncture, the mild inconvenience in undergoing a chest X-ray, or other annoyances inherent in almost any type of investigative study, some net gain has accrued. The fact that fewer tests mean fewer false positive findings implies an additional saving. Some patients will be spared further investigations or treatments that are often uncomfortable, occasionally harmful, and almost always costly.

By any standard, then, zero-benefit activities can be categorized as "wasteful" and "unnecessary." Clinical experience, and a careful look at the available evidence, strongly suggest, however, that these useless activities contribute a relatively small proportion to the total health care bill. Moreover, it seems improbable that increases in the volume of such activities contribute significantly to the ever-rising costs of hospital care. A recent study provides support for this view.[3]

Production Inefficiencies. Production inefficiencies, which are obviously "wasteful," have been widely identified as a major target in the effort to control expenditures. The incentives provided by competition can be expected to address this problem: Providers will be stimulated to offer service of a given quality at the lowest possible cost.

Policy makers and the public have long believed that a leading contributor to production inefficiency is duplicated hospital facilities. For this reason, the Health Resources Administration (HRA) has established guidelines for number of hospital beds, volume of cases to be carried out in open-heart surgical units, and a variety of other activities. But this regulatory strategy, which was expected to reduce unnecessary expenditures, has had little success. In fact, there is no evidence that certificate of need, the leading policy instrument, has reduced hospital costs significantly, although it may have shifted expenditures and distorted investment patterns.[4]

In a truly competitive environment, without regulation, one might reasonably expect many duplicated facilities to be eliminated. Yet, even if the system responded as anticipated, the effect on hospital costs would be small. This discouraging result comes from a recent study designed to estimate the potential savings from meeting the HRA guidelines.[5] Taking the present demand for care as fixed, the study asked how large a saving could be achieved under the guidelines, and what offsetting costs would be incurred in the process of consolidation. The estimated savings can be interpreted in one of two ways. They represent the amounts that would have been saved had the utilization standards been in effect for many years. Equivalently, they predict the saving that could be achieved in the future by forcing the system to grow into the existing capacity until HRA guidelines are achieved.

The areas examined were the "villains" of facility duplication: computerized axial-tomographic (CAT) scanners, open-heart surgery, cardiac catheterization units, megavoltage radiation units, and general hospital beds. The findings indicated that the theoretical savings from consolidation would be about $1 billion a year. They also indicated, however, that, if this goal were achieved by regulation, offsetting administrative and social costs would eradicate the saving or reduce it to only several hundred million dollars a year. Even in a competitive, nonregulatory environment, dollar and social costs would reduce the potential saving considerably. Moreover, if facilities were reduced in number and were less widely dispersed, some patients would have to travel longer distances for both diagnosis and treatment. They and their families would incur additional travel and costs, and very ill patients would suffer additional discomfort caused by travel. Quality of care would also be impaired. Consider, for example, the patient with a head injury who must be transferred some distance to a CAT scanning unit. The resultant loss of time until a diagnosis was made would, in some instances, be life-threatening. Thus, even in an environment that does not incur regulatory costs, the theoretical saving from eliminating duplication would likely be reduced to a net value of no more than a half billion dollars. This number is not trivial, but its impact on the national hospital expenditures would be slight. An additional small saving might be achieved by consolidating certain other services such as laboratories or laundries, but the magnitude would probably be small and have a negligible impact on overall costs.

Equally important, perhaps, is the fact that much of this gain consists of a one-shot saving. Eliminating excess beds, for example, either by closing hospitals or by forgoing new construction, would reduce the base level of expenditures but would not reduce expenses year after year. After the first year, the reduction would have a minimal effect on the annual rate of increase, the statistic of greatest public concern.

17

Opportunities for reducing production inefficiencies beyond those already considered do, of course, exist. If competition, for instance, led to a shift of additional patients from the inpatient to the outpatient sector, dollars would be saved. Competitive pressures might also be expected to exert downward pressure on the wages and salaries of health care personnel. Organizational slack would presumably be lessened as well. It is far from clear, however, that the resultant saving would be substantial.

To summarize, though competition should reduce production inefficiencies, the saving would most likely not have a major effect on rising hospital costs.

Consumption Inefficiencies. Competition will be effective in controlling hospital costs only if some medical benefits are forgone. Each year brings new technological advances on the medical scene. CAT scanners, open-heart surgery, dialysis, intensive care, and total parenteral nutrition emerged during the 1970s as major contributors to patient care and to medical expenditures. Each of these procedures provides enormous benefits to a few patients, moderate benefits to a further group, and slight benefits to many others. Because the cost is typically high even for the marginal group, a dilemma must be faced. If large numbers of dollars are to be saved by the new cost-consciousness, then much of the high-cost, low-benefit care now being provided will be done away with. Put in different terms, not all care that has positive value will be provided. Cost-benefit analysis will enter the decision-making process, just as it did thirty or forty years ago when few people had health insurance.

Who decides what is provided will depend on whether the patient faces a coinsurance provision or is a member of an HMO. With coinsurance, the patient will decide, along with his doctor, whether the diagnostic study or treatment is worth the expense. In the case of the HMO, the patient is virtually removed from the decision-making process. Instead, the physician will determine whether the benefits are worth the costs, always bearing in mind the effect on the HMO's competitive position. The patient is not likely to be aware that such a cost-benefit analysis is being carried out.

Consider some of the situations facing the cost-conscious consumer or provider. A patient with headaches, for example, consults his doctor, who asks careful questions, conducts an examination and a few simple tests, and, on the basis of this information, diagnoses tension headaches. A CAT scan, which would cost several hundred dollars, could help to rule out the highly unlikely possibility of a serious, treatable cause of the headaches. The doctor explains that the procedure is relatively quick, completely painless, and without risk. If the patient's policy contains an unsatisfied coinsurance or deductible feature, he now has to make a decision. Is the procedure worth the out-of-pocket cost given that the doctor doubts it will show anything? The patient's decision might well be to abandon a course of action that offers only a minute likelihood of yielding useful information.

This list could easily be extended. If a patient has a severe skin rash, the greatest chance for prompt relief of symptoms and quick recovery will often be through consultation with a dermatologist. But some patients will not find the benefit worth the expense and fewer consultations will be sought.

The physician in an HMO faces analogous decisions, made even more difficult by the fact that the group practice must absorb the full cost of the diagnostic procedure and of referring patients to specialists outside the group. In many instances, the physician will reasonably decide that the cost far exceeds any conceivable benefit.

This sort of problem will also face physicians and patients in the domain of therapy. Consider the use of a whole range of therapeutic procedures for a near-terminal illness: a patient found to have metastatic disease at operation, after which serious complications develop. In such a patient, expenditures on an intensive care bed, X-ray studies, laboratory tests, respiratory therapy, dialysis, hyperalimentation, and repeated surgery for various complications might easily amount to $50,000 or $100,000 or more, even when there is no hope of extending his life more than briefly. Moreover, the extra days or weeks of survival are often characterized by pain, discomfort, and deep emotional anguish. In some instances, the patient will be in a coma throughout the terminal care. Each of the treatments is, of course, of great value when used in the appropriate setting. But are the costs of such therapies justified in the circumstances just described?

Similar decisions must be faced in deciding whether to hospitalize. Take, for instance, the patient with an acute kidney infection and a high fever who is seen in the emergency room. Such an individual might be evaluated and treated on an ambulatory basis at low cost and with very small risk, but the likelihood of a serious complication could be further reduced by an expensive admission to the hospital.

Decisions within the hospital will also be affected as the marginal benefits diminish. For example, some patients will have a slightly higher chance of dying if they are transferred out of the intensive care unit early than if they remain under constant, specialized observation. But the costs of reducing an already low likelihood of death may well be enormous.

Cost-consciousness and its effect on health care assume particular importance given the nature of the technological revolution taking place in medicine. In the past, the bulk of expensive diagnostic procedures involved some significant risk to the patient or caused appreciable discomfort or pain. The patient and doctor were thus forced to weigh risks against the potential gain in information and in many instances found that, on medical grounds alone, the procedure could not be justified. Consequently, many diagnostic techniques were limited in use. This has all changed in recent years. Most new tests entail no risk and produce no discomfort, and many of them replace older procedures that were hazardous or painful. As a result, risk-benefit analysis is frequently no longer necessary; the only restraint on their use is dollar cost.

To summarize, the terms "unnecessary" and "wasteful" are meaningful only when defined in both medical terms and economic terms. Clearly, zero-benefit activities and production inefficiencies are unnecessary and wasteful. But the situation is more complicated when care yields some medical benefits. Such care is not wasteful in medical terms; in a world of no resource constraints it would, therefore, be worth providing. But much of what is medically effective does not meet standards of economic efficiency.

Limiting expenditures on health services will doubtless lower the quality of care below what can technically be attained. Incorrect diagnoses will be more frequent, and proper treatment will thus be forgone. Many people are uncomfortable with this prospect. They feel that it is improper, even immoral, to put a dollar price on health or life. In fact, however, we as individuals constantly balance dollars or pleasure against the risk of injury, illness, or death. Collectively, we make such decisions all the time, such as when we decide how much radar equipment to buy for an airport, or whether to regulate smokestack emissions. If we as a society choose to limit the amount of money we spend on health care, we must do so knowing that treatment will not be provided to everyone who might benefit from it.

Notes

1. How much effect coinsurance would have will, of course, depend on the level at which a cap on annual out-of-pocket expenditures is set.

2. See Joseph P. Newhouse and others, "Some Interim Results from a Controlled Trial of Cost Sharing in Health Insurance," *New England Journal of Medicine,* vol. 305 (1981), pp. 1501–7; and Harold S. Luft, "How Do Health-Maintenance Organizations Achieve Their Savings? Rhetoric and Evidence," *New England Journal of Medicine,* vol. 298 (1978), pp. 1336–43.

3. J. A. Showstack, S. A. Schroeder, and M. F. Matsumoto, "Changes in the Use of Medical Technologies, 1972–1977: A Study of 10 Inpatient Diagnoses," *New England Journal of Medicine,* vol. 306 (1982), pp. 706–12.

4. William B. Schwartz, "The Regulation Strategy for Controlling Hospital Costs: Problems and Prospects," *New England Journal of Medicine,* vol. 305 (1981), pp. 1249–55.

5. William B. Schwartz and Paul L. Joskow, "Duplicated Hospital Facilities: How Much Can We Save by Consolidating Them?" *New England Journal of Medicine,* vol. 303 (1980), pp. 1449–57.

2

Decentralizing Decision Making: Private Contract versus Professional Norms

Clark C. Havighurst

Until recently, little in the health policy debate challenged the prevalent assumption that the health care system must operate under prescriptive standards of acceptable care and appropriate spending. Instead, the issue debated was whether the medical profession alone should define these performance limits or whether government should exert an influence. When the advocates of competition entered the discussion, however, they rejected both professional self-regulation and government command-and-control methods as mechanisms for resolving medical-economic issues. Their scenario opened the possibility that consumers would have a chance to decide for themselves in the marketplace what standards of medical practice best suited their preferences and pocketbooks. In essence, the market reformers contemplated that decision-making responsibility could be shifted to the numerous actors on the demand side of the market and that consumers could safely be encouraged to do business with health plans and providers whose practices departed from accepted norms. In particular, procompetition strategists anticipated that cost considerations would be given greater weight in medical decision making if those paying the bills were given a wider range of choice.

One way in which the market-reform advocates could go wrong, however, is by assuming too readily that interacting private parties and institutions would be free and uninhibited in their competitive efforts to translate consumer cost concerns into economizing behavior by providers. In fact, many efficiency-dictated reductions in the quantity,

NOTE: Work on this chapter was supported by Grant No. HS04089 from the National Center for Health Services Research, U.S. Department of Health and Human Services.

quality, and cost of inputs, in utilization levels, and in insurance coverage for marginally beneficial services are quite possibly now inhibited by much more than just the system's weak cost-consciousness. Thus, policy measures strengthening cost-consciousness may fail to trigger the desired economizing reforms. A complete policy analysis must consider the strength of these inhibiting factors and the prospects for their relaxation.

This chapter identifies some possible obstacles to economizing innovation that lie largely outside the realm of public law and regulation and are thus apt to escape the notice of policy makers. The specific concern is the flexibility of the private contract and its utility as a vehicle for introducing new standards in the health care industry. Doctrines of private law—the law of torts and contracts—may impose on private parties duties that are inconsistent with both efficiency and the parties' contractually specified obligations. If such legal doctrines, originally designed to prevent economically powerful interests from overreaching the consumer, stand in the way of departures from prevailing standards of care and practice in the medical care field, market reformers' hopes of seeing consumers offered a full range of choice are doomed to frustration. One purpose of this chapter is to encourage courts to tolerate departures from conventional standards. An analysis of cases construing health insurance policies and enforcing consumers' contracts with organized health plans leads to the conclusion that, if precautions are taken, responsible departures from prevailing standards will probably be upheld. Nevertheless, there is still a serious question whether enough freedom of contract prevails to allow competition to bring about in fact all of the reforms in health care financing and delivery that competition theorists expect it to yield.

The Tyranny of Professional Norms and Standards

Medical-economic decision making reflects surprisingly widespread acceptance, by both government and private parties, of professional standards as determinants of health care spending. Such standards are of two kinds, which together delimit the range of acceptable professional practice. Standards of adequate treatment, which define the minimum level of care that ethical and competent practitioners are expected to provide, represent the lower boundary of this range. The upper end of the spectrum is currently delineated by standards of medical necessity, which purport to distinguish appropriate services from those representing wasteful overutilization of resources. Because both kinds of standards affect the allocation of society's limited resources to medical care, they are of immense public importance. If professionally deter-

23

mined standards cannot reasonably be expected to reflect sensible priorities with respect to resource use, a case can be made for tolerating and even encouraging responsible departures from such standards.

The Nature and Unreliability of Professional Norms. Minimum standards of adequate treatment are imposed on practitioners primarily through the law of medical malpractice. Because the courts draw the standards of care used in detecting professional negligence almost exclusively from prevailing professional custom and practice,[1] individual professionals are under substantial pressure to adhere to the standards of their peers. Indeed, a physician departs from such standards only at the peril of becoming an absolute guarantor against any bad result. From an efficiency standpoint, such rigorous enforcement of adherence to prevailing standards is unwise because customary practice is distorted by third-party financing, a mode of payment that encourages practitioners systematically to discount the cost consequences of their treatment decisions. Many practitioners complain that medical-legal considerations force them to practice "defensive medicine" by ordering tests, X-rays, and other measures that, in their professional judgment, are not cost-effective or necessary for the patient's welfare. Moreover, because physicians are apt to be conservative in judging what care is economically dispensable, the economizing omissions inappropriately deterred by the legal system are probably not limited to measures that doctors regard as defensive. The evidence indicates that physicians and patients should probably be allowed, within limits, to agree upon different standards of care in particular cases or otherwise to mitigate privately the cost-escalating impact of the prevailing standards of adequate treatment.

The other professional norms that are of interest here relate to the appropriateness of spending and generally govern the availability of financing. Private health insurance policies commonly cover all "medically necessary" care or the equivalent, and the Medicare legislation commits the government to pay for care that is "reasonable and necessary." Inevitably, determinations of medical necessity and reasonableness are made by reference to current medical practice, and here again, because of the weakness of economic constraints on medical decision making, prevailing practice may not reflect appropriate attention to the marginal tradeoffs between the benefits derivable and the costs incurred. Physicians treating patients who need not be concerned about the cost of care are free to spend large amounts of money pursuing highly speculative benefits, and they naturally feel ethically obligated to do everything possible to help the patient and not to spare expense simply to protect an insurer or a government program. Because prevailing standards of medical practice do not reflect constrained public or private judgments about spending priorities, private health plans and insurers might reasonably be encouraged to look elsewhere for spending guidance and to draw new lines between covered and non-covered services.

Professional organizations have sometimes explicitly developed professional standards. The most obvious example of such direct self-regulation is the federal program creating Professional Standards Review Organizations (PSROs), by which Congress sought to control the otherwise uncontrollable costs of Medicare and Medicaid entitlements. PSROs are profession-sponsored entities that are assigned statutory responsibility for judging on a case-by-case basis whether care rendered to federal beneficiaries conforms to "appropriate professional standards" and is "medically necessary." [2] This delegation to professional organizations of decisions about the extent of government's payment obligations is a striking demonstration of public acceptance of professionally defined standards.[3] Similarly, committees of local medical associations have long been used by private insurers to resolve disputes over medical necessity and the reasonableness of fees. In addition, PSROs have recently had some success in offering their utilization review services to private payers.

The deference shown to the medical profession as a source of wisdom on medical-economic issues is surprising. Norms drawn from prevailing practice are suspect not only because of the demand distortions introduced by third-party payment but also because of deficiencies in the processes by which clinical practice is shaped. In a recent article, Dr. David M. Eddy states, "Unfortunately, there is reason to believe that there are flaws in the process by which the profession generates clinical policies." [4] He then identifies a large number of problems, in the way clinical policies evolve—specifically, problems in the perspective and methods of researchers, in clinicians' uses of empiricism, and in incentive systems. This catalog of problems suggests, at a minimum, that the profession's customary practices should not be automatically converted into legally binding standards. Surprisingly, few of the accepted methods of clinical practice achieved their status through a scientific demonstration of their superiority in all relevant respects over other methods.[5]

Although individual professionals should be urged to improve their methods of developing, recommending, adopting, and using what Eddy calls clinical policies, profession-sponsored groups seem ultimately unpromising as rectifiers of the errors and inefficiencies embodied in prevailing standards. For one thing, peer-review organizations begin with a strong presumption in favor of existing practice. As representatives of the medical profession, they also have interests directly in conflict with the interests of the public on many of the questions at issue, which concern nothing less than the value that society should place on medical services. Medical organizations also lack much of the expertise and data needed to calculate benefit/cost ratios for society as a whole or otherwise to evaluate particular allocations of society's resources. Entities controlled by the medical profession are therefore unlikely to reduce spending to optimal levels. Although such mechanisms have sometimes induced economizing, these reforms have usually appeared only in response to threats of regulation or competition. Such concessions should thus be viewed more as strategic professional retreats in the face of external pressure than as demonstrations that the profession can subordinate its self-interest and accept economizing as legitimate even when it may sacrifice an arguable increment of quality.

Centralization of medical-economic decisions in the hands of the medical profession imparts to the highly diverse and fragmented health care industry an essentially monopolistic character that should raise further doubts about its economic efficiency. Unlike the typical monopoly, the health care system has not dedicated itself primarily to reducing output in order to raise prices. Instead, the providers of care have striven to prevent financing entities from acting as independent decision makers competing to provide more cost-effective coverage to consumers.[6] To the extent that the passive financing system thus fostered has spared them from having to confront a demand curve reflecting consumers' true willingness to pay, providers have been able to increase output without reducing prices. Thus, in contrast to the usual monopoly problem, the welfare loss attributable to noncompetitive conditions in the medical marketplace has taken the form of an overallocation, rather than an underallocation, of resources to the industry. The problem is thus precisely the one suggested above—namely, that under professionally determined standards the health care industry will provide too many costly services. Because professional norms, whether drawn from prevailing practice or promulgated by profession-sponsored organizations, are questionable guides for social spending, they would seem to deserve substantially less credibility and deference than they currently appear to enjoy.

The Consensus Supporting Centralized Decision Making. Far from struggling against the monopolistic features of the health care industry, the public appears to have accepted them. This acquiescence is reflected in the common tendency to speak of health care as the product of a unitary system rather than an industry. In general, much of what goes on both publicly and privately in the health care sector flows naturally from a deep-seated assumption that monopoly is inevitable and that the medical profession must be looked to as the ultimate decision maker. Although there are signs of increasing willingness to approach the industry differently, old habits of deference die hard.

To a surprising degree, both government and private actors continue to view and to treat the health care industry as a single entity. The acceptance of health maintenance organizations (HMOs) as "alternative delivery systems" implies that they compete against a single dominant system and thus perpetuates the unitary view of the fee-for-service sector. At the same time, numerous specific public and private actions continue to affirm the view that the fee-for-service sector must be dealt with as a monopoly—unless an alternative delivery system can be found. Thus, government and private actors constantly "jawbone" the industry, urging it to improve its collective performance. These interests also look with favor upon such industry-wide cost-containment initiatives as the much vaunted Voluntary Effort to control hospital costs and the development by local medical societies of individual practice associations and foundations for medical care. Local employer coalitions, currently being organized to contain community health care costs, are most often conceived by their founders as exercises in "countervailing power"—that is, as mobilizations to confront and bargain with the system as a single entity rather than as a competitive industry. The numerous employers and insurers who are turning increasingly to PSROs for utilization review services and who are referring disputes over fees and medical necessity to local peer review committees are likewise demonstrating their continued acceptance of the monopoly model of the fee-for-service sector.

In addition to having its standards and its decision-making mechanisms generally accepted by public and private payers, the medical profession has also had great success in getting its essentially monopolistic view of medical practice accepted by its main antagonists in health policy debates. During the 1970s, for example, there was general agreement that the system had to be approached and reformed as a single entity. Not only did the PSRO program reflect the view that a single professionally determined local standard should govern practice under Medicare and Medicaid, but the regulatory programs proposed to control private health care costs embodied a similar unitary view. Thus, advocates of regulation did not propose to dictate medical practice to professionals. Instead, regulation was aimed at rationing care indirectly by limiting the availability of facilities and services (through certificate-of-need laws) and the revenues of hospitals (through rate-setting legislation). It was apparently believed that, under conditions of enforced stringency, practitioners would develop new and more cost-effective standards of practice, thus distributing services equitably in accordance with medical need.

27

Government's choice of this method of rationing reflected not only its own inability or reluctance to ration care directly but also an acceptance of the assumption that standards must be developed through professional processes and imposed on a systemwide basis.

Central in the thinking of regulation advocates has long been an egalitarian impulse calling for a public policy that promises an equivalent standard of care for all citizens. Although achieving this goal would require both drastic rationing and a substantial narrowing (from both ends) of the range of acceptable medical practice, it would require no revision of the conventional conception that medical practice should, in the last analysis, be centrally governed. Indeed, the desire of regulation advocates for equality fits in rather well with the medical profession's view that the health care system should be viewed as a single entity providing a single professionally designed product of uniformly high quality to all citizens. Egalitarian concerns have thus given the medical profession some surprising allies in its effort to maintain ultimate authority over the standards of medical practice. Moreover, the political debate has tended to define perceptions in the private sector, contributing to the development of a strong entitlement mentality in employer-sponsored health plans and to the general agreement of employers and insurers with the medical profession's views on the nature of the system and the appropriateness of centralized decision making.

Implications of the Competition Strategy

The competition strategy represents a direct challenge to the conception of the health care industry as a monolithic system offering a single class of service. Specifically, it rejects the medical profession's view that, subject only to limited economic constraints such as cost sharing, practitioners should be guaranteed clinical freedom within a broad range of acceptable practice delineated by standards derived either by observing professional practice or by consulting informed professional opinion. The theory underlying the competition strategy is also incompatible with the egalitarian model of the health care system, though it in no way precludes (and indeed contemplates) government subsidies to ensure the availability of good quality care to needy citizens. In sum, the procompetition movement proposes to substitute a demand-side reform strategy for strategies premised upon the view that the health care system is a single entity that must be managed and reformed by some combination of professional self-discipline and government regulation.

Viewing health services as the product of a competitive industry that can reasonably be expected to respond to consumer demand, competition advocates counsel reliance on consumer choice among a variety of independent financing and delivery systems as the means to ensure efficiency in resource use. Their advocacy of reforms aimed at strengthening consumer cost-consciousness assumes that reforms in the financing system can eventually ensure that signals from the demand side of the market are effectively transmitted to the supply side. Competition proponents limit their concerns on the supply side of the market to removing restraints on the ability of insurers and providers to respond to the consumer preferences being communicated. They thus object to most regulatory prescriptions concerning the organization and financing of services and favor antitrust enforcement to eliminate profession-sponsored restraints on innovation in these areas. Implicit in the competition advocates' message is the idea that there is no single right way to organize health care delivery or to treat particular diseases and that, with accountability to consumers ensured in the marketplace, decisions on such sensitive and significant matters can safely be entrusted to private actors. In place of the prevalent assumption that change can occur legitimately only by altering professional standards across the board, these theorists welcome the prospect of diversity and deviations from professional consensus.

Although traditional health insurers compete intensely in some respects, they have to date made little progress in forcing providers into a competitive mode. For reasons that are exceedingly complex,[7] competing insurers have lacked, or have been unwilling to exercise, the independence needed to challenge the monolithic system and the professionally dictated standards that ultimately govern its performance. Competition adherents believe, however, that insurers have the potential to act as aggressive purchasers rather than passive reimbursers of costs incurred by providers or by their insureds, and that insurers can introduce price sensitivity and competition by tailoring their benefits and coverage in ways enhancing the cost-effectiveness of the coverage provided.[8] In time, competition advocates believe, payment systems will be driven by competitive pressures to change in ways that force providers into price competition, thus finally invalidating the economic assumptions on which cost-containment regulation has historically been based.

Progress in breaking down the system's general acceptance of professional norms and standards may be slow because of the credibility and apparent legitimacy those norms and standards enjoy. Interestingly, group-practice HMOs, the vanguard of the competition movement, may owe their past success to their ability to introduce efficiency without having explicitly to declare their independence from the tyranny of professional standards. Although their contracts with subscribers provide coverage at least as comprehensive as that of private health insurance, such HMOs' integration of delivery and financing precludes open conflicts with providers—such as insurers encounter—over the appropriateness of particular outlays. Thus, group-practice HMOs can readily limit coverage to those services that their own physicians deem essential without having to justify their refusal to cover the more extensive or costly care dictated by dominant norms. Although HMOs may still not be as independent as a competition advocate might wish, they have apparently succeeded in replacing profession-dictated standards of medical necessity and appropriateness with standards of their own. A lesson from their success may be that innovations in the style of medical practice are easier if they are not explicitly presented as departures from prevailing standards. The same public that has tolerated and even applauded the reluctance of HMOs to hospitalize their patients would probably be slow to accept the use by insurers of internal rather than profession-sponsored committees to review the hospitalization decisions of independent physicians.

The competition strategy may not bear much immediate fruit because of inertia born of long acceptance of the monopoly model and acquiescence in professional norms and standards. Nevertheless, the antitrust laws are gradually breaking down the industry's monopolistic features, removing many of the self-regulatory controls that the system has hitherto used in responding to pressures to control costs.[9] Once industry-sponsored cost containment is seen to be unlawful, private purchasers will be forced to consider how to solve their own cost problems, and they can be expected to approach insurers and providers more and more as cost-conscious buyers approach competing sellers. Important benefits are likely to flow from thus opening the door to privately negotiated change. Even if the deviations from established patterns are infrequent and tentative, much might be learned from them. Thus, if innovators discover that they can provide the same quality of care as the dominant system for a lower cost, or better quality care for the same price, their market shares will expand, and others will be encouraged to embark on similar paths. Whether some consumers would be willing to sacrifice bits of arguable quality in order to obtain cash savings cannot be known until the choice is offered, but decisions to economize by forgoing some measures are not irrational on their face. As braver souls discover that certain kinds of economizing do not carry grave risks, others will follow, ultimately causing the symbolic significance of professional standards to decline. The competitive marketplace, in which unreasonable demands and unexamined preferences may carry higher price tags, is the best arena in which to educate consumers and others to the high cost of accepting professionally developed norms and standards.

Although we cannot know for certain that too much is currently being spent on health care or that money is being spent in the wrong ways, we do know that the professionally dominated system, which has yielded the present level and pattern of spending, cannot be depended upon to reflect consumers' wishes about how their resources are employed. A competitive market provides the basis for a strong presumption that the allocation of resources prevailing at any point fairly reflects consumers' desires. The essential prerequisite for establishing such a competitive regime in medical care is the decentralization of decision making on the standards of medical practice and the scope of health care financing. Progress on this front has begun but could be blocked in many ways. The remainder of this chapter considers the risk that the judiciary will fail to respect private economizing choices and will refuse to enforce private contracts that explicitly depart from accepted standards.

Varying Professional Standards of Adequate Care

As noted earlier, the standard of care enforced by the tort system is not demonstrably efficient. It reflects medical practice under a financing system that does little to discourage inappropriate spending and incorporates many defensive practices undertaken not for the patient's benefit but in anticipation of possible litigation. Moreover, much medical practice has never been subjected to careful scrutiny for efficaciousness, let alone cost-effectiveness. As a result, customary practice probably incorporates many procedures that could readily be avoided without harm to the patient. Many other procedures, though positively beneficial to the patient, may not be enough so in statistical terms to warrant incurring the expense as a social cost—though a patient, with professional advice, might elect to purchase the service himself. For these reasons, deviations from professional norms of practice may frequently be desirable. By the same token, judicial insistence on adherence to such norms may be destructive.

The question for consideration here is whether courts will enforce contractual provisions in which a patient authorizes a physician to depart from customary practice or absolves the physician of the usual legal consequences of such a departure. The answer to this question may illuminate the true extent of society's submission to professional norms and standards as determinants of medical-economic issues. A finding that courts would be unwilling to enforce reasonable contractual provisions under which patients give up the presumed protections of the tort system would diminish the prospects for achieving efficiency through competition.

Contractual Waivers of Malpractice Rights. The case for relying more on private contract and less on judicially developed tort rules in the medical malpractice field has been argued by Richard A. Epstein of the University of Chicago Law School as follows:

31

When malpractice cases are treated as though they raise only tort [as opposed to contract] issues, there is the unmistakable tendency to treat the judicial rules as the inflexible commands of positive law. It becomes, therefore, a natural if unfortunate tendency for courts to overlook the possibility, indeed the desirability, of having the rules that they have laid down varied by the agreements between the parties. Where the situation is looked upon as contractual, the basic rules governing the relationship between physician and patient are then best understood as approximations of the rules which the parties themselves would choose to govern their own relationship. . . . The problem with medical malpractice is that the legal relationships fashioned by the courts do not begin to approximate on many points the contractual solutions that the parties would choose, or have chosen, for themselves. The problem with much of the modern approach to medical malpractice lies in the great willingness, even eagerness, of both courts and legislatures to respond to private law problems with public policy solutions. . . . And the rules that have been adopted and proposed, whether concerned with informed consent, the place of custom in setting the standard of care, the measure of damages, or any of the other issues discussed in the body of this paper, are very poor substitutes [for contractual rules] indeed. We need in the context of medical malpractice less government, and not more government; we need greater respect for private initiative and control; and we need a return to the passive virtues of both judicial and legislative statesmanship.[10]

Arguing that contractual variations on the common-law allocation of risks should not be viewed with suspicion, Epstein goes so far as to contend that patients' agreements to waive their malpractice rights altogether should generally be enforced.[11]

Despite Epstein's logic and the widespread dissatisfaction with the law of medical malpractice, courts are reluctant to allow patients to waive their rights under the tort system. Indeed, in the recent case of *Emory University* v. *Porubiansky,* the Georgia Supreme Court refused to enforce an exculpatory clause even though the service, provided by a university dental clinic, was obtained for a lower price.[12] Without reaching the question whether the plaintiff had been misled or overreached in some way, the court held that the clause violated public policy as expressed in a statute authorizing recovery for a dentist's failure to exercise "a reasonable degree of care and skill." Other courts have also consistently refused to give effect to exculpatory clauses waiving professional liability.[13]

The *Emory University* case involved an attempt to economize by shifting the entire risk of the defendant's incompetence to the plaintiff and to escape liability for a broken jaw suffered in the course of dental treatment. It is therefore arguable that the decision might not govern an explicit attempt to contract, not for complete immunity, but for a reduced standard of care—that is, a standard different from the one supplied by tort doctrine in the absence of a contractual delineation of rights. Thus, a contract that limits liability to cases of gross negligence, or one that acknowledges the provider's right to depart in good faith from conventional standards, or one that seeks to define a "reasonable degree of care and skill" (in the terms of the Georgia statute) might be viewed more tolerantly than an exculpatory clause.[14] The question is what it would take to persuade a court to accept the contract's test for liability in lieu of the legal/professional standard.

The case for tolerating contractual departures from prevailing norms rests on much more than Epstein's general theories of tort law and his preference for "a return to a legal regime with enough faith in the intelligence and good will of its people."[15] Epstein fails, for example, to make the argument that, where third-party payment prevails, customary practice is poor evidence of what competing sellers and cost-conscious buyers would actually agree upon and is thus not a presumptively valid guide to efficient resource use. Furthermore, the protection given to consumers by the tort system is probably not what contracting parties would elect for themselves—which is another way of saying that it is not worth its high cost. In effect, malpractice law supplies patients with a kind of insurance that protects them against only a few of the many injuries they may suffer, duplicates coverage (life, disability, and health insurance) that most of them already possess, and is very costly to administer. It is thus far from obvious that such protection should be compulsory—that is, that consumers should be denied the right to reject that protection and to substitute a different allocation of risks. The discussion below suggests that at least some contractual variations on tort doctrine have enough merit and apparent legitimacy that courts should accept them.

An HMO's Dilemma. A helpful and realistic illustration of the need for some contractual freedom emerged in a conversation this writer once had with an HMO administrator who reported that his plan's physicians felt compelled to provide fetal monitoring for all pregnant women because that was the standard of care prevailing in the community. The other member of our party, Professor Alain Enthoven, rightly observed that this practice is not good medicine because fetal monitoring has been shown to be of no benefit and some risk in a majority of cases.[16] Nevertheless, we elected to approach the matter on the

33

more controversial basis that the service, even if beneficial, should be dispensed with whenever it is not worth its cost.

Our discussion then focused on how the HMO could go about altering its practice without paying a malpractice claim whenever a jury thought that a bad outcome might have been prevented. We first considered some malpractice defenses that might work, among them the doctrine permitting a practitioner to adhere to the standards of a "reputable minority" or a separate "school of practice" that might exist within the profession.[17] Although the idea that HMOs might be subject to their own national standard of care as a reputable minority or separate school has apparently not been tested, its judicial acceptance would go some way toward recognizing the virtues of diversity. It would not, however, establish that private contracts alone can define the standard of care. Unless contracts could vary from the relevant standard, experimentation would be penalized and parties would be denied the chance to develop, in Epstein's phrase, "individuated responses to their practical problems."[18]

Our conversation next turned to whether the HMO's subscriber contracts should be written to exclude fetal monitoring as a covered service in the absence of specified clinical circumstances. Although contractual fine print alone might not be enough to deter a court from imposing liability for omitting the service, the contract might be enforced if it were backed by expert testimony showing that the standard was reasonable. Obviously, however, the HMO would wish to avoid having to litigate the standard's reasonableness. Indeed, it might be willing to change its practice only if it was assured by its lawyers that the contract raised at least a presumption of validity.

In order for the contract to be presumptively enforceable, a court would have to be satisfied that subscribers had knowledge of the limits of the plan's obligations and an opportunity to bargain about them. In this connection, we considered whether it would help to ask the consumer advisory panel maintained by the plan to approve the omission of the service in appropriate cases. (We were told that the head of this panel was a feminist with an antitechnology bias who would undoubtedly oppose fetal monitoring.) Such ratification would obviously strengthen the legitimacy of a contract provision by demonstrating the plan's conscientiousness and willingness to bargain. Moreover, in the case of minor deviations from accepted practice or complex departures that would be hard to spell out in the contract, consultation with an advisory committee would show that the plan's practices were negotiable and not unilaterally imposed.

The clear desirability of allowing this HMO to limit its use of fetal montioring demonstrates why private decision makers should be allowed to determine their own obligations, rights, and conduct.[19] Nevertheless, a court asked to rectify a hardship encountered by some individual will not easily be convinced that the individual voluntarily assumed that particular risk. Contractual provisions are not necessarily conclusive, particularly if bargaining power was arguably unequal, if disclosure was arguably incomplete, or if no other option was offered or readily available. As a result, private health plans not only must be careful to define and limit their obligations clearly but also must be prepared to demonstrate that the contracting process gave adequate assurance that the bargain struck accommodated the interests of both parties. Although broad waivers of liability are likely to be too much for most courts to swallow, less sweeping and less seemingly unilateral departures from the dictates of the tort system should be defensible if steps are carefully taken and a proper record is made. Thus, an organized health plan acting in good faith and meeting its responsibilities for disclosure can probably avoid malpractice suits based on nothing more than deviation from prevailing standards. Unfortunately, this conclusion is not entirely secure because of a lack of legal precedents. Nevertheless, the legal doctrines discussed below indicate that private arrangements meeting reasonable requirements will usually be upheld.

Contracting Out of the Tort System. There are several theories under which courts evaluate contractual provisions that derogate in some respect from the patient's right to sue for medical malpractice. The initial inquiry is likely to be to determine whether the contract in question is a "contract of adhesion"—that is, an agreement imposed on the patient under circumstances limiting the patient's opportunity to bargain for a different arrangement or to choose an alternative provider.[20] Although an adhesion contract may be enforced, a court can be expected to take special pains to assure itself that the terms of the contract are equitable. Moreover, even if a contract is not an adhesion contract, a court may still refuse to enforce a term that it finds unconscionable[21] or that violates public policy in some respect. As noted earlier, blanket exculpatory clauses have been found to be inconsistent with general public policy toward professionals and thus held unenforceable regardless of whether the contracts containing them were adhesive. Courts are less likely to use these doctrines to invalidate a contract term, however, if they are satisfied by all the circumstances that the agreement was arrived at fairly.

Some help in identifying adhesion contracts comes from a series of California cases involving the enforceability of agreements to arbitrate future medical malpractice claims.[22] Though notoriously plaintiff-oriented, the California Supreme Court has required malpractice plaintiffs lacking actual knowledge of the arbitration clause to submit to

35

unwanted arbitration in accordance with their HMO subscriber contracts. The leading case is *Madden* v. *Kaiser Foundation Hospitals*.[23] In that case, the state, acting as the plaintiff's employer, had agreed to the arbitration clause, and the plaintiff had selected the HMO from a list of alternative plans, including some that did not require arbitration. The court upheld the clause, finding that the contract was not one of adhesion and that the state had implied authority to agree to the clause in question. In other cases, California courts have refused to enforce arbitration clauses because of differences in the bargaining circumstances.[24] In one such case, the court refused because of the one-sided nature of the clause, which bound only the subscriber to arbitration.[25]

Although the *Madden* decision allowed the parties to alter an important feature of the tort system by contract, a future plaintiff could easily distinguish that case from one involving an attempted variation of the applicable standard of care. The court's decision rested firmly on the public policy favoring the use of arbitration to resolve disputes, a policy based on efficiency considerations. Thus, unless a future court could be independently persuaded of the possible desirability of substituting a different standard of care for the judicially set standard, it might refuse to enforce a clause purporting to establish a reduced standard or to omit some customary practice. Indeed, the court in *Madden* emphasized that the arbitration clause "does not detract from Kaiser's duty to use reasonable care in treating patients, nor limit its liability for breach of this duty, but merely substitutes one forum for another."[26] Despite this technical distinction, however, an arbitration clause can affect substantive outcomes and cannot be entirely disassociated from other contractual specifications of the parties' rights and duties.[27] Thus, willingness to enforce arbitration bodes well for the enforceability of other private agreements.

In upholding the arbitration clause, the *Madden* court emphasized that, in addition to bearing "equally on Kaiser and the members," it benefited the latter by "facilitat[ing] the adjudication of minor malpractice claims which cannot economically be resolved in a judicial forum."[28] A court looking for comparable mutuality of benefit in each discrete provision of a contract would be troubled by the seeming one-sidedness of a provision relaxing the standard of care. Indeed, unless it was willing to assume, on the basis of satisfactory bargaining circumstances, that the patients had received compensating benefits in the form of a reduced price or otherwise, such a court would inevitably refuse to enforce any simple relaxation of judicially set standards. Nevertheless, such paternalism might well be tempered upon a showing that the contracting process gave consumers adequate opportunities to protect themselves. In any event, many courts are less paternalistic than California's and should be willing to adopt "the contractarian view."

Given judicial concern about apparent mutuality, a private health plan might feel that its best bet for obtaining relief would lie in offering an explicit quid pro quo in the form of an alternative injury compensation system based on no-fault principles.[29] Thus, the plan might offer to insure the patient against certain adverse medical outcomes—"designated compensable events"[30]—without regard to the existence of fault. Because elimination of the fault issue would save large administrative costs, the plan should be able, without additional expense, to offer its members adequate, predictable protection against a wider class of risks than the tort system currently covers. Moreover, the plan would continue to have an incentive to prevent the occurrence of compensable events, thus obviating the most serious public policy objection to exculpatory clauses. As long as the bargaining process supplied protections similar to those in the *Madden* case, a court should be satisfied that the consumer's interest is protected. Although the mechanics of a no-fault scheme have not been fully developed, enough work has been done to suggest its feasibility.[31] Moreover, no better solution to the malpractice problem has appeared.[32] The tantalizing prospect of achieving fundamental reform of the tort system through private contract nicely demonstrates the potential power of competition as a vehicle of change in the health care industry.

Because the plaintiff in the *Madden* case had the protection of both his employer's representation of his interests and an opportunity to reject the HMO, it might be asked whether the absence of either of these two forms of protection—sophisticated representation and individual choice—would change the result. This is an important question, since different versions of the procompetition strategy would locate the responsibility for choice in different places. Some competition advocates, for example, wish to see the employer's decision-making role strengthened.[33] Others, however, contemplate the elimination of the employer as intermediary and the offering to all citizens of an opportunity to choose from a government-maintained list of plans.[34] The set of proposals most in keeping with the *Madden* case would mandate that each employer offer "multiple choice" among several plans that it initially selects.[35] Even in the absence of such a mandate, of course, an employer might prefer to let individual employees make the final choice to avoid the charge that it was shortchanging the workers.[36] Although courts should probably accept the consequences of an economizing decision made either by the consumer himself or by someone representing his interests, the closer one could come to the *Madden* paradigm the better the prospect that a contractual innovation would be enforced. Some additional reasons for adopting multiple choice, equally applicable here, appear in the discussion below.

37

Varying Professional Standards of Medical Necessity and Appropriateness of Spending

Health care plans vary in the degree to which they are independent, integrated providers of care maintaining internal quality and cost controls. An example of a tightly integrated plan is a group practice HMO, which offers a single standard of care to all patients and leaves no room for subscribers to purchase more or less service than the plan provides.[37] Thus, in the conversation described above, the idea of making fetal monitoring optional (for an extra fee) in all but high-risk cases was rejected because it violated the HMO's conception of itself as a fully integrated plan committed to providing a single style of prepaid care. This refusal to countenance choice within the HMO system, in addition to being an echo of the larger system's adherence to a single set of professionally designed standards, points up both the value of the HMO model in offering a clear-cut alternative to the dominant system and its drawback in limiting further choice.

An arguable advantage of less integrated health plans—both service-benefit and pure insurance arrangements—is that, since they do not hold themselves out as providers, they are potentially in a position to offer consumers a range of choice, including self-payment options of the kind the HMO was reluctant to provide in the fetal-monitoring case. Thus, instead of underwriting all "medically necessary" care, an insurer might exclude from coverage certain services that are of questionable value in many cases.[38] Nevertheless, the use of such exclusions to induce cost-conscious choice in grey areas is inhibited by the widespread acceptance of the view that insurers should pay for any service that falls within the range of professionally acceptable practice. Whereas previous discussion considered the validity of contractual arrangements altering the malpractice standard of care applicable to a provider, this discussion examines the enforceability of contract provisions by which insurers seek to avoid having to reimburse subscribers for any service a physician can prescribe without facing professional sanction.

The effect of excluding desirable but nonessential services from insurance coverage would be to encourage doctors and patients to economize within the professionally accepted range of practice. As noted earlier, HMOs have succeeded in part because they accomplish such economizing implicitly. On the other hand, explicit exclusion of desirable services from coverage raises more questions in people's minds than an HMO's less visible economizing. Unlike HMOs, however, insurers do not altogether foreclose consumer choice when they refuse coverage of marginally beneficial care. Thus, precisely because HMOs cannot or will not respond well to differing individual preferences, it is desirable to facilitate privately initiated reforms in third-party insurance. These reforms will lead to a greater diversity of health plans and to increased opportunities for cost-conscious choice in the fee-for-service sector. A truly competitive market that is responsive to consumers' individual concerns and circumstances cannot be said to exist if HMOs represent the only economizing option and if the fee-for-service sector must continue to operate, however clumsily, as a single economic unit. Thus, procompetition strategists need to consider whether insurers' contractual limitations on their payment obligations will be enforced by the courts so that cost-consciousness can be restored in doctor-patient decision making.

Because insurance policies usually have all the earmarks of adhesion contracts, the law of insurance is an extreme case of judicial reluctance to enforce contractual fine print. Issues of insurance coverage are generally addressed under the doctrine of "reasonable expectations," which allows courts to enforce insurer-induced expectations rather than the language of the insurance policy. Professor Kenneth Abraham has observed that the doctrine has two aspects, the first designed to rectify misleading impressions that the insurer may have created and the other designed to eliminate unfair gaps in coverage.[39] Only the second branch of the doctrine threatens conclusively to defeat health insurers' efforts to employ selective coverage as a cost-containment strategy. The first element of the expectations doctrine, while posing certain problems, promises to make the administration of selective health insurance coverage more tolerable than it would otherwise be.

Obviously, an insurer should not be allowed to mislead its policyholders concerning the coverage provided.[40] Where there is a discrepancy between the sales literature and the policy, the former should certainly be binding since that is likely to be all the insured ever reads. A legal rule holding an insurer strictly to the representations it makes and to the impressions it creates will induce full disclosure, thus making the competitive market work better. Furthermore, the courts could usefully require affirmative disclosure to overcome mistaken assumptions that the insured might reasonably harbor. Thus, the mere act of selling "health insurance" without affirmatively disclosing unusual gaps in coverage could itself be deemed misleading.

If the policy exclusions were at all technical or complex, merely giving a brochure to the insured would not necessarily satisfy the insurer's obligation to overcome the policyholder's misconceptions. Indeed, because the insured patient cannot reasonably be expected to control his own medical treatment, nothing short of notifying the physician of specific coverage limitations would effectively offset the natural expectation of both the treating physician and the patient that all "medically necessary" services would be paid for.[41] On the other hand, an insurer could fairly insist on compliance with preconditions of coverage that are easily disclosed and understood.[42] Thus, an insured who was given reasonable notice would probably be bound by a policy that covered nonemergency care only if it was rendered or prescribed by a "participating" provider (as in a primary care network) or only if the insurer certified coverage in advance (as in the case of plans requiring preadmission certification or predetermination of benefits). In addition to meeting a court's concern about induced reliance on false impressions, provisions like these would probably prove to be the most practical and acceptable methods of effecting selective coverage and of putting physicians and patients in the position of making informed, cost-conscious choices about noncovered care.

The other facet of the reasonable expectations doctrine, however, threatens to undercut the possibilities for translating consumer demand into competitively stimulated change. The specific danger is that a court might refuse to honor contractual exclusions from health insurance coverage simply because it perceived them to be harsh and unfair. Such a holding would presumably reflect a judgment that the insurance policy was a contract of adhesion and that the exclusions represented an unconscionable overreaching of weak and ignorant consumers. If a court so regarded it, the policy would be subject to judicial rewriting in the light of community standards—in this case professionally defined norms of medical necessity and appropriateness.[43]

Because group health insurance is purchased by a knowledgeable employer in a large and competitive insurance market, it is not obvious that such insurance should, like individually purchased policies, trigger protective doctrines designed to rectify perceived inequalities in sophistication and bargaining power. Nevertheless, employer-employee relationships are in some respects adversarial, and an employer purchasing a health plan to be included in a fringe benefits package could fairly be treated, in the absence of a union, as imposing an adhesion contract on its employees. Thus, a group insurance plan that seemed niggardly by conventional standards could well strike a court as calling for cavalier treatment of contractual language.

This result would not be inevitable, however. If an employer made full disclosure and arranged for the plan's coverage restrictions to apply only prospectively, so that reimbursement would not be denied for expenses already incurred in reliance on the plan, an employee's appeal for broader coverage should fail. Any other legal rule would have the undesirable effect of forcing employers to offer either a costly traditional plan covering all medically necessary care or no plan at all. Because employers are ultimately accountable to employees in the labor market, an employer who takes steps to disabuse wrong assumptions and to avoid induced hardship should have its choice of a health plan respected by the courts.

An even more certain solution to the employer's problem is suggested by Abraham's observation that, although courts have sometimes mandated coverage where it seems desirable, they

> have engaged most frequently in this kind of activity where the omitted coverage is otherwise unavailable from other sources. In cases where such coverage is available, the courts do not find a fictional expectation in order to create coverage where in fact it does not exist.[44]

In view of such judicial recognition of the legitimizing value of consumer choice, it would seem that an employer could avoid having its limited-benefit plan implicitly treated as a contract of adhesion by offering it as an option in a multiple-choice situation. With a traditional plan offering comprehensive benefits also available (for an extra cost), an employee could not complain that his expectations were unfairly disappointed, and the courts should feel secure in enforcing the bargain. Competition advocates should be reassured to find that they and the courts share similar views concerning the conditions under which consumer choice is appropriately exercised.

Conclusion

Important signs point to an accelerating breakdown in the historically wide acceptance, by governmental, private, and professional actors alike, of professionally defined standards governing medical practice and medical care spending. The federal government has begun to emphasize the virtues of consumer choice both in its own programs and in the private sector and, by eschewing regulation, has shifted the burden of controlling private costs to private parties. Employers and insurers have begun to recognize both the existence of major economizing opportunities within the broad range of professionally acceptable practice and the difficulty of trying, without credible sanctions, to persuade the system to alter its standards across the board. Moreover, the antitrust laws, by inhibiting efforts of the profession-dominated system to manage itself more efficiently, are causing those who might have been content with whatever concessions they could wring from the profession to pursue procompetitive options instead. Finally, the egalitarian ideal, embodying the same unitary conception of the health care system that the medical profession has sought to maintain, has lost much of its luster as a practically and politically attainable goal. In general, both government and private parties are looking more to their own interests and less to reform

41

of the entire system in defining the cost problem and seeking solutions. If this climate continues for an appreciable period, a final breakdown of the profession's dominant authority in medical-economic decision making is inevitable—if the courts do not unduly impede private implementation of responsible departures from accepted practice.

In the areas of tort, contract, and insurance law canvassed in this chapter, the courts appear to be primarily concerned with ensuring the integrity of the contracting process. They should thus not impose insuperable obstacles to private initiation of efficient changes in medical practice. To the extent that the law does pose problems for employers, HMOs, and insurers seeking to implement such changes, it promises to move them in directions that are entirely compatible with the competition strategy, and to be helpful both in clarifying and expanding consumer choices and in protecting consumers against abuse and unwarranted hardship. This demonstration that judicial protections of consumer interests can appropriately operate in a competitive health care system should reassure not only the advocates of competition but also those observers who claim to fear consequences of making consumers fend for themselves in the health care marketplace.

Notes

1. See William L. Prosser, *Handbook of the Law of Torts* (St. Paul, Minn.: West Publishing Co., 1971), pp. 165–68; Allan H. McCoid, "The Care Required of Medical Practitioners," *Vanderbilt Law Review,* vol. 12 (June 1959), pp. 558–75.

2. 42 U.S.C. § 1320c (1976).

3. See Clark C. Havighurst and James F. Blumstein, "Coping with Quality/Cost Tradeoffs in Medical Care: The Role of PSROs," *Northwestern University Law Review,* vol. 70 (March-April 1975), pp. 6–68. Budget legislation enacted in 1982 extended the concept of professional-sponsored peer review with some changes.

4. David M. Eddy, "Clinical Policies and the Quality of Clinical Practice," *New England Journal of Medicine,* vol. 307 (August 5, 1982), pp. 343–47.

5. See, for example, Eddy, "Clinical Policies"; John P. Bunker, Benjamin A. Barnes, and Frederick Mosteller, *Costs, Risks, and Benefits of Surgery* (New York: Oxford University Press, 1977); A. L. Cochrane, *Effectiveness and Efficiency—Random Reflections on Health Services* (Great Britain: Nuffield Prov. Hospital Trust, 1972); Office of Technology Assessment, *The Implications of Cost-Effectiveness Analysis of Medical Technology* (Washington, D.C., 1980).

6. See Clark C. Havighurst, "Professional Restraints on Innovation in Health Care Financing," *Duke Law Journal,* vol. 1978 (May 1978), pp. 303–87.

7. Ibid., pp. 319–43.
8. See Clark C. Havighurst and Glenn M. Hackbarth, "Private Cost Containment," *New England Journal of Medicine,* vol. 300 (June 7, 1979), pp. 1298–1305.
9. See Clark C. Havighurst, "The Contributions of Antitrust Law to a Procompetitive Health Policy," chapter 15 in this volume.
10. Richard A. Epstein, "Medical Malpractice: The Case for Contract," *American Bar Foundation Research Journal,* vol. 1 (January 1976), pp. 94–95.
11. Richard A. Epstein, "Medical Malpractice: Its Cause and Cure," in Simon Rottenberg, ed., *The Economics of Medical Malpractice* (Washington, D.C.: American Enterprise Institute, 1978), pp. 254–57.
12. 282 S.E.2d 903 (Ga. 1981).
13. See, for example, Olson v. Molzen, 558 S.W.2d 429 (Tenn. 1977); Meiman v. Rehabilitation Center, Inc., 444 S.W.2d 78 (Ky. 1969); Tatham v. Hoke, 469 F. Supp. 914 (W.D.N.C. 1979), affirmed, 622 F.2d 584 and 587 (4th Cir. 1980).
14. It is important to observe the difficulty of drafting a clause that spells out an alternative standard of care with enough clarity to be readily enforceable and to satisfy a court that the patients knew what they were buying. Although courts should recognize these difficulties and make allowances for them, the drafting problem may prove a greater obstacle to private innovation than the judicial doctrines canvassed here. Perhaps nothing short of a clear-cut alternative compensation scheme based on no-fault principles (see the text) will succeed.
15. Epstein, "Medical Malpractice: The Case for Contract," p. 149.
16. Raymond Neutra, Stephen Fienberg, Sander Greenland, and Emanuel Friedman, "Effect of Fetal Monitoring on Neonatal Death Rates," *New England Journal of Medicine,* vol. 299 (August 17, 1978), pp. 324–26.
17. Prosser, *Handbook of the Law of Torts,* pp. 163–64; McCoid, "The Care Required of Medical Practitioners," p. 565. Bovbjerg argues cogently for a variation on these doctrines that would look to "HMO custom." Randall Bovbjerg, "The Medical Malpractice Standard of Care: HMOs and Customary Practice," *Duke Law Journal,* vol. 1975 (January 1976), pp. 1375–1414.
18. Epstein, "Medical Malpractice: The Case for Contract," p. 95.
19. See Carl Stevens, "Medical Malpractice: Some Implications of Contract and Arbitration in HMOs," *Milbank Memorial Fund Quarterly/Health and Society,* vol. 59 (Winter 1981), pp. 59–88; Bovbjerg, "The Medical Malpractice Standard of Care," pp. 1375–1414.
20. See, for example, Tunkl v. Regents of University of California, 60 Cal.2d 92, 383 P.2d 441, 32 Cal. Rptr. 33 (1963); Henningsen v. Bloomfield Motors, Inc., 32 N.J. 358, 161 A.2d 69 (1959).
21. The doctrine of unconscionability allows a court wide discretion in deciding whether it can in good conscience enforce a contract term. Restatement (Second) of Contracts §208 (1981); Uniform Commercial Code

§2-302. Such "substantive unconscionability" has been contrasted with "procedural unconscionability," which involves defects in the bargaining process similar to those leading to characterization of a contract as a contract of adhesion. Arthur A. Leff, "Unconscionability and the Code—The Emperor's New Clause," *University of Pennsylvania Law Review,* vol. 115 (February 1967), pp. 485–559.

22. On the subject of medical malpractice arbitration agreements, see generally George H. Friedman, "Medical Malpractice Arbitration: Time for a Model Act," *Rutgers Law Review,* vol. 33 (Winter 1981), pp. 454–501; Stanley D. Henderson, "Contractual Problems in the Enforcement of Agreements to Arbitrate Medical Malpractice," *Virginia Law Review,* vol. 58 (September 1972), pp. 947–98.

23. 17 Cal.3d 699, 552 P.2d 1178, 131 Cal. Rptr. 882 (1976).

24. See, for example, Wheeler v. St. Joseph Hospital, 64 Cal. App.3d 345, 357–69, 133 Cal. Rptr. 775, 783–91 (1976).

25. Beynon v. Garden Grove Medical Group, 100 Cal. App.3d 659, 161 Cal. Rptr. 146 (1980).

26. 17 Cal.3d at 711, 552 P.2d at 1186, 131 Cal. Rptr. at 890. See also Doyle v. Giuliucci, 401 P.2d 1, 43 Cal. Rptr. 697 (1965).

27. Stevens argues that the arbitration clause may be a crucial ingredient in the move from a tort-based system of HMO liability to a contract-based system. Stevens, "Medical Malpractice," pp. 64, 78–82.

28. 17 Cal.3d at 712, 552 P.2d at 1186, 131 Cal. Rptr. at 890.

29. See, for example, Clark C. Havighurst, " 'Medical Adversity Insurance'—Has Its Time Come?" *Duke Law Journal,* vol. 1975 (January 1976), pp. 1233–80; Clark C. Havighurst and Laurence R. Tancredi, " 'Medical Adversity Insurance'—A No-Fault Approach to Medical Malpractice and Quality Assurance," *Milbank Memorial Fund Quarter/Health and Society,* vol. 51 (Spring 1973), pp. 125–68; American Bar Association, Commission on Medical Professional Liability, *Designated Compensable Event System: A Feasibility Study* (Chicago, Ill.: American Bar Association, 1979); Jeffrey O'Connell, "An Alternative to Abandoning Tort Liability: Elective No-Fault Insurance for Many Kinds of Injuries," *Minnesota Law Review,* vol. 60 (February 1976), pp. 501–65; Jeffrey O'Connell, *Ending Insult to Injury: No-Fault Insurance for Products and Services* (Chicago, Ill.: University of Illinois Press, 1975).

30. American Bar Association, *Designated Compensable Event System.*

31. Ibid.

32. For criticisms of the no-fault approach, see Guido Calabresi, "The Problem of Malpractice—Trying to Round Out the Circle," in Rottenberg, ed., *The Economics of Medical Malpractice,* pp. 239–43; Epstein, "Medical Malpractice: Its Cause and Cure," pp. 257–67.

33. See Clark C. Havighurst, *Deregulating the Health Care Industry* (Cambridge, Mass.: Ballinger Publishing Co., 1982), pp. 406–16.

34. See Alain Enthoven, *Health Plan: The Only Practical Solution to the Soaring Cost of Medical Care* (Reading, Mass., and Menlo Park, Calif.:

Addison-Wesley Publishing Co., 1980), pp. 114–44; Alain Enthoven, "Consumer-Centered v. Job-Centered Health Insurance," *Harvard Business Review*, vol. 57 (January-February 1979), pp. 141–52; H.R. 850, 97th Congress, 1st Session (1981), introduced by Congressman Richard A. Gephardt.

35. See, for example, S. 433, 97th Congress, 1st Session (1981), introduced by Senator David Durenberger; S. 139, 97th Congress, 1st Session (1981), introduced by Senator Orrin G. Hatch.

36. See Havighurst, *Deregulating the Health Care Industry*, pp. 409–16.

37. Of course, subscribers, on their own initiative, may purchase additional care outside the plan.

38. See Havighurst and Hackbarth, "Private Cost Containment."

39. Kenneth S. Abraham, "Judge-Made Law and Judge-Made Insurance: Honoring the Reasonable Expectations of the Insured," *Virginia Law Review*, vol. 67 (September 1981), pp. 1151–99.

40. Health insurance cases that give effect to insurer-induced misimpressions include Little v. Blue Cross of Western New York, Inc., 424 N.Y.S.2d 553 (N.Y. App. Div. 1980); Kemp v. Republic National Life Insurance Co., 649 F.2d 337 (5th Cir. 1981); Abernathy v. Prudential Insurance Company of America, 264 S.E.2d 836 (S.C. 1980); Van Vactor v. Blue Cross Association, 365 N.E.2d 638 (Ill. 1977).

41. It has been suggested that, once notified, the physician should be held liable to the insured for any noncovered services he prescribes without informing the insured that the services are not covered. J. M. Eisenberg and Arnold J. Rosoff, "Physician Responsibility for the Cost of Unnecessary Medical Services," *New England Journal of Medicine*, vol. 299 (July 13, 1978), pp. 76–80.

42. See, for example, Gulf Atlantic Life Insurance Company v. Disbro, 613 S.W.2d 511 (Tex. Civ. App. 1981); Franks v. Louisiana Health Services & Indemnity Co., 382 So.2d 1064 (La. Ct. App. 1980); Group Hospitalization, Inc. v. Westley, 350 A.2d 745 (D.C. 1976); South Dakota Medical Service, Inc. v. Minnesota Mutual Fire & Casualty Co., 303 N.W.2d 358 (S.D. 1980); Papanicolas v. Group Hospitalization, Inc., 434 A.2d 403 (D.C. 1981).

43. The test for substantive unconscionability is unclear, but presumably a court would look to industry custom. This article argues strenuously that departures from professionally defined norms should raise no presumption of unconscionability.

44. Abraham, "Judge-Made Law and Judge-Made Insurance," p. 1155.

3

How Will Increased Competition Affect the Costs of Health Care?

Warren Greenberg

In an effort to slow escalating health care costs, several legislative proposals that rely on competition among insurers and alternative delivery systems have been introduced into the Congress. One type of "competition" bill would offer vouchers to individuals enrolled in Medicare and Medicaid that they could use to purchase qualified private health plans.[1]

In this paper, I will first describe the thrust of the major competition bills, including those that call for vouchers. Second, I will outline how the implementation of the competition bills may make the market for health insurance and the market for health services more efficient. I suggest that the most important impediment to greater efficiency is the conflict in values between economic efficiency and medical efficacy that William Schwartz and Paul Joskow described nearly three years ago.[2] In addition, I evaluate the requirement that employers offer at least three health plans, the potential effects of adverse risk selection, and the structure of the health industry and health services markets, to assess their implications for economic efficiency. Finally, I suggest that a link exists between efficiency and the escalation of health care costs which might allow, after the enactment of competition legislation, a one-time decline in the rate of escalation, with a slight slackening in the rate (adjusted by the age mix of the population) thereafter.

Thrust of Major Competition Bills

The common denominator of the major competition bills, including those that provide for vouchers for individuals enrolled in Medicare and Medicaid, is that insurer-based competition—that is, among third-party insurers, alternative delivery systems, limited-provider groups, and health maintenance organizations (HMOs)—is the most viable, if not the only, form

46

of competition in health care. Currently, the advocates of insured-based competition argue, the market for health services is flawed because of excessive insurance, which allows the patient to demand services when the real societal costs are greater than the benefits. In addition, the market for health services is imperfect even without the presence of insurance, since an asymmetry of information exists between the patient and physician, which may lead to overutilization.[3]

A choice of health care plans is expected to result in a greater growth of the more cost-effective plans, presumably the HMOs. It has been suggested that costs might decline between 10 percent and 40 percent for those enrolled in HMOs.[4] The competition bills have not contained any estimates of how the *escalation* in costs might be affected by increased HMO enrollment.[5] Quality, access, and availability of care are apparently not affected adversely in this competitive environment. It has not been suggested that costs will be curtailed under the competition bills; it is presumed, however, that utilization will be curtailed when expected benefits are zero.

Incentives for the formation of cost-conscious health insurance plans would stem, first, from a change in the tax laws requiring that employer contributions above a certain amount be taxable to the employee just as ordinary income is taxable. Second, the employer would be required to offer a multiple choice of plans and to contribute the same amount to each of the plans; if the chosen plan's premium was less than the employer contribution, the employee would receive a tax-free rebate for the difference.[6]

The bills directed toward Medicare and Medicaid recipients differ, in general, from those directed toward employer groups insofar as the employer plays no role in the offering of plans; rather, competing health plans are offered directly to the individual. One variation of the bills directed toward Medicare beneficiaries would "prospectively reimburse HMOs enrolling Medicare beneficiaries at a rate equal to 95 percent of the amount spent by Medicare for the average beneficiary in the area (the average area per capita cost or AAPCC)."[7]

Toward Economic Efficiency

My assumption is that the insurer-based competition bills are intended to create a more efficient market for health insurance as well as for health services, and thereby to reduce the escalation in health care costs. In this section, first, I briefly comment on the efficiency of the market for private health insurance by stressing the importance of information in choosing among plans. Second, in the health services market, I suggest that the most important advantage of increased competition among insurers, alternative delivery systems, and HMOs is the increased incentive to utilize information that can be gathered from the health services industry to contain costs.[8] Third, I suggest that, as a result of information in the health services market, the increased incentives to exert leverage over providers would also be a product of the insurer-based competition bills.

Information and the Market for Health Insurance. Currently, in the market for most private health insurance, information is transmitted by the employer to the employee. That is, the employer, by offering one or more health benefit plans to retain employees, has substantial incentives to offer a plan or plans that coincide with the majority of the employees' desires. The employer generally has professional benefit managers on his staff to review potential legal loopholes and benefit inconsistencies in the plans offered. The most cost-effective insurer can be selected by the individual who has ample time to gather information before his or her decision. If the employer is to offer a greater array of benefit packages or a different structure of benefit packages under procompetition legislation, one would expect the employer to become an even more important source of information to the employee.

Information and the Market for Health Services. In general, an individual either does not know or is not concerned about the prices of physician and hospital services, the "appropriate" number of ambulatory procedures and lengths-of-stay in hospitals, or the "appropriate" number of hospital beds or types of sophisticated equipment in an area.[9] Third-party insurers (Blue Cross and the commercial insurers) and alternative delivery systems, however, know the prices of physician and hospital services and may well know the appropriate number of ambulatory procedures and lengths-of-stay in hospitals as well as the appropriate number of hospital beds or types of sophisticated equipment in an area. "Appropriate" is defined here as the point beyond which marginal benefits of health services are zero.

In addition, third-party insurers and HMOs clearly already have incentives to contain costs. Among third-party insurers, for example, generally vigorous competition in dental insurance has resulted in extensive pre-treatment review of dental procedures. Firms that are more successful in reducing the escalation of costs in dental care will be able to secure more business from the employer.[10] The incentives that HMOs already have to contain costs have been described elsewhere.[11] Furthermore, the fact that hospital prices are not still higher suggests that there are some limits to what third parties will pay or to the level at which providers will set their prices.

48

Cost containment involves certain costs, however, especially from the viewpoint of the traditional third-party insurer. These include the transaction costs of designing and carrying out the program, of ascertaining what appropriate medical procedures are, and of negotiating with the providers and potentially alienating the patients.

How might a third-party insurer with increased incentives use information to contain costs to a greater extent than at present? With a large number of enrollees and with physicians as consultants on its staff, the third-party insurer can examine more closely procedures or tests that exceed the point beyond which marginal benefits are zero. It can also question fees for procedures that exceed the mean for a group of enrollees in a particular location. A recent study of a small "administrative services only" firm that attempts to collect this information and subsequently use it to deter unnecessary utilization and higher than average fees found that the firm enjoyed some success in curbing higher fees as well as prohibiting procedures beyond which marginal benefits are zero. In instances where the marginal benefits were positive, the firm was less successful.[12]

This seems to be consistent with Kenneth Arrow's notion that "an insurance company can improve the allocation of resources to all concerned by a policy which rations the amount of medical services it will support under the insurance policy."[13] Arrow then suggests that

> there might be a detailed examination by the insurance company of individual cost items allowing those that are regarded "normal" and disallowing others, where normality means roughly what would have been bought in the absence of insurance.[14]

Third-party insurers might also generate and utilize information based on an entire health care market. An analysis might be made of the appropriate number of hospitals and beds within a hospital, as well as the appropriate number of sophisticated technologies. Insurers would then refuse to pay for that capital configuration beyond which the marginal benefits are zero.[15]

A third party will not, however, attempt to contain costs for the entire health care market unless the firm has a substantial market share. A firm incurs certain expenses in setting up a cost containment program, including the design and administration of such a program. At the same time, these cost containment efforts are subject to the free-rider effect. Other insurer-competitors in the same market would also benefit if cost containment efforts were successful. In order to provide an incentive for an insurer's efforts at cost containment, which may potentially affect the entire health care market (a public good), a tax credit might be provided to internalize some of the benefits.[16]

Not only do HMOs have the same types of information available to them as health insurers, but, because of their incentive structure, they can use this information to contain costs. Physicians who are paid on a salary basis have no incentives to provide services beyond which the marginal benefits are zero. The salaries of physicians and paraprofessional personnel need not be higher than their opportunity costs. The HMO, however, generally does not engage in the types of global cost containment that limit the number of hospital beds or sophisticated technical equipment.[17]

Insurer Leverage and Providers. Unlike an individual with little or no bargaining power, insurers may be able to exert leverage or monopsonistic power in order to contain costs.

Indeed, monopsonistic bargaining power has been the issue in a number of cases that have progressed to litigation. The U.S. Federal Trade Commission, for example, recently secured a consent agreement with the Indiana Dental Association, whose dentists have objected to insurer interference in the dentist-patient relationship. The dentists were objecting to pre-authorization review by a number of commercial insurance companies.[18] In addition, Blue Cross/Blue Shield of Michigan attempted to institute a new reimbursement policy for physician services in 1977. The most important element of such a program was to establish a uniform maximum payment regardless of geographic area of practice and regardless of whether a physician is a specialist or a generalist. It was hoped that this payment method would encourage physicians to practice in areas that are underserved because of traditional low reimbursement and would put a lid on physician payment.[19] Efforts by the Michigan State Medical Society to engage in "concerted action" to regulate cost-containment and reimbursement policies of Blue Cross/Blue Shield of Michigan were subsequently judged to be illegal by an administrative law judge of the Federal Trade Commission.[20]

The bargaining power of insurers may result in real cost savings, or it may result instead in a transfer of costs to another third party. Reduction in the number of dental procedures may result in real cost savings, while lids on reimbursement may simply shift costs from one third-party payer to another. The much-discussed Blue Cross discount may be another example in which costs are reduced for one insurer but increased for others.[21]

HMOs may be able to exert their bargaining power before health services are performed. As an informed buyer, the HMO can carefully consider the salaries of physicians and auxiliary personnel, as well as the sophisticated equipment and types of hospitals that it will use.

Conflict between Economic Efficiency
and Medical Efficacy

Given that the asymmetry of information and the lack of bargaining power between the patient and providers has been reduced by the accumulation of information (and the willingness to use such information) by third-party insurers and HMOs, to what extent might one expect costs to be controlled? Suppose, with perfect information and no uncertainty, one was able to assess the potential benefits of a particular procedure as equal to $100. Yet assume that the costs of a particular procedure are $200.[22] Medical efficacy would dictate proceeding, while economic efficiency considerations would not allow the procedure to continue. Schwartz and Joskow, in fact, suggest that "most" health care expenditures engender some positive benefits.[23]

It would take substantial incentives to induce individuals to select insurers that are willing to contain costs up to the point at which economic efficiency equaled medical efficacy. Indeed, given the substantial current incentives of HMOs, how many forgo procedures when there are marginal benefits to be gained? Luft's evidence that HMOs do not reduce admissions disproportionately in "discretionary" or "unnecessary" categories might provide further support to those who believe that HMOs would be reluctant to forgo procedures where there is some marginal benefit.[24] Other observers have also raised doubts about the ability of health insurance plans to "cope with the imperatives of the medical profession."[25]

Third-party insurers might possibly be able to contain costs closer to the point at which economic efficiency and medical efficacy are equated in two instances. First, when attempts are made to contain costs in the entire health care market, such as attempts to reduce the number of beds, medical efficacy concerns are not directly related to the well-being of a particular individual. Therefore, insurers can avoid bearing any antagonisms from the physician and/or patient. Second, when third-party insurers compete over deductibles and copayments, medical efficacy and economic efficiency might move closer together. In this instance, however, one might lose some of the advantage of information and bargaining power described above.

In summary, I suggest that the difficulty of overcoming the stumbling block of medical efficacy will be considerable. Even with regard to the HMO, the extent to which physicians' imperatives are violated is a major question. Nevertheless, given appropriate incentives, one would expect traditional health insurers along with HMOs to contain costs when marginal benefits are zero.

Information and Economic Efficiency:
Voucher System

Under a voucher system for Medicaid and Medicare recipients, employer-based information for the purchase of health insurance does not exist. There are no information efficiencies of experienced benefit counselors who may advertise, highlight, and market health insurance plans to employees. An alternative to employer marketing is a minimum benefit package specified by the government. The government, however, is always pressured by many different groups to include their services in the minimum benefit package. Another alternative is to set a minimum benefit package equal to, say, the package of the average of the 500 largest U.S. corporations. Also, benefit packages would have to be marketed to individuals, which would increase costs to all participating insurers and HMOs.

To what extent can a Medicaid and Medicare voucher system affect costs in the health services market? People over sixty-five with present Medicare coverage constitute a group that would appear to be quite risk averse in the purchase of a health insurance package—that is, they are likely to choose a package with comprehensive coverage. Alain Enthoven has reported that "about 17 million of the 23 million people aged sixty-five and over in 1975 carried private insurance in addition to Medicare."[26] If open enrollments are held too infrequently, this might stimulate even greater enrollment in the comprehensive plans, since I believe that one's willingness to take risks will be inversely related to the time before one can switch plans. Therefore, for this group of individuals, it would appear that even more substantial incentives are needed to encourage the purchase of health insurance so that costs are contained at the point where economic efficiency equals medical efficacy.

Finally, a large variance in income appears to exist in the Medicare-Medicaid groups, indicating that many Medicaid enrollees would select health care coverage far below that of some higher-income Medicare individuals. Some income adjustment in addition to a health status adjustment would thus seem to be necessary for the Medicare-Medicaid voucher system.

I believe that, if information can be transmitted efficiently to the Medicare-Medicaid enrollees, the voucher system can approach economic efficiency in the health insurance market. However, improvements in the efficiency of the health services industry depend on the issue of adverse selection to be discussed below.

Some Complexities of Procompetition Legislation

Two prominent objections to the procompetition legislation have been raised that may affect the cost savings to be obtained from increased competition.

The first is the requirement that an employer offer at least three health plans.[27] Employers will apparently offer benefit packages up to the point where the marginal costs (including transaction costs and publication costs) are equal to the marginal gains (including the probability that the employee will enroll in a lower-cost plan, thus reducing the employer's payroll costs). Since most employers today do not offer a choice of health plans, the costs presumably outweigh the benefits. With procompetition legislation, a greater diversity of plans is possible, perhaps making it cost-effective for the employer to offer the multiple-plan option. If the employer elects to offer only one plan, however, one would expect that it would approximate the mean of the demands of the employee population. Presumably, this mean would be less than the current mean since more of the employee population would desire a lower-cost alternative. Indeed, to the extent that the employer offers only one plan, it can alleviate the problem of intensified adverse risk selection that could occur when multiple plans are provided for consumer choice.

The second objection is that the problems of adverse risk selection will be exacerbated when procompetition bills are effectuated. Even today, however, comprehensive plans with open-enrollment periods are subject to an influx of poorer risks. In 1976, for example, the hospitalization rate per 1,000 Blue Cross enrollees was 1,040 days for nongroup enrollees (many of whom enroll during open-enrollment periods) and 769 for group enrollees.[28] The commercial insurers ignore completely the more costly nongroups. Indeed, in response to competition from HMOs, Blue Cross has elected to enroll fewer nongroup individuals.[29] Blue Cross has reported that, under the Federal Employees Health Benefit Program, enrollment increases substantially in their high-option plan before hospitalization.[30] In contrast, the current Mendocino County (California) teacher's plan discriminates against those who are in ill health. Under this plan, a beneficiary whose claims are less than $500 receives a credit for the unspent balance, without any allowance for those who might be in ill health.[31]

Under procompetition legislation, with probably a greater diversity of health insurance plans from which to choose, one might expect that self-selection of plans to fit one's health status would be intensified. The costs of the more comprehensive plans will grow relative to the less comprehensive, which will mean correspondingly higher payments for those in ill health. Competition, in part, will be based not on saving real resources, but on marketing to the better risks. It is difficult to understand how this "market failure" can be solved other than by some sort of government regulation or intervention, such as mandatory open enrollment and community rating for all plans. In addition, a scale of reimbursement, based on the health status of individuals enrolled, would also have to be provided to health insurance firms.

53

There are currently substantial costs of regulation, however, in part because of adverse risk selection. In nearly every state, for example, Blue Cross is regulated so that rates can be kept lower for individual enrollees who generate proportionately higher costs.[32]

Finally, I would like to suggest that the scale of reimbursement based on health status is crucial and that the optimum reimbursement would depend, in part, on how insurers would behave under procompetition legislation. Suppose, for example, insurers compete for the business of the employer or under a Medicare-Medicaid voucher plan in the following way. Suppose a high-deductible, high-copayment insurer enters the market. A more comprehensive insurer that enters the market is likely to have higher costs because of its complete insurance coverage in addition to its attraction to high-risk individuals. In addition to rebate advantages, the gap between the less comprehensive and the more comprehensive insurers would widen considerably. Therefore, the comprehensive insurer might desire to enter with coverage closer to the high-deductible insurer. In fact, this state of less insurance would approach the goal of many economists.

Structure of the Health Insurance Industry

In 1978, private health insurance included 674 commercial carriers, 69 Blue Cross plans, 70 Blue Shield plans, and 203 HMOs. Also included in the private insurance segment are a growing number of corporations that self-insure their employees' health care expenses while using third-party administrators to process benefit claims. Total private health insurance benefit payments were more than $50 billion in 1978. In addition, public health insurance expenditures, consisting primarily of the Medicare program for the elderly and the Medicaid program for the poor, were more than $78 billion in 1978.

Although the health insurance industry includes a large number of firms, the relatively large share of the market of the combined Blue Cross/Blue Shield plans (nearly 50 percent of the private health insurance industry) suggests that there might be imperfections in competition among health insurers. The nonprofit status of the Blue Cross/Blue Shield plans, for example, exempts them from property and income taxes as well as premium taxes in most states. It appears, however, that Blue Cross/Blue Shield plans may be subject to greater state and local regulation than those of commercial firms. Blue Cross/Blue Shield may be required to hold an open-enrollment period during which individuals can enroll regardless of physical condition. Blue Cross/Blue Shield might also be required to community-rate its members, so that those with poor medical histories need not pay higher premiums.

Whether the advantages that Blue Cross/Blue Shield enjoys are off-set by additional regulatory requirements is not known. Blue Cross/Blue Shield may also have certain recognition or trademark advantages, or it may simply be more effective in controlling costs and providing better service than the commercial firms. To the extent that there are imper-fections in competition at the insurer level, one cannot say that cost containment is greater or lesser than it would be in the absence of these imperfections. As has been pointed out, however, there may be econ-omies of scale in cost-containment efforts as well as potential monopso-nistic power by firms with a large number of enrollees and a large market share.[33]

With the large number of health insurers and various types of alternative delivery systems, one might suggest that entry into this industry is generally easy (although if Blue Cross or the commercial health insurers enjoy cost advantages, entry is impeded to this extent), making the possibility of collusion among health insurers and HMOs remote.[34]

After procompetition legislation is enacted, how might health insurers and HMOs compete? Previous analysis has cast doubt on whether increased competition from HMOs might, in fact, mean lower costs.[35] If there are sufficient incentives created to choose lower-cost plans, however, I can only assert that competition among health insurers and HMOs will shift toward attempts to reduce the rate of escalation of costs. Firms that do not make greater attempts at cost control might find that higher costs are being passed on to them by providers.

Structure of the Health Services Industry

Thus far, the procompetition legislation has not emphasized the supply side of the health services industry. Supply-side restrictions, however, could possibly be eliminated without a conflict between economic effi-ciency and medical efficacy. Eliminating restrictions on advertising by dentists and physicians, for example, might help to lower costs without impinging on the quality of care. This would especially be the case if the heightened competition among health insurers resulted in increased copayments, which would in turn increase the individual's incentive to search. Increased information might also be helpful in hospital advertis-ing, an area not investigated by the antitrust authorities.[36] If it filters down to the patient, however, increased information—such as about the number of various types of procedures performed in a hospital—may increase the quality of care as well as reduce costs, even though the physician is the one who admits the patient to the hospital.[37]

Further restrictions on the supply of health services are enumerated in a recent paper by Rosemary Gibson and John Reiss.[38] The vast differences in state regulations on licensing within states, reciprocal licensing, and supervision of auxiliary manpower suggest that some of these restrictions can be removed without a significant reduction in quality.

A number of imperfections in the health services industry may remain unaffected by procompetition legislation. Frank Sloan and Bruce Steinwald have suggested three examples: (1) the non-profit nature of the majority of hospitals which may not lead to an efficient output; (2) the local monopoly nature of "many" hospitals; and (3) medical-staffing privileges, which "severely limit patient and physician choice of hospital."[39]

A Link between Efficiency and the Escalation of Costs?

Removing the tax-based distortions in the purchase of health insurance would substantially improve the efficiency in the purchase of health insurance since employees, utilizing the information passed on by employers, would be able to choose an insurance plan without major distortions by the tax laws.

One might also see a one-time decline in the escalation of costs. I assume the following:

• Existing HMOs will continue to control costs at their current rate—that is, when expected marginal benefits are zero.

• Additional third-party insurers, motivated by changes in the tax laws, will contain costs when marginal benefits are zero.

• Because of a change in the tax laws, the number of HMOs will increase, which should result in greater production efficiencies (reduced hospitalization, better use of health manpower, and so on).

• Price competition between third-party insurers and HMOs will intensify because the consumer is more cost-conscious in selecting a health insurance plan.

The extent of the decline in the escalation of costs will depend on the willingness of society to balance medical efficacy and economic efficiency. That is, the decline will vary directly with the size of the tax rebate. I believe, for example, that procedures, especially in HMOs, may not be allowed where marginal benefits are far outweighed by their marginal costs. It is doubtful, however, that society will pick a point at which medical efficacy is substantially eroded.

What will happen after a one-time decline in the escalation of costs? In the case of HMOs, Harold Luft's paper is quite useful.[40] In examining data from the Federal Employees Health Benefit Program, California

State Employees, and Kaiser-Oregon, Luft found that "costs per unit of service (e.g., per hospital patient day) . . . are generally comparable to national trends, as are measures of factor inputs." Luft concludes that "the rate of growth in total costs (including out-of-pocket expenses) is only slightly lower for persons in HMOs"—relative to those patients with conventional insurance coverage.[41] Luft further suggests "that the cost advantages of HMOs are almost entirely attributable to utilization patterns, rather than the ability to provide specific services less expensively."[42]

As Luft acknowledges, only a small sample of HMOs was used, which might not be representative of the trend in costs of HMOs in general. Yet the results are somewhat disturbing for those who believe that HMOs can stem physician imperatives. Although subject to many factors including differences in population mix and benefit packages, the observation that trends in hospital patient-day costs are about the same in HMOs as in fee-for-service suggests that even HMOs must respect the pressures of medical efficacy.

I believe, however, that the escalation of costs will be slightly mitigated for the following reasons:

1. Increasing costs of health care should lead to new entry of alternative delivery systems, which should increase the degree of competition among plans. As health care costs have increased rapidly in the past few years, new plans such as Safeco, many new HMOs, and new initiatives by Blue Cross have come into being. One should be cautious, however, about projecting any large increases in HMO growth. HMO enrollment under the Federal Employees Health Benefit Plan is still less than 10 percent of the federal work force. Increases in HMO growth, outside the states of California and Minnesota, have not been great. Even a tripling of HMO growth will still leave less than 15 percent of the population covered under these plans.

2. To the extent that providers are able to shift costs to the less vigilant insurers, the costs of these insurers will rise relative to those of the more active insurers. This may put more pressure on the less vigilant insurers to increase their cost consciousness.

3. A predicted "oversupply" of physicians might induce providers to enter into less costly relationships with cost-conscious insurers or HMOs. Such relationships might provide competitive advantages to these insurer groups.

I believe, therefore, that the enactment of procompetition legislation will mean a one-time drop in the escalation of costs, with costs continuing to rise, but at a slightly lower rate, thereafter.

A more definitive answer about how costs will be affected after the

57

enactment of procompetition legislation depends on a better understanding of how much of current health care services provide little or no benefit. If, as Schwartz and Joskow suggest, most health care provides some benefit, then the government would have to present an attractive tax package to achieve a slowdown in the escalation of health care costs.

Notes

1. Two bills that have included provisions for vouchers are the National Health Care Reform Act of 1981, H.R. 850, introduced by Congressmen Richard A. Gephardt (Democrat, Missouri) and David Stockman (Republican, Michigan), and the Competitive Health and Medical Plan (CHAMP) Act of 1981, S. 1509, introduced by Senator John Heinz (Republican, Pennsylvania).

2. See William B. Schwartz and Paul L. Joskow, "Medical Efficacy versus Economic Efficiency: A Conflict in Values," *The New England Journal of Medicine,* vol. 299 (December 28, 1978), pp. 1462–64.

3. See Mark V. Pauly, "Is Medical Care Different?" in Warren Greenberg, ed., *Competition in the Health Care Sector* (Aspen Systems Corp., Germantown, Md., 1978). Pauly, himself, is somewhat skeptical of the argument that suggests that lack of information leads to excessive utilization, although he suggests that the lack of information in medical care is what differentiates this industry from others.

4. See Alain C. Enthoven, "Consumer-Choice Health Plan," *New England Journal of Medicine,* vol. 298 (March 30, 1978), p. 717.

5. See, however, Harold S. Luft, "Trends in Medical Care Costs: Do HMOs Lower the Rate of Growth?" *Medical Care,* vol. 18 (January 1980), pp. 1–16, and n. 5.

6. See Paul B. Ginsburg, "Altering the Tax Treatment of Employment-Based Health Plans," *Milbank Memorial Fund Quarterly,* vol. 59 (Spring 1981), p. 226.

7. See *Washington Report on Medicine and Health: Perspectives,* August 17, 1981, unpaged.

8. In the remainder of this paper, I shall include alternative delivery systems such as Northwest Healthcare, in which physicians generally bear the risk for laboratory tests or hospitalization, in the term "health maintenance organization."

9. Prices of services that are purchased relatively frequently and are uninsured may be known by the patient. See Pauly, "Is Medical Care Different?" p. 12. In addition, individuals may through extensive search secure increased information, but this is not costless.

10. See Warren Greenberg, "Provider-Influenced Insurance Plans and Their Impact on Competition: Lessons from Dentistry," in Mancur Olson, ed., *A New Approach to the Economics of Health Care* (Washington, D.C.:

American Enterprise Institute, 1981). Greenberg also offers some reasons why it is more difficult to control medical costs than dental costs.

11. Paul M. Ellwood and Walter McClure, *Health Delivery Reform*, rev. ed. (Excelsior, Minn.: Interstudy, November 17, 1976).

12. See George A. Goldberg and Warren Greenberg, "Third-Party Cost Containment and the Physician-Patient Relationship: A Case Study," *Journal of Community Health*, vol. 7 (Spring 1982), pp. 215–30.

13. See Kenneth J. Arrow, "The Economics of Moral Hazard: Further Comment," *American Economic Review*, vol. 53 (June 1968), p. 538.

14. Ibid. Arrow's definition of "normality" is not equivalent to what I have termed "appropriate."

15. When the entire health care market is examined, however, the standard for the appropriate hospitals, beds, and technologies may differ somewhat from the standard for individual medical interventions.

16. The health insurer not only would receive the benefits of a tax credit, but also would garner the benefits of lower costs if its cost-containment efforts proved successful. For an additional perspective on cost containment for the entire market, see Roger Feldman and Warren Greenberg, "Blue Cross Market Share, Economies of Scale, and Cost Containment Efforts," *Health Services Research*, Summer 1981, pp. 175–83.

17. Some HMOs such as Kaiser-Permanente and Group Health Cooperative of Puget Sound on the West Coast own their hospital. In this case, the number of beds in the community ceases to be a cost factor for them.

18. See "FTC Charges Indiana Dental Groups with Restricting Insurers' Cost Containment Efforts," *FTC News* (November 15, 1978).

19. Blue Cross/Blue Shield of Michigan, News Release (August 11, 1977).

20. See Federal Trade Commission, News Summary (July 3, 1981), p. 1.

21. See Roger Feldman and Warren Greenberg, "The Relation Between the Blue Cross Market Share and the Blue Cross 'Discount' on Hospital Charges," *Journal of Risk and Insurance*, vol. 48 (June 1981), pp. 235–46.

22. It is, of course, well established in the literature that the measurement of expected costs and benefits of most medical procedures is exceedingly difficult.

23. Schwartz and Joskow, "Medical Efficacy versus Economic Efficiency," p. 1464. Pauly has also suggested that, in general, most surgery has some potential benefits. See Mark V. Pauly, "What Is Unnecessary Surgery?" *Milbank Memorial Fund Quarterly*, vol. 57 (Winter 1979), pp. 95–111, especially p. 103. In contrast, Enthoven suggests that a "great deal of . . . health care resources are being used in ways that yield very little or no discernible health benefit." See Alain C. Enthoven, *Health Plan, Addison Wesley*, (Reading, Mass.: 1981), especially p. 46.

24. Harold S. Luft, "How Do Health Maintenance Organizations Achieve Their 'Savings?' " *New England Journal of Medicine*, vol. 298 (June 15, 1978), pp. 1336–43.

25. See Louis A. De Niro, review of *Health Plan*, in *Journal of Economic Literature*, vol. 59 (September 1981), pp. 1129–32.

26. See Enthoven, *Health Plan*, p. 18.

27. Enthoven, for example, has suggested that "to create real competition, we need multiple choice for each consumer." See Alain C. Enthoven, "Consumer-Centered v. Job-Centered Health Insurance," *Harvard Business Review*, vol. 57 (January-February 1979), p. 150.

28. See Blue Cross Association, *Enrollment and Utilization Data of Blue Cross Plans* (Fourth Quarter 1976), Table IX, p. 37.

29. See Philip Fanara, Jr., and Warren Greenberg, "The Impact of Competition on Blue Cross Risk Selection," mimeographed (Washington, D.C.: March 1982).

30. Stanley Jones, "Competition in the Health Care Sector," mimeographed (Washington, D.C.: Blue Cross and Blue Shield Association, September 18, 1981).

31. See "Greater Price Competition in Health Care Sought by Reagan in Bid to Pare Expenses," *Wall Street Journal*, August 25, 1981, p. 52.

32. National Association of Life Underwriters, "Survey of Extent of Regulation and Taxation of Blue Cross-Blue Shield Plans," mimeographed (Washington, D.C.: June 1, 1981).

33. See Feldman and Greenberg, "Blue Cross Market Share, Economies of Scale, and Cost Containment Efforts."

34. See Warren Greenberg and Lawrence G. Goldberg, "The Determinants of HMO Enrollment and Growth," *Health Services Research*, vol. 16 (Winter 1981), pp. 421–38. The authors suggest that entry generally corresponds to what would occur in a competitive market.

35. See Alain C. Enthoven, "Competition among Alternative Delivery Systems," in Greenberg ed., *Competition in the Health Care Sector*, pp. 255–78, and Harold S. Luft, "HMOs and the Medical Care Market," in *Socioeconomic Issues of Health* (Chicago: American Medical Association, 1980), pp. 85–102.

36. One reason might be the prohibition in the Federal Trade Commission Act against litigation involving nonprofit firms.

37. See Harold S. Luft, John P. Bunker, and Alain C. Enthoven, "Should Operations Be Regionalized? The Empirical Relation between Surgical Volume and Mortality," *New England Journal of Medicine*, vol. 301 (December 20, 1979), pp. 1364–69.

38. See chapter 13 of this volume.

39. Frank A. Sloan and Bruce Steinwald, "Effects of Regulations on Hospital Costs and Input Use," *Journal of Law and Economics*, vol. 23 (April, 1980), p. 81.

40. Harold S. Luft, "Trends in Medical Care Costs, Do HMOs Lower the Rate of Growth?" *Medical Care*, vol. 18 (January 1980), pp. 1–16.

41. Ibid., p. 1.

42. Ibid., p. 2.

4

Competition in Health Care:
A Cautionary View

Burton A. Weisbrod

You can fool all the people some of the time and some of the people all the time, but competition prevents you from fooling all the people all the time. Economists' confidence in competition is not unbounded, but it is surely of the first magnitude. How, then, can an economist argue seriously that increased competition may not be desirable—indeed, that it may be inefficient?

In markets for ordinary commodities, competition is generally thought of as an unmitigated blessing. Noncompetitive markets normally imply "market failures." Competition increases options for consumers and leads producers, as if by an "invisible hand," to minimize production costs and to maximize economic efficiency—all in their pursuit of profit. The result, at least in equilibrium, is that individual self-interest—utility maximization for consumers and profit maximization for producers—coincides with the maximization of social welfare.

The meaning of "competition," however, deserves attention. It may refer to (1) the number of sellers (or buyers—but I focus here only on the supply side of the market), (2) the degree of independent, non-collusive action among sellers, (3) the variety of goods or services offered, or (4) the variety of pricing arrangements available. Given that our subject is the desirability of increased competition in health care, it is important that we be clear about precisely which dimensions of competition are being considered. It is a theme of this chapter, for example, that greater competition in any or all of dimensions (1), (2), and (3) may well be unproductive or even counterproductive if certain conditions hold with respect to dimension (4). Moreover, whatever the conditions regarding dimension (4), the ability of consumers to take advantage of

I thank Elaine Gilby, Mark Schlesinger, and Barbara Wolfe for helpful comments.

increases in dimensions (1), (2), and (3) remains an important issue—and more so in the health care area than in most markets.

Is the market for health care different from other markets? If it is, what is the role of competition in that industry? Without arguing that health care is unique, I want to emphasize that some basic assumptions underlying economists' confidence in competition do not hold in much of the health care industry. As a result, our confidence in the ability of competition to optimize price, quantity, and quality may not hold. Why not? There are three principle reasons: consumers' lack of information, inefficient pricing, and the influence of private nonprofit and governmental providers.

Information

First, the standard competitive model assumes that consumers are well informed or, what is equivalent, that they can and do learn quickly and at low cost. Consider, for example, the market for chocolate chip cookies. A consumer typically purchases cookies frequently enough to learn from experience which variety or brand of cookie he or she prefers. For medical care, the situation is typically different; because it is obtained infrequently, in a wide variety of forms, and for a wide variety of symptoms, it is difficult for the consumer to judge quality. That is, the consumer is not purchasing a standardized commodity consumed under standardized conditions; so learning from experience is more complex.

Another aspect of the assumption of full information is that the consumer is able to judge the effect of a particular purchase—that is, able to compare his or her utility level with and without the specific purchase, for it is this comparison that determines the consumer's willingness to pay. The consumer has little difficulty determining his or her utility with and without cookies. But for medical care, judging the "counterfactual"—what would happen if the consumer did not obtain the care compared with what would happen if he or she did obtain it—is often dramatically difficult. The main reason is the ability of the human body to correct problems without external intervention. Physicians seem to have little doubt that at least 90 percent of all visits by patients with symptoms are "unnecessary" in the sense that the patient would have recovered fully without seeing the physician. The uncertainty about the effectiveness of medical care gives this class of services an unusual character.

Answering the question of how one's welfare will be affected by the consumption of a particular good or service is more difficult for medical care than for most goods and services not only because body mechanisms fight disease independently of medical interventions but also because evidence of the effectiveness and side effects of the medical intervention is frequently delayed for days, weeks, or even decades. An example is the recent discovery of an abnormal frequency of cervical cancer among women whose *mothers* ingested a particular drug during pregnancy. It is frequently difficult to disentangle these forces to determine the incremental effect of the medical input. Health care, we must remember, is the field that made the term "quackery" famous. This is the economic sector that gave us the violetta, a high-voltage generator that allegedly "could treat 86 ailments, ranging from abscesses to writer's cramp," and this is the sector that brought forth a hand-held vibrator that promised to "remove cobwebs from the brain" and the spectro-chrome, which treated heart disease with red and purple lights while the patient faced north, in the nude.[1]

In many markets, consumers' information is enhanced through producers' advertising of prices and quality. The virtual absence of advertising in the health care area is noteworthy. It suggests not that competition is absent but that the industry is highly unusual, so that conventional models of organization behavior may have limited applicability. What is the significance of medical societies' success in preventing price advertising by physicians? What is the importance of the fact that one does not find physicians advertising the price of a standard office visit or hospitals advertising their high quality, low prices, or special "sale" prices on surgery performed during periods of off-peak demand? Price advertising is so rare that a recent example of it was deemed worthy of being reported on a radio broadcast: Milwaukee County Hospital recently advertised a flat-fee obstetrical service of $999, its "usual" price being $2,500.[2]

Consumers' awareness of their inability to judge the effectiveness of medical attention leads to another sense in which medical care is special, though by no means unique: consumers are likely to turn to agents for advice. Perhaps nowhere is the use of agents more widespread than in medical care, where physicians are in many cases delegated virtually full decision-making authority for patients, not merely an advisory role.

The use of an agent generally carries the risk that the agent may have a conflict of interest, possibly serving his or her self-interest rather than the interest of the consumer-patient for whom he or she is agent—or, for that matter, the interests of society. When a physician recommends return office visits, care in a hospital of which he or she is an owner, or use of a costly new diagnostic technology that has been installed in the office, the consumer-patient may find it difficult to know whether the physician is or is not serving the patient's best interest. Such agent-principal problems are associated with situations characterized by "informational asymmetry," in which buyers and sellers are unequally informed. Similar situations are found in other industries, such as legal services, education and child care, and, in varying degree, throughout the business world. The same phenomenon occurs with respect to the honesty and completeness of information in corporate reports to stockholders. The point is not that medical care is a unique industry but that it has characteristics that make inappropriate certain common assumptions—such as that of well-informed consumers—and that therefore raise doubts about the economic consequences of increased competition.

Another aspect of the agent-principal relationship deserves attention. Our current medical care system, by establishing the physician as its linchpin, relies on the physician to determine the "appropriate" medical care to be provided, including whether hospitalization is required, for what period, with what level of service, with what specialists, and with what technology. One matter that seems to have been overlooked is that the current system places physicians in a position of dual and conflicting responsibility: acting as (1) agent for the ill-informed patient—doing what the patient would do if he or she possessed the medical expertise of a physician—and simultaneously as (2) agent for the government— taking into account the fact that consumer-patients, given the low private cost of medical care, sometimes have incentives to act in a privately rational but socially inefficient manner. Pressure may be brought on the physician, for example, to admit an elderly parent into a hospital so as to reduce the burden on the family. The physician's ethics code, which is frequently seen by economists as anticompetitive, seems to be oriented toward the physician-patient relationship rather than the physician-government relationship. We need to understand much better than we do now how this ethics code affects the behavior of physicians, hospitals, and patients. Given that the code restricts competition in the physician's direct sphere of influence, it is not apparent what the effects would be of increased competition in closely related parts of the medical care industry —including the markets for nurses, psychiatric social workers, and health care insurance.

Despite these various mechanisms for coping with informational asymmetries in health care, even quite sophisticated consumers are often poorly informed about options that are important to them.

Thirty years ago Tibor Scitovsky wrote an influential article that, though not dealing explicitly with the health care market, is relevant to its informational problems. In "Ignorance as a Source of Oligopoly Power," he showed that when consumers find it costly to judge quality, their lack of information restricts the effectiveness of competition and enhances monopoly power.[3] Just a few years ago, Mark Satterthwaite analyzed the physician market in the context of consumers' information problems.[4] He showed that an increase in the supply of physicians could

64

increase the cost to consumers of searching for an appropriate physician. By raising search costs, the increased supply would make the demand for each physician's services more inelastic, thereby augmenting the physician's monopoly power. Mark Schlesinger pointed out that the same argument could apply to nursing homes. Increased supply could lead to higher prices, not lower, as a conventional model of competition would imply. Still more recently, Joseph Stiglitz showed other conditions under which "increases in competition may lower welfare."[5] It is not difficult to see that in a "second-best" world, where markets are imperfect and information is differentially costly for buyers and sellers, increased competition may well decrease economic welfare.

Pricing in Health Care

In this discussion I emphasize the role of competition in terms of increased numbers of suppliers. If, however, measures were taken to increase competition by encouraging changes in pricing practices, some of the remarks in this section would not hold. At the same time it should be recognized that increased numbers of competitors would not necessarily bring increased price competition; moreover, increased price competition would have uncertain effects, given the informational problems discussed in the preceding section.

The health care industry is unusual not only in the degree to which its consumers are ill informed but also in its pricing practices. The economist's idealized competitive model assumes that prices reflect marginal social costs of production; consumers who face these prices will purchase the commodity only if its marginal value to them exceeds its marginal cost of production. But the economist's model of pricing is at best caricatured in the health care industry. With 90 percent or more of the U.S. population having some form of health insurance, the price to the patient of additional medical care is often zero, even though the social cost is far higher. Moreover, because employer-financed health insurance is not subject to income taxation, the purchase of health insurance is subsidized. Finally, the health care coverage under governmental Medicare and Medicaid programs acts further to drive a wedge between the real cost of medical care and the price to the consumer.

Whenever consumers of any good confront a price that is below social cost, excessive consumption is likely. Add to this effect a pricing system in which hospitals, physicians, and other providers are often paid by governmental and private insurers on the basis of actual costs, so that there is little incentive for holding those costs down, and on the basis of average, not marginal, costs, and we see a pricing system that at every point fails to confront decision makers with the true social costs of their decisions. This is far from the economist's model, in which having more

65

competitors promotes allocative efficiency. If, of course, pricing practices were changed at the same time that consumers were given more alternatives, the combined effect could be significant.

Prices serve as incentives. Prices that do not provide efficient choices permeate the medical care market. One element of nonoptimal pricing that has received little attention involves medical research. In most industries research is responsive to perceived opportunities either to reduce costs or to develop new and profitable products. These incentives do apply to research in the proprietary segment of the medical care market—for example, in the pharmaceutical industry—but they do not necessarily apply to the billions of dollars of research sponsored annually by the government through the National Institutes of Health. The peer-review grant system rewards research that is regarded as scientifically promising; the fruits of such research may well be expensive "halfway" technologies[6] that would receive less attention were it not for the medical insurance and reimbursement arrangements that provide incentives to adopt technological improvements almost regardless of cost.[7]

With virtually every hospital wanting, for example, the latest type of CAT scanner—at a purchase price now over $1 million—one cannot help doubting the consequences of increased competition if that meant having CAT scanners in more hospitals, clinics, or physicians' offices. Unless the health insurance and medical care pricing systems are altered, it is by no means clear that an increase in the supply of medical resources will cut costs or increase social welfare.

Moreover, given the prevailing institutional structure, in which only certain physicians may treat patients in any particular hospital and only a physician can admit a patient to a hospital, it is also not clear what increased competition in the form of greater freedom of entry into the hospital industry would bring about. It is likely, however, that the results would include more excess capacity and commensurately higher average costs.

All these pricing problems and interrelated institutional constraints limit our conventional reliance on competition among producers and freedom of entry to allocate medical care resources efficiently. Still another important sense in which the health care industry is unusual that raises doubts about the wisdom of applying the familiar prescription of competition for the industry's ailments is its "mixed industry" character. This is the subject of the next section.

The Influence of Governmental and Private Nonprofit Firms

So far I have tried to show that the medical care market violates two fundamental assumptions of the economic model in which more competition is better: well-informed consumers and prices that reflect the real marginal cost of production. A third important dimension in which the medical care market is unusual (though, again, not unique) in deviating from the model in which competition contributes to efficiency is the substantial role of nonproprietary producers—governmental and private nonprofit. In the short-stay hospital industry, for example, 28 percent of the beds are in governmental hospitals (city, county, state, federal), and 64 percent are in private nonprofit hospitals, and 8 percent are in proprietary hospitals (figure 4–1). In the nursing home industry, 10 percent of the beds are in homes run by governments (typically county), 23 percent are in private nonprofit homes, and 67 percent are in proprietary homes (figure 4–1).

The significance of this mixed industry character may well be profound. In a market comprising only profit-maximizing firms, increased competition will tend to promote allocative efficiency and low prices (if there are no distortions resulting from informational, pricing, or other sources of "private market failure"). Will the same be true of markets dominated by governmental and private nonprofit firms? The answer is not clear. Our present ability to understand and predict how such firms respond to increased competition is limited indeed.

The point is this: if one talks about the effects of increased competition in the health care sector, one is implying that it makes little or no difference whether the increased competition is from proprietary firms, church-owned nonprofit organizations, other nonprofit organizations, governmental institutions, or some other form of institution. Yet the assumption that all these institutions behave in essentially the same way is not suggested either by prevailing theory or by empirical evidence. There is some reason to believe, for example, that nonprofit hospitals concentrate on "high quality" service to a greater extent than proprietary hospitals.[8] If this is so, the effects of an increase in the number of hospital competitors will depend on the institutional form of those competitors. More nonprofit hospitals might well lead to increased costs, associated with the higher quality; more proprietary hospitals might bring about decreased costs and quality. The main point is not that we can assert confidently how the various institutional forms of hospitals and nursing homes compare in quality and efficiency, but rather that it is likely that they differ, that they are not perfect substitutes in all relevant respects. Institutional form counts, but we know little about how.[9]

Public policy measures affect not only the amount of competition in health care but also its institutional forms: entry of nonprofit organizations depends significantly on congressional legislation on tax-exempt nonprofit organizations and on the Internal Revenue Service's administration of that legislation; entry of governmental organizations is deter-

FIGURE 4-1
THE "MIXED" HEALTH CARE INDUSTRY

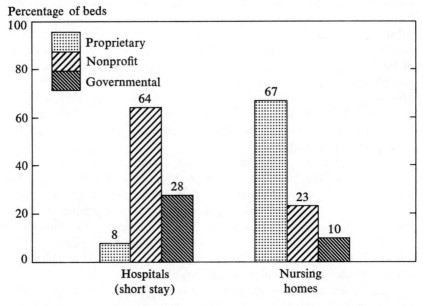

NOTE: Data on hospitals are for 1979; data on nursing homes are for 1976.
SOURCES: Hospitals—*Health: United States, 1981* (U.S. Department of Health and Human Services, National Center for Health Statistics, December 1981), p. 251; nursing homes—*Health: United States, 1978* (U.S. Department of Health and Human Services, National Center for Health Statistics, December 1978), p. 373.

mined explicitly by legislatures; and entry of proprietary firms depends similarly on governmental policies involving taxation, subsidization, and regulation of expenditures, minimum service quality, and prices. There are, in short, many restrictions on entry and competition; changes in some or even all will affect both the numbers of suppliers and the institutional composition, with consequences that are not entirely foreseeable. The principal reason is that we do not have satisfactory theoretic models for predicting the behavior of governmental and private nonprofit organizations (church-owned or otherwise), models that specify objectives (such as profit maximization in the proprietary sector) and constraints (such as market demand). More specifically, we know little about how various types of organizations respond to such stimuli as taxes, subsidies, expenditure ceilings, regulatory constraints, and increased or decreased competition.

Although formal theory may be weak, there are widespread opinions about the comparative behavior of nonprofit, governmental, and proprietary organizations. A New York State regulatory commission report recently recommended that the government "gradually phase out proprietary nursing facilities in New York . . . [and] substitute voluntary, nonprofit institutions as the mainstay of this industry."[10] Another study —this of children's day care—stated: "There appears to be near-consensus among persons who write about day care that private for-profit enterprises and the 'market' is an unsatisfactory way of organizing this activity." Turning to the health care sector, the authors observed that "relatedly, there is a deep suspicion of for-profit nursing homes and hospitals. Clearly, profit is being mentally associated with exploitation rather than responsible service."[11] Such alleged exploitation is possible because of the informational asymmetry discussed above.

In a study of the nursing home industry I have under way in collaboration with Mark Schlesinger, we seek to shed light on the question whether institutional form matters in health care—whether, in particular, nursing homes owned by proprietary firms, by church-run nonprofit organizations, by other nonprofit organizations, and by governments behave differently. Specifically, we ask whether they violate regulatory codes with different frequency and whether they give rise to different numbers of formal complaints to the state. Our findings: controlling for size and a number of locational and quality variables, (1) proprietary homes have significantly fewer violations of regulatory codes, but (2) church-run nonprofit organizations have significantly fewer complaints.[12] At least in adherence to regulatory codes, the various ownership types do behave differently, and consumers do seem to perceive some differences. Such findings do not necessarily imply differences in quality that are medically relevant, but they do highlight the likelihood that it makes a difference whether increased competition comes from one institutional form or another.

Conclusion

I have focused on three important ways in which the health care industry is unusual: the limited information available to consumers, the prevalence of prices that bear little relation to real costs of services, and the prominence of governmental and private nonprofit firms in competition with proprietary firms. Our conventional confidence in competitive markets grows largely from a model in which consumers are well informed, prices reflect real marginal costs, and firms are profit maximizers. Thus the consequences and the virtues of increased competition in the health care sector are not self-evident. In general, when some conditions required for efficiency do not hold, fulfilling other conditions does not enhance efficiency.

I have barely touched on other characteristics of the health care market that make it unusual: that life itself is sometimes at stake, that the industry is heavily regulated and much of the regulation (particularly by the Food and Drug Administration when approving new drugs) ignores prices and costs, and that equity—equal access or at least some substantial minimum level of access to health care for everyone, poor and nonpoor—is as important as efficiency.

A coherent health care policy remains a distant vision in the United States. Given the system we now have—some call it a nonsystem—we should be cautious about relying heavily on competition, on an increase in the supply and variety of health-care providers and facilities, to optimize the level and distribution of health care resources. Changes in pricing and reimbursement practices may help, if combined with other measures to encourage competition, but the unusual informational problems of the industry and its reliance on nonprofit institutions combine to pose serious questions about our conventional faith in competition.

I do not wish to close, however, by unduly dramatizing the uniqueness of health care. In many ways it is similar to the legal services and education markets, for example, where output is also difficult to monitor, consumers are often poorly informed, prices are often inefficient, and professional suppliers are powerful. More broadly, the health care market is not immune to the competitive pressures and tensions that characterize interactions between buyers and sellers in all markets. The point on which I will close is this: we cannot construct wise public policy on health care by applying elementary economic analysis. Competition does have a role to play. Yet the markets for health care and for chocolate chip cookies *are* different.

Notes

1. *Wall Street Journal*, May 29, 1981, p. 23.
2. Ralph Andreano, "Hospitals on TV," Radio Station WHA, Madison, Wisconsin, "Morning People" program, April 23, 1981.
3. *American Economic Review*, vol. 40, no. 2 (May 1950), pp. 48-53.
4. "The Effect of Increased Supply on Equilibrium Price: A Theory for the Strange Case of Physicians' Services," mimeographed, n.d. (circa 1977).
5. *American Economic Review*, vol. 71, no. 2 (May 1981), pp. 184-89, at p. 189.
6. Lewis Thomas, *The Lives of a Cell* (New York: Bantam Books, 1975).
7. John Goddeeris and Burton A. Weisbrod, "Medical Progress and Health Care Expenditures: The Uneasy Marriage," *Viewpoints* (Hoffmann-LaRoche, 1980).
8. Joseph P. Newhouse, "Towards a Theory of Nonprofit Institutions:

An Economic Model of a Hospital," *American Economic Review,* vol. 60, no. 1 (March 1970), pp. 64-74; and A. James Lee and Burton A. Weisbrod, "Collective Goods and the Voluntary Sector: The Case of the Hospital Industry," in Weisbrod, *The Voluntary Nonprofit Sector* (Lexington, Mass.: D.C. Heath & Co., Lexington Books, 1978).

9. For a recent study comparing the behavior of proprietary, governmental, and private nonprofit organizations, with particular emphasis on nursing homes, see Burton A. Weisbrod and Mark Schlesinger, "Comparative Institutional Behavior in Markets with Asymmetric Information: An Application to Nursing Homes," mimeograph, University of Wisconsin-Madison, Institute for Research on Poverty, October 1981.

10. *Long Term Care Regulation: Past Lapses, Future Prospects, Summary Report,* New York State Moreland Act Commission on Nursing Home and Residential Facilities (Albany, April 1975), p. 13.

11. Richard Nelson and Richard Krashinsky, "Two Major Issues of Public Policy: Public Subsidy and the Organization of Supply," in Dennis Young and Richard Nelson, eds., *Public Policy for Day Care of Young Children* (Lexington, Mass.: Lexington Books, 1973).

12. See citation in note 9, above.

Part Two
New Frontiers in Cost Containment

5

Quiet Revolutions in Medicaid

Rosemary Gibson

The thrust of the incentives-based approach to health care reform has not come to fruition in federal legislation. Despite the absence of legislative reforms in health policy discussed elsewhere in this volume, a number of state and local governments are significantly altering the traditional approach to delivering and financing health services. These changes, which are representative of recent trends, indicate that the U.S. health care system is undergoing a gradual but steady change. Both the private and the public sectors are beginning to formulate rules that reward cost-conscious buyers and efficient sellers in the medical service markets. Some of the private sector initiatives identified in chapter 8 by Patricia Samors and Sean Sullivan are attempting to change the incentives that influence decisions by consumers, providers, employers, insurers, and employees on the use and financing of medical services. These initiatives include preferred provider plans, alternative benefit packages, and utilization review. In public sector programs, especially Medicaid, long-range, structural changes are being made that parallel the private sector activity and alter the incentives for providers and consumers. Thus, consumers' incentives to choose efficient health care plans and providers' incentives to reduce costs are affected by both new initiatives of private employers and insurers and the gradually developing policies of government at all levels.

This discussion highlights state and county initiatives in Medicaid programs that attempt to encourage cost consciousness on the part of providers and recipients, as well as the states and counties themselves. Specifically, examples of initiatives in developing primary care networks (PCNs), case management systems, and alternatives to institutional long-term care are examined. These initiatives are contrasted with, and may help avoid, cuts in Medicaid eligibility and benefits and controls on fees and charges that address the symptoms of spiraling medical costs rather than the sources. These innovative approaches reflect the growing interest among the states and counties in designing medical care delivery and financing systems. Therefore, in addition to the legal, economic, and medical questions that policy makers need to consider as part of any federal health legislation, the burgeoning role of state and local governments needs to be emphasized and examined. The success of any federal initiative to promote changes in the incentives in the health care delivery and financing system is contingent upon the policies and programs of other levels of government.

Background

Before the enactment of the Medicaid program in 1965, state and local governments spent more for health purposes than the federal government did.[1] In the 1970s, the federal role grew to the extent that total federal health expenditures grew to be more than twice as large as state and local expenditures combined.[2] In the 1980s, the states are reemerging in health policy making at a time when the "New Federalism" has placed more responsibility on the states to design, implement, and finance health care programs. Block grants and new regulations for the Medicaid program offer states more flexibility in structuring and administering their programs. This flexibility, however, appears to be overshadowed by budget constraints. Along with their enhanced policy and administrative functions, states are faced with increasing health care costs and diminishing federal support.

Between 1970 and 1980, total federal health expenditures quadrupled, while total state and local health expenditures more than tripled. Medicaid constitutes the fastest growing portion of state budgets. Whereas in 1970 Medicaid accounted for one-third of state health budgets, by 1978 it constituted one-half of these budgets.[3] In the Medicaid program itself, federal and state expenditures grew at an average rate of 15 percent a year from 1975 to 1980 and increased 21 percent from 1980 to 1981.

Medicaid program expenditures continue to soar for the federal government, even though federal matching for the Medicaid program has been reduced. Expenditure growth was reduced by $3.4 billion in the fiscal year (FY) 1982 budget and will be reduced further in the FY 1983 budget. In spite of these reductions, federal program expenditures (excluding administrative expenses) are expected to grow at an annual rate of more than 10 percent in 1983 and 1984, and by more than 15 percent in 1985.

These factors, together with the fact that state laws generally prohibit deficits, severely pressure the states to solve immediate budget problems by cutting benefits or eligibility rather than by developing structural reforms. Although short-term responses to a budget crunch are

76

inevitable, they do not constitute a firm basis for developing long-range cost-containment policies and programs to provide quality care to those in need. It is therefore important to address the long-term evolution of state policies in health care delivery and financing.

Examination of long-term state initiatives comes at a crucial time not only in budgetary matters but also in the development of health policy. Existing and proposed federal policies indicate that a new approach to the economics of medical care is emerging. This approach incorporates incentives to encourage consumers, providers, employers, and insurers to be conscious of cost and quality in their choice and provision of health insurance and medical care. Several bills—H.R. 850, introduced by Congressman Richard A. Gephardt (Democrat, Missouri); S. 139, by Senator Orrin Hatch (Republican, Utah); and S. 433, by Senator David Durenberger (Republican, Minnesota)—would alter the existing tax incentives that encourage the purchase of first-dollar health insurance coverage. The Hatch and Durenberger bills would require employers to offer their employees a choice of health plans. Other proposals have been introduced that encourage the development of alternative forms of financing and providing long-term care, the largest component in Medicaid. Legislation introduced by Senator Hatch (S. 234) would offer a tax credit of up to $500 to families who take care of elderly dependents.

The success of market reform, however, depends upon state laws and policies. Some state laws governing premium taxes and financial requirements prevent different insurers from competing on an equal footing. Other state laws serve as barriers to entry, especially occupational licensing which delineates the scope of practice of new, emerging groups of medical service providers. Such constraints may inhibit the development of alternative delivery mechanisms that could utilize these new providers effectively. Thus, in some instances, there is an insufficient nexus between proposed market-oriented federal policies and state policies. Many of these potential barriers to a competitive health care market are discussed in chapter 13 of this volume by Rosemary Gibson and John Reiss. The purpose of this chapter is to describe and evaluate other areas of state and local government health policies in the Medicaid program that parallel proposed federal policies designed to encourage cost-effective use of medical services by providers and consumers.

Medicaid

Medicaid is a joint federal-state program administered by the states under federal guidelines. Eligibility for Medicaid benefits extends to certain categories of low-income persons who are eligible for cash assistance under the Aid to Families with Dependent Children (AFDC) program. States, however, have considerable freedom to set the income levels for AFDC eligibility, thereby varying Medicaid eligibility among the states. In addition, most recipients of Supplemental Security Income (SSI), a federal program for the aged, blind, and disabled, are eligible. Because states had the option to provide Medicaid to the increased SSI population when the federal government assumed responsibility for the program in 1972, not all SSI eligibles are automatically eligible for Medicaid. Income limits for SSI, unlike the AFDC program, are set by the federal government. AFDC beneficiaries number about 63.6 percent of all Medicaid recipients but generate only 27.8 percent of program expenditures. In contrast, SSI recipients make up 28.4 percent of total Medicaid recipients but account for 67.8 percent of program expenditures.

States have the option of providing coverage to the medically needy who are categorically eligible—that is, the aged, blind, and disabled, as well as members of families with dependent children whose income, though low, is too high to qualify for AFDC or SSI. Families with monthly incomes greater than the cash assistance level but less than 133⅓ percent of that standard are eligible for medically needy assistance. Moreover, through spend-down provisions, medically needy eligibility extends to those who have incomes above the 133⅓ percent level, but whose medical expenses reduce their income below that standard.

Certain basic services that must be offered in any state Medicaid program include inpatient hospital care, outpatient care, laboratory and X-ray services, and skilled nursing facility and physician services. States, however, may limit the scope of coverage for the required services—for example, by limiting the number of inpatient hospital days or outpatient visits that Medicaid will cover. Optional services include dental services, prescribed drugs, and private nursing, which also are subject to limitations.

Federal and State Medicaid Budgets. Because Medicaid is a jointly funded and administered program, state Medicaid policies are contingent on federal budgets and regulations, which set the framework within which states operate their programs. Recent federal budget changes, as well as current economic conditions, have affected the thrust of long- and short-term policies for state programs. Currently, the federal share of state Medicaid expenditures, based on the per capita income in each state, ranges between 50 and 78 percent and averages 54.5 percent nationwide. The reductions in the federal match in the Omnibus Budget Reconciliation Act of 1981 are projected to decrease the current federal share in Medicaid (see table 5–1). Moreover, the Reagan administration's FY

TABLE 5–1

PROJECTED FEDERAL AND STATE MEDICAID EXPENDITURES,

1981–1984

(billions of dollars)

Fiscal Year	Federal Expenditures	State Expenditures	Federal Expenditures as a Percentage of Total Expenditures
1981	17.1	13.9	55.16
1982	18.3	15.5	54.14
1983	19.9	17.0	53.92
1984	21.9	18.8	53.08

NOTE: As of the Omnibus Budget Reconciliation Act of 1981.
SOURCE: U.S. Office of Management and Budget.

1983 Medicaid budget proposals incorporated a number of measures that would have further reduced the federal matching in Medicaid by $2 billion for 1983, $2.3 billion in 1984, and $3.7 billion in 1985. The Congress, however, rejected many of the proposed cuts.

One of the major provisions in the administration's 1983 budget proposal that was accepted by the Congress in the Tax Equity and Fiscal Responsibility Act of 1982 allows states to charge all Medicaid beneficiaries nominal copayments for certain mandatory and optional services. States cannot, however, impose copayments on categorically needy children under eighteen, and on services related to pregnancy, categorically needy patients in skilled nursing and intermediate care facilities, emergency and family planning services, and categorically needy persons enrolled in a health maintenance organization (HMO). The copayment provision is estimated to decrease federal Medicaid expenditures by $45 million in 1983, $50 million in 1984, and $56 million in 1985.

These budget changes in Medicaid for FY 1983 are in addition to the 1981 Reconciliation Act changes for FY 1982. Federal Medicaid matching rates to the states will be reduced by 3 percent in 1982, 4 percent in 1983, and 4.5 percent in 1984, although these percentages vary if a state meets certain stipulations. A state receives a one-percentage-point increase in federal payments if it has a qualified hospital cost review program, or if it has an unemployment rate 50 percent higher than the national average, or if the recoveries from fraud and abuse are greater than or equal to 1 percent of the quarterly federal payments to the states. States may also receive relief from the 3 percent reduction by keeping federal Medicaid reimbursement in FY 1982 from growing more than 9 percent over federal FY 1981 levels. If federal reimbursement grows less than 9 percent, a state qualifies for a dollar-for-dollar offset of the difference between actual federal spending and the 9 percent target growth rate.

AFDC Budget. In addition to addressing the Medicaid program directly, the 1981 Reconciliation Act incorporated changes in the AFDC program that affect Medicaid eligibility. The act changed AFDC eligibility and hence the number of Medicaid recipients by tightening the requirements for cash assistance. The act imposed an eligibility limit restricting benefit payments to families whose gross income does not exceed 150 percent of the states' need standards. The act also tightened the limit on family resources by lowering the cap on assets (other than a home and one car) from $2,000 to $1,000 and by allowing states to consider as income the value of food stamps and rent or housing subsidies to the extent that these amounts duplicate food or housing components in the state standard of need.

Also, Congress accepted in the 1981 Reconciliation Act an administration proposal to end a child's eligibility for AFDC on his eighteenth birthday, unless the state chooses to extend the limit to age nineteen for those expected to complete secondary school by that age. This provision is estimated to remove up to 25,000 families from AFDC.

In total, the administration estimated that the 1981 act ended AFDC benefits and automatic Medicaid eligibility for those who are categorically needy for more than 400,000 families, or 10.5 percent of the present total. These cuts in eligibility, however, do not automatically translate into decreasing Medicaid eligibility. For example, individuals who are no longer eligible for AFDC, but who have medical expenditures that reduce available income below designated levels, may be eligible for medically needy Medicaid assistance instead of categorically needy assistance, if the state offers a medically needy program.

The Tax Equity Act of 1982 made comparatively minor changes in AFDC. It required states to round both their AFDC need standard and actual monthly benefit amounts to the next lower whole dollar. A more substantial change requires that AFDC benefits be no longer payable to families if the parent is absent solely because of active duty in the uniformed services. The 1982 act is estimated to eliminate AFDC eligibility for 15,000 families with a corresponding savings for Medicaid estimated to be $12.6 million in FY 1983.

Regulatory Changes. In addition to budget changes, the 1981 Reconciliation Act incorporated significant regulatory changes that allow states the flexibility to experiment in the Medicaid program. For instance, states are authorized to purchase laboratory services and medical devices through competitive bidding arrangements. States may also "lock-out" or suspend the participation of a physician that a state finds has provided services that do not meet professionally recognized standards of care. Beneficiaries found to overuse services may be "locked-in" to particular providers. This provision, in effect, legitimizes what some states have already been doing with selected Medicaid recipients.

The statute also allows states to request the U.S. Department of Health and Human Services (HHS) to waive federal requirements to enable them to manage their Medicaid programs more cost-effectively. States may request waivers to restrict beneficiaries to receive services (in nonemergency circumstances) only from cost-effective providers. States also may set up arrangements whereby beneficiaries share in the savings resulting from their use of more cost-effective care in the form of additional benefits. Under a waiver, local jurisdictions may act as central brokers in helping beneficiaries select among competing health care plans. The statute also authorizes Medicaid reimbursement for home and community-based services, beyond what is already reimbursed, for beneficiaries who are otherwise eligible for admission to long-term care institutions.

State Responses to Budget and Regulatory Changes

State Medicaid programs are responding to the budget and regulatory climate in two ways. Several states are limiting the scope of services and restricting eligibility as a way to control Medicaid budgets. Given the severity of budgetary pressures in many states, these immediate steps are perceived to be the only way to stave off impending budget crises.

Other states, however, are attempting to undertake major restructuring and reorientation in their Medicaid programs to encourage providers, consumers, and the states themselves to provide and finance more cost-effective care. The restructuring of the program is being attempted by establishing primary care networks and case management and by instituting cost sharing. Moreover, some states are making legislative changes that encourage their state health departments to act as prudent purchasers of Medicaid services. The reorientation of the program is taking place in states that are encouraging the development of noninstitutional, community-based alternatives in long-term care.

Short-Term Changes. In response to spiraling costs, decreased federal support, and increasing pressure from other social service programs, many states are focusing on short-term budget considerations in assessing their Medicaid program expenditures. Since most states are prohibited by state law from having deficits, and since there is a limit on the states' ability to "hide" deficits, states have pressing needs to balance their budgets. One of the most obvious areas for budget cutbacks is the fastest growing part of the state budgets—Medicaid.

A study of state laws governing the Medicaid program indicates that 1980 may have been "the last year for some time in which state Medicaid programs show a net expansion of services and eligibility."[4] Although in 1980 most of the laws dealt with broadening the scope of benefits, "reports on 1981 legislation and departmental activities indicate that this trend, for the most part, has reversed."[5]

Virginia, for example, is projecting a Medicaid deficit of $122 million for the two-year period 1983–1984.[6] In response to these deficits, the state has focused on cutbacks in eligibility, benefits, and reimbursement levels. Services to AFDC medically needy adults will be limited to prenatal and delivery services for pregnant women. AFDC medically needy children will have their benefits curtailed to include only ambulatory care services. All coverage would be discontinued for AFDC-related children eighteen years of age and older and their caretakers who have no children under eighteen in their care. This change coincides with the amended AFDC cash assistance program instituted under the 1981 Reconciliation Act. The aged, blind, and disabled who are medically needy also would have their benefits discontinued. Savings are estimated to be $34 million if the Virginia proposal is accepted by the State Board of Health.

In addition to eligibility cutbacks, services would also be curtailed under the proposed Virginia plan. The maximum number of days covered per inpatient hospital admission would be cut from 21 to 10. Under current policy, 18–20 percent of hospital stays exceed 10 days, and the average length of stay is 16.6 days. The proposed policy would result in a reduction of 65,000–70,000 covered days, thereby reducing expenditures by an estimated $13 million. The proposal would further limit the number of covered inpatient hospital days per recipient to 21 per year, whereas under current policy there is no annual limit. This will lead to an estimated savings of $12.6 million. In its cutbacks on reimbursement, the state would limit the annual cost increase allowed to hospitals to 9 percent.

In another example, California has passed legislation that would make eligibility requirements for Medi-Cal, the state's Medicaid program, more strict.[7] Beginning in January 1983, eligibility for coverage as medically indigent will be limited to children under twenty-one years of age and adults residing in skilled nursing facilities and intermediate-care facilities. Moreover, whereas the earlier law set the income limitation at 115 percent of the AFDC program's highest payments, the new legislation reduces the standard to the lowest levels at which federal financial participation will still be provided.

In 1982, fourteen states limited the scope of mandatory services. Some reductions are relatively less extreme; for example, New Hampshire's benefits will no longer include cosmetic surgery. Other states, such as South Carolina and West Virginia, however, have limited covered inpatient hospital days—to a total of twelve to twenty days per year, depending upon the state. Thirteen states have begun charging small fees for services such as dentistry and optometry. Eleven states have tightened eligibility criteria, limiting coverage of welfare recipients between eighteen and twenty-one years.

Several problems arise, however, when states attempt to cut back eligibility and benefits. There is a history of court action that has had the effect of blocking or delaying states' initiatives or policies aimed at controlling their Medicaid costs.[8] One of the most common actions preventing states from implementing cost-saving modifications involves alleged violations of the notice and fair-hearing requirements before benefits are reduced or terminated. Moreover, federal regulations provide that states cannot deny or reduce the amount or duration of services solely on the basis of diagnosis, type of illness, or condition. In 1979, for example, Florida's limit on physician services to three visits per month was permanently enjoined by a U.S. district court, in part because the limit was contrary to those regulations. Upon appeal, the decision was reversed because, under Florida's limits, no particular medical condition had been singled out for unique treatment.

In other examples, Washington attempted to terminate its medically needy programs in 1981, but was enjoined from doing so by the federal district court on procedural grounds. West Virginia was similarly enjoined in July 1981. Thus, if states choose to pursue restricting their Medicaid benefits and eligibility, legal impediments may be more the rule than the exception.

Another result of short-term changes in Medicaid eligibility benefits and reimbursement rates is significant cost shifting from public to private payers. The lower reimbursement rates under Medicaid as well as Medicare, which do not account for hospital bad debts, teaching and research functions, and charity care provided by the hospitals, encourage providers to shift costs to private payers rather than to economize to meet lower payment schedules. Moreover, when states limit eligibility and cut benefits, individuals no longer covered may be taken as bad debts or treated as charity care patients, which are not accounted for in public program reimbursement. According to some estimates, the total shift from Medicare and Medicaid amounted to $4.8 billion in 1981.[9] This cost shift is expected to be exacerbated by proposed reductions in provider reimbursement in federal and state budgets.

The cost shift is a clear indication that there are no real cost savings in limiting reimbursement to providers; rather, the costs are "hidden" as they are shifted to other payers. Moreover, by limiting eligibility and scope of benefits in Medicaid, states do not address the inefficient and ineffective structures that exacerbate the program cost spiral. The cost-based reimbursement system, which fuels the unrestrained use of the system by consumers and providers, remains intact. Thus, any substantive change in the Medicaid program requires a restructuring of the program itself and a change in the way in which health care delivery is organized and financed.

Primary Care Networks and Case Management. Because the states are faced with both the limited potential of short-term approaches to holding down Medicaid costs and the leeway afforded by recent federal regulations to develop alternative means of providing care, several states and counties have proposed to move toward a restructuring of their Medicaid programs. A key component of this restructuring is to reverse costly financial incentives in the fee-for-service system by establishing primary care networks and case management.

Unlike the short-term changes in the Medicaid program, the PCN and case management approach alters the behavior of providers, consumers, and the state, county, or administering body itself. PCNs are composed mostly of primary care physicians in solo or group practices who serve as "gatekeepers" for patients enrolled in the networks. PCNs incorporate case management by having the physician, as is done in HMOs, refer and review all medical care that the patient requires. Case management, which is an integral part of PCNs, could involve hospitals, rather than primary care physicians, as case managers.

PCNs place the primary care physician at varying degrees of risk, depending upon the arrangements made by the physicians and the public body or other organization administering Medicaid. To enable the physician to serve as an effective gatekeeper, the primary physician may receive an account of all services provided to the patients by specialists and hospitals. The physician can then identify where, adjusting for case mix, cost savings can be realized.

Consumer behavior is also affected by PCNs since costly and unnecessary use of services can be curtailed. Primary care physicians provide nonemergency services in primary care centers rather than emergency rooms, which yields considerable savings. Also, PCNs eliminate excessive patient self-referrals to medical services, with the added advantage of allowing continuity of patient care. Moreover, PCNs can alleviate patients' difficulty in locating a primary care physician who will take responsibility for the patients, assuming that the physician performs the case management function judiciously.

The state or administering body for PCNs can also be exposed to changed incentives. In the Arizona Health Care Cost Containment System (AHCCCS) program, for example, the state receives a capitated amount of federal money per eligible indigent enrollee, which puts the state at risk. In turn, the state contracts with an administrative intermediary, which is also at risk. Thus, PCNs remove the open-ended nature of the health system that creates disincentives for providers as well as the states; moreover, PCNs eliminate the unlimited availability of services to recipients. These altered incentives are the key to long-run efficiencies in the health system because they try to respond to the demands of both medical efficacy and economic efficiency. In this way, the growing tension between unlimited demand for care and the shrinking growth of available resources can be reconciled by the participants in the system rather than by legislative or executive fiat.

One of the major features of PCNs, besides the primary care physician as gatekeeper, is the limitation on free choice of provider. This limit in PCNs is representative of a trend in the private sector where the growth of preferred provider organizations (PPOs) and prepaid plans indicates an acceptance of limits on choice of provider.[10]

For the states, the freedom-of-choice requirement in the Medicaid program greatly restricts their ability to contain costs. States have argued that they have been "precluded by federal law from acting as prudent purchasers of care."[11] States have perceived a need to be able "to contract with physicians, hospitals, and other providers in a manner that establishes a point of responsibility and accountability for total medical costs."[12]

Supporters of freedom of choice contend that patients, rather than the states, are in the best position to judge quality of care. Although states may monitor quality of care, patterns of abuse may not become immediately evident. Instances when abuse has been cited—for example, in California's Medi-Cal program in the 1970s—have inhibited efforts to curtail freedom of choice. Supporters also argue that access to care may be limited if the state contracts with too few providers or if the providers are not conveniently located. The Colorado Medicaid program, for example, has instituted its own form of PCN, but has been prevented from carrying out the plan until it can ensure sufficient access to care.

Others have argued forcefully, however, that the freedom-of-choice requirement is the main source of overspending on health care. Preferred provider plans, which segment the physician market by rewarding the

85

more efficient providers, would curtail the tendency for consumers and medical providers to have "the freedom to choose the most expensive of the available alternatives without having to pay extra for it."[13] The current system of reimbursement, under private or public insurance, takes away incentives for consumers to choose less costly providers. As Mancur Olson argues:

> The patient [has] an incentive to seek the best and most comfortable care, since it does not cost him any extra money; the providers have an incentive to compete with one another in providing more costly care, even if the extra dollars spent are worth only pennies to the patient. The situation is usually much the same for those whose medical care is paid for by the government; thus even the poorest people often have an incentive to choose the most costly care.[14]

Some states that have incorporated PCNs and case management in their Medicaid programs point to specific examples of inappropriate or unnecessary utilization of services. The Massachusetts Department of Public Welfare, in its FY 1983 budget proposal, maintained that

> with few exceptions, Medicaid does not limit recipient use of services. It also does not determine the setting in which recipients obtain care. Further, according to the Department of Public Welfare, Medicaid reimburses for each service provided which creates an economic incentive for using more intensive services. The result is that Medicaid patients receive more services and more costly services in more expensive settings than is required.[15]

The department estimated that up to 5 percent of the acute inpatient hospital days for which it pays are not medically necessary; payments for these days cost approximately $12 million in FY 1981. Another department study of approximately 300 randomly chosen visits to one hospital's emergency room found that 47 percent of the costs incurred were inappropriate—that the recipients could have obtained the care they required for 50 to 75 percent less than the cost in an emergency room.

Although there are incentives to overutilize services in a fee-for-service system, there are incentives to underutilize services in a prepaid or capitation scheme in PCNs, HMOs, or PPOs where providers are generally paid prospectively a set amount for each patient. Olson argues convincingly:

> to the extent competitive pressures and consumer ignorance allow, the fee-for-service physician can provide unnecessarily

costly services. Equally, to the extent the competitive pressures and consumer ignorance allow, the prepaid group can provide less services or poorer services than the consumer has paid for. Thus, there is no inherent superiority of prepaid group practice over fee-for-service.[16]

But, Olson adds, prepaid group practices provide "practically the only existing alternative to the so-called freedom of choice rule for those who want health insurance."[17]

Models of State Initiatives

A number of states and counties are attempting to control and project their Medicaid costs better through a variety of systems that limit free choice of provider and incorporate alternatives to the open-ended reimbursement system. Some states have received federal waivers, whereas others have made their own changes in their state legislatures. Currently, eleven states have received waivers from the freedom-of-choice requirement in Medicaid and are establishing variations on case management. The following are sketches of several state and local initiatives involving both federal waivers and state legislative action.

Oregon. One of the pioneering efforts in offering medical care to the medically indigent through prepaid health plans is Project Health in Multnomah County, Oregon. The founders of Project Health were intent upon following the consumer choice model closely identified with Alain Enthoven. The project is therefore relevant to the current regulatory environment, which encourages states to incorporate incentives for providers and recipients in the Medicaid programs.

The project began in 1976 as a five-year demonstration program and involved a government agency acting as a broker to contract with prepaid health plans. Enrollees were given a choice among six plans, all of which offered a standard comprehensive benefit package. The enrollees also could choose to receive care through a fee-for-service program, in which high-risk patients were placed. A key component in the system, unlike the more recent case management programs, was the beneficiaries' monthly contributions to "enrollment fees," which were adjusted according to ability to pay and the cost of the different plans.

One problem encountered by Project Health was adverse selection, which is a stumbling block for market-oriented approaches in general. Adverse selection caused a disproportionate share of high-risk beneficiaries to enroll in the open panel plans, where patients have a wider ranging choice of providers than in closed panel plans. One apparent

87

reason for this is that those who would want most to preserve an existing relationship with a physician through an open panel have had ongoing treatments for illness. Consequently, the open panel plans attracted a less healthy population. As a result, one of the open panel plans opted to withdraw from the project, whereas the remaining open panel plan requested and received a rate increase as an alternative to withdrawing.

Despite the adverse selection problem, Project Health achieved some notable successes. A final evaluation of the program found that, for most of the five years, the project had lower health care costs than conventional medically needy programs in California and Washington.[18] The cost savings are primarily attributed to the fact that 25 percent of the recipients enrolled in the Kaiser Health Plan, which had significantly lower premiums than those of other plans. Moreover, cost sharing on the part of beneficiaries was found to be one of the essential components of the project.

Project Health has evolved from a demonstration project to a program that pools public and private funds and brokers private plans for most of the five years, the project had lower health care costs As in the demonstration project phase of Project Health, the client selects a plan and shares in the cost of the premium based on income, family size, and plan selected.

As a counterpart to Project Health, the county has established and funded Multicare, a primary care/case management system. The system responds to the adverse selection problem encountered in Project Health by screening medically indigent applicants and placing the highest-risk clients in Multicare. By screening the highest-risk patients into the county PCN, Project Health may be able to control for adverse selection, thereby preserving the participation of private health plans in the project.

While Multnomah County is a unique area, given the prior existence of several prepaid health plans, key factors in the success of the program were the spreading of financial risk to include providers and consumers and the use of enrollment counseling to isolate the high risks and prevent "cream skimming" by the health plans. Clearly, one of the lessons learned from Project Health is the advantage of organized delivery systems in providing care to Medicaid recipients who were financial participants in the system. Consequently, the greater flexibility in the 1981 Reconciliation Act allowing the states to set up their own organized delivery systems is a potential milestone in the Medicaid program.

Massachusetts. In Massachusetts, which proposed to cut back state Medicaid funding by 25 percent, a group of Boston teaching hospitals and clinics has formed the Commonwealth Health Care Corporation (CHCC). This plan is unique in that it is a private sector initiative which will be assuming some of the major functions of a public program. The corporation would serve as an intermediary and contract with case-management-oriented providers to offer coordinated care to Medicaid recipients. The corporation would assume most aspects of Medicaid management, including claims processing and utilization review, which the state currently performs. Medicaid patients would choose among a number of plans offered by neighborhood health centers, HMOs, and hospitals. As in the other states with case management, the recipients would be locked-in to their choice of provider for all nonemergency services.

The teaching hospitals perceived two advantages of the corporation model as financial and administrative intermediary. First, it has the potential to provide overall coordination of the program because the member organizations will be providing the bulk of the services offered by the corporation. Providers will thus have a more direct role in the operation of the plan. The second reason is that data management, claims processing, and utilization review are not available in the individual provider institutions. These information systems are vital for evaluating and maximizing the efficiency of resource use.

The corporation would identify participating health plans and offer a uniform benefit package. Medicaid recipients would choose among primary care sites, and within each site, among primary care physicians. The CHCC would receive a per capita amount from the state and negotiate a fair capitation rate for each provider plan. Unlike other state plans, each plan would not be at risk financially for its own enrollees. Risk would be shared on an aggregate basis in the sense that all providers would share in any surplus or deficit left at the end of the year.

This program is being planned against a backdrop of other efforts in Massachusetts to set up case management systems. An initial Massachusetts case management demonstration project sponsored by HHS was aimed at reducing unnecessary inpatient care, visits to hospital emergency rooms and outpatient departments, and excess laboratory tests and X-rays by enrolling Medicaid recipients in single sites through which they were to receive all their care. The pilot project enrolled 6,000 AFDC Medicaid eligibles at three community health centers and one hospital-based ambulatory care center. The sites were to coordinate their medical care, though enrollees could go elsewhere for care. This experiment failed to demonstrate net savings, although one center did achieve cost savings through reducing some unnecessary visits to hospital outpatient departments and emergency rooms. Yearly medical costs actually rose by as much as $500 per Medicaid family. The state did correct some of the deficiencies in the program with administrative changes—for example, by providing recipients with Medicaid cards that would prevent them from receiving unauthorized care outside their designated sites.

Although the state experienced administrative pitfalls with managed care, it is planning to increase significantly the number of recipients enrolled in managed health care plans. Savings are anticipated in the long run from shifting care to less costly, more appropriate settings.

Kentucky. The Citicare program is a proposed plan for Louisville that aims to incorporate a capitation payment program for AFDC-eligible Medicaid recipients. The plan is currently under negotiation. An initial plan that was discussed but not implemented was designed so that patients would sign up with a primary care physician who would receive part of the capitation fee, to be based on age, sex, and family size. The rest of the capitation would have been reserved for a pool of specialists who were to be reimbursed on a fee-for-service basis. If a loss occurred in the pool, the specialists would have been reimbursed on a prorated basis. The advantage of this type of project is that the specialists as well as the primary care physicians have incentives to monitor their use of medical services. Under other case management arrangements, the system tends to exert direct leverage over the primary care physicians, but not the specialists. Thus, in the initial plan, the state would have been putting direct leverage on both primary care physicians and specialists to contain costs.

The renegotiated plan, however, has taken a different form. Primary care physicians will receive a capitated monthly fee, of which one-half is designated to cover all physician services and the other half is designated for hospital care, including outpatient surgery and home health care. In the first year, Citicare will assume all risk for losses, whereas in subsequent years the primary care physicians will be at risk for losses up to 5 percent of their total capitation. Copayments of $10 and $2, respectively, are incorporated in Citicare (subject to federal waiver approval) to give incentives to patients to substitute primary care for the use of emergency rooms.

New York. New York's Metropolitan Comprehensive Care Program is a demonstration project that has been operating for two years, providing comprehensive health care services to the residents of parts of Manhattan including East Harlem. The Citycaid plan is the city's first move to restrict Medicaid recipients to specific health facilities. The long-range plan is to require all of the city's 1,250,000 Medicaid recipients to receive health care from the municipal hospital or facility nearest their home. The five-year pilot project offers services in a manner similar to HMOs. Physicians are currently reimbursed on a fee-for-service basis, but this will eventually change to a capitation system, so that the program will work strictly like an HMO. Enrollees can choose among three patient care teams, comprising two physicians, a nurse practitioner, a registered nurse, a nutritionist, and a social worker. One of the physicians is assigned as the patient's primary care provider.

The medically needy are locked into the system to the extent that they receive medical care financed by the city. The categorically needy, however, have the option to receive care from a municipal hospital or other providers. The unique feature of this plan is that both the categorically and the medically needy can disenroll at any time. The incentive for patients to choose case management, however, is that continuity of care is provided by a medical team.

Importantly, competitive elements are emerging, as some physicians are requested by patients more than are others; these physicians have an increased patient load and increased payments. Thus, under managed care, where recipients have a choice among different providers, new incentives for physicians are emerging.

Michigan. Michigan, which has had a 15 percent unemployment rate and growing numbers of Medicaid recipients, has been experiencing increasing pressure on its state budget. Wayne County alone, which includes Detroit, has more Medicaid recipients than thirty-seven of the states. Consequently, the state applied for and received a waiver from HHS to restructure its Medicaid program, using the Physician Primary Sponsor plan developed by the Michigan State Medical Society and the Michigan Department of Social Services. This plan involves a primary care network in which primary care physicians receive an administrative service fee for authorizing and arranging all the medical services for the patient and making all referrals to specialists. Both the primary and the specialist physicians are reimbursed on a fee-for-service basis. Recipients may continue with their existing physicians or choose a physician from a list of participating providers.

The key cost-saving component is based on the premise that physicians are often unaware of the costs of medical services. Each quarter, the primary care physician will receive a record of services he authorized and if, after two quarters, a particular physician's cost of services is in the highest 5 percent, compared with other physician's services, the administrative service fee is held in escrow until costs and quality are within an acceptable range. The control system will facilitate identifying high- and low-cost utilizers, thereby allowing the primary physicians and the state to locate the more cost-conscious providers.

Implementation problems have arisen, however, which illustrate the legal and administrative obstacles a state must overcome in developing

91

a new program. The Physician Primary Sponsor plan was blocked for several months by a temporary restraining order on the grounds that physicians who would be identified as high utilizers and dismissed from plan participation would be given insufficient recourse to appeal the decision. In addition, some physicians have challenged the program provision that limits the number of Medicaid patients per participating physician to 1,500. These administrative and legal barriers represent potential pitfalls for any of the states undertaking new program initiatives.

Colorado. Another variation on case management is found in a Colorado initiative in which the state requested and received a waiver to enroll Medicaid eligibles in a case management program. It is a statewide effort that will offer all Medicaid eligibles a choice between HMOs and PCNs. An earlier waiver had been received to conduct a more limited experiment enrolling Medicaid recipients in rural Mesa County in an HMO. But because physicians and Medicaid recipients opposed the plan as not affording sufficient access to care, it was terminated in favor of a more encompassing scheme.

Currently, physicians serving Medicaid recipients are reimbursed 55 percent of billed charges. Under the new plan, the physicians will be reimbursed 75 percent of billed charges if they achieve savings targets on hospital utilization. The twenty-percentage-point difference between current and proposed reimbursement will be pooled and, to the extent that the physicians meet the targets, they will have the opportunity to earn more than they would under current reimbursement rates. Thus, whereas physicians might possibly gain financially, there is no possibility of loss below the existing levels. Reimbursement will still be on a fee-for-service basis, as with the Michigan plan, and enrollees are required to remain with the designated physician until open enrollment. Because the proposal for this program came from the Colorado Medical Society, good physician participation is expected.

Arizona. The Arizona Health Care Cost Containment System (AHCCCS) is an established statewide health care system for private and public employers as well as the state's indigent population.

A unique part of the Arizona program is the participation of the state, as well as that of providers and consumers, in bearing a portion of the financial risk in providing services. Unlike the open-ended federal matching in the Medicaid program, the state will bear part of the financial risk through a capitation payment model. The capitation rates will be set at no more than 95 percent of the estimated cost of services currently delivered in Arizona under conventional fee-for-service arrangements. Another unique aspect of the program is the competitive bidding process whereby private and county hospitals and HMOs will submit bids to provide services in a given county. Where there are insufficient bids for a given county, capped fee-for-service arrangements will be established with providers. One goal of the competitive bidding process, established in lieu of the negotiation process with providers that characterizes other states' organized health delivery systems, is to attract at least two competing qualified bidders in each county.

Like the primary care networks being set up in other states, the AHCCCS program incorporates limitations on freedom of choice. Enrollees will select from among several plans the particular group in which to enroll as well as the primary care physician in the group. When enrollees join a plan, they will be required to remain for a designated period.

Unlike other states' plans, however, consumers will be required to share in the cost of their care through nominal copayments. While public and private employees and employers make full premium payments, the medically needy contribute to the cost of their premiums on a sliding scale. The total required contribution for the indigent will be based on actuarial principles such that the contributions equal 10 percent of the cost of covered services to all medically needy persons.

Obstacles to Implementation and Cost Savings

Implementation of primary care/case management systems, which alter provider, employer, government, and consumer behavior in medical care markets, will face numerous obstacles. For example, organizing diverse health care providers into formal networks, making employers and consumers "buyers" of insurance and medical services, and making providers "sellers" of services is a significant task. Reimbursement mechanisms and risk-sharing arrangements need to be negotiated and stated in contractual terms. The lack of available data to serve as the basis for reimbursement rates can be a stumbling block to implementation.

Moreover, a number of the proposed plans in the states incorporate only the AFDC-eligible Medicaid population. Given the more costly and complex nature of the SSI-eligible Medicaid population, states are starting with the AFDC population, which offers case management a greater likelihood of success. Yet, since SSI Medicaid recipients account for more than two-thirds of Medicaid expenditures nationally, a significant component of the Medicaid program remains untouched. Moreover, since demographic trends indicate that in the 1970s the number of Americans over sixty-five grew by 28 percent, compared with an 11.5 percent rise in the total population, and that the fastest growing age

93

group consists of those aged seventy-five and older, the potential SSI population may yield significant growth in Medicaid expenditures.

Yet the possibility of per unit cost savings in Medicaid under managed care programs is borne out in a General Accounting Office (GAO) study which indicates that restricting a recipient's freedom of choice for nonemergency hospital services could potentially result in significant Medicaid savings.[19] The GAO did, however, point out practical problems that could erode savings. Some of the hospitals surveyed, for example, expressed concern that they would be stigmatized if they were a Medicaid hospital and that this would cause other patients to seek care elsewhere. Other hospitals expressed concern about increased Medicaid patient load because government reimbursement is low relative to that of other third-party payers.

Another cost-related issue is the extent to which Medicaid eligibles who have not been receiving medical services decide to avail themselves of care under case management once they realize that they have a group of physicians ready to take them on as patients. The increased access to care afforded the "new-found eligibles" can yield an increase in costs, further tempering the overall cost-saving potential.

Administrative issues also arise regarding identification of eligible recipients. In the Massachusetts case management program described above, when recipients were not properly identified as being in a case management program and therefore not limited in their self-referrals, problems of out-of-system care and high costs resulted. Yet since some case management plans do not provide the full benefit packages, recipients will still be receiving services from out-of-plan physicians. Thus, the recipients need proper identification to receive both case management and out-of-plan services.

A related and crucial need is for providers to abide by the system and, in nonemergency services, deny self-referral care and indicate to the patient the appropriate place to receive treatment. Still another issue for the states is how to distinguish true emergencies from nonemergencies. Moreover, managed care programs require the support of providers who are key decision makers in the medical delivery system. Although physician services account for only 18.9 percent of health expenditures, physician decisions determine up to 75 percent of all health care expenditures.[20] A related issue is the extent to which physicians are willing to participate in the programs and whether they are located in areas that facilitate patient access. A crucial issue is the extent to which the administrative and financial structures established by the states and counties will alter the ways in which providers and consumers participate in the program.

Another issue is the extent to which case management actually contributes to greater efficiency than open-ended reimbursement systems. Harold Luft's work indicates that savings do accrue from coordinated care in HMOs.[21] One estimate of the savings from HMOs indicates that total health costs for those enrolled in Kaiser plans in California were 10–40 percent lower than for those with third-party conventional insurance. There are, however, several mitigating factors affecting the cost savings. For example, lower expenditures for current HMO enrollees were found to be a function of the number and mix of services provided rather than more efficiency in the way care is provided. Lower hospitalization costs, for example, are attributed to lower rates of hospitalization rather than shorter lengths of stay. Moreover, the lower rates of hospitalization occur among discretionary and nondiscretionary services alike. Thus, the cost savings are not attributed to a disproportionate decrease in discretionary or unnecessary services. Importantly, Luft also found that HMOs, while having lower cost levels, do not slow the rate of growth in health costs. Another mitigating factor is self-selection since those who join prepaid plans tend to be relatively low users of medical services. Thus, HMO case management does not appear to hold any monopoly on ongoing cost control.

In spite of the obstacles to implementing a primary care network and case management system, these initiatives represent efforts by the states to make significant and needed changes in how medical care is provided and financed under Medicaid. The initiatives are a major step in encouraging providers and consumers, as well as the states themselves, to become financially knowledgeable sellers and consumers of medical services.

Cost Sharing

In some of the primary care/case management programs discussed above, such as AHCCCS and Project Health, states are incorporating nominal cost sharing to encourage patients to use services judiciously. There are states that view the collection of copayments as an administrative burden, especially for physicians who would be required to collect the payments. Yet overall, a number of states have expressed interest in expanding the use of cost sharing in the Medicaid program. The 1972 Amendments to the Social Security Act allowed states to require nominal copayments on optional services for the categorically needy and for any care for medically needy recipients. Currently, for example, fifteen states have some form of copayment on prescription drugs, vision and dental services, and other optional services for the medically needy. Some states, however, have requested federal waiver authority to allow them to incorporate more cost sharing. Their attempts have been ineffective, however, since under Medicaid greater cost sharing requires a legislative rather than regulatory change.

In response to this growing interest, the Tax Equity and Fiscal Responsibility Act of 1982 expands the ability of the states to require cost sharing. The act allows states to charge nominal copayment for mandatory services, such as hospital days and physician care, to the categorically needy. States are precluded, however, from imposing copayments on children under eighteen, services related to pregnancy, patients in skilled nursing and intermediate care facilities, emergency service, and family planning services. In addition, nominal copayments for nonemergency services delivered in an emergency room could be waived by the secretary of HHS in favor of higher copayments.

State Legislation

In addition to incorporating primary care networks, case management, and greater cost sharing in Medicaid, some of the states are undertaking their own internal initiatives that encourage long-run structural changes in how care is provided and financed under Medicaid. Some states are facilitating the restructuring of their Medicaid programs by state legislation. The California legislature, for example, recently passed a bill affecting both the private and the public sectors. It makes an exception to the California law requiring that an individual have the right to free choice of hospital and physician under private health insurance plans. The bill allows a health plan to negotiate alternative rates of payment with different providers, with the plan offering benefits of the alternative rates to those who select such providers. Essentially, the law allows consumers to share in the benefits from more cost-effective and less elaborate styles of care. Moreover, the law applies to private insurers and beneficiaries, which signifies a trend in the private sector market paralleling the emphasis in the public sector on limiting consumer choice of physician and hospital services.

The public sector counterpart to the California law allows the state to consider a number of options for arranging for health services under Medi-Cal. The Department of Health Services (DHS) has the authority to enter into contracts with individual and group providers or primary care physicians to organize case management. Medi-Cal, for example, can contract with hospitals on an individual or group basis through competitive bidding or other negotiations, or with counties that would conduct their own programs.

In addition, the law provides greater incentives to participate in HMOs and prepaid plans in Medi-Cal. The DHS is authorized to grant rate differentials to cost-effective HMOs and prepaid plans and to provide services beyond those required under Medi-Cal.

In another example of state initiatives in Medicaid, the Illinois Department of Public Aid is developing a plan whereby it would cooperate with hospitals, teaching institutions, and other interested parties to establish alternatives to the Medicaid system. One potential alternative is a hospital-based management system in which a hospital would manage a mix of services of Medicaid recipients. This proposal represents a shift to the hospitals, rather than the primary care physicians, as a focal point in case management. The state is also considering a competitive bidding process among hospitals to serve as providers of care to Medicaid recipients.

In another example, the Minnesota legislature passed a bill in its 1982–1983 session to encourage counties to enroll their Medicaid recipients in HMOs. The state share of the cost would increase from 90 to 95 percent, with counties assuming the other 5 percent. HMOs would be encouraged to enroll Medicaid recipients through a provision that would guarantee enrollment for six months, relieving HMOs of administrative costs of turnover with Medicaid patients whose fluctuations in monthly income inhibit sustained eligibility, and therefore enrollment, in HMOs under Medicaid.

Long-Term Care

Some states are beginning to provide alternatives to institutionally based long-term care as an attempt to alleviate the rate of growth in Medicaid costs. While freedom-of-choice waivers, cost sharing, and state legislative changes represent ways to restructure the Medicaid program, state waiver requests to encourage alternatives to institutionally based long-term care represent more of a reorientation in Medicaid.

The 1981 Reconciliation Act encourages this reorientation by allowing states to request waivers that enable them to provide more extensive home and community-based services for persons who would otherwise need institutional care. Until the 1981 act, the Medicaid program provided little coverage for long-term care services in a noninstitutional setting while offering full or partial coverage for such care in an institution. If the waivers are granted, homemaker services, respite care, and "other services" can be provided with a federal match under Medicaid. States are required to show that average per capita expenditures under community-based services are less than in an institutional setting. In this way, individuals whose needs qualify them for institutional care would have a choice of alternative types of services that could be more cost effective and could enhance the quality of life.

97

The need to address alternatives and more appropriate forms of long-term care is an immediately pressing one because long-term care benefit expenditures amounted to 42 percent of all Medicaid program spending in 1981 and is the major expenditure item in the program. In some states, long-term nursing home care amounts to more than 60 percent of total Medicaid expenditures. Moreover, nursing home expenditures under Medicaid increased at an annual rate of 20.2 percent between 1970 and 1979 compared with 14.2 percent for hospital services and 12.9 percent for physician services.

Evidence indicates that 10 to 20 percent of skilled nursing facility patients and 20 to 45 percent of intermediate care facility residents are receiving inappropriately high levels of service.[22] Although these figures do not represent exactly the patient demand for home or community-based care, they do indicate that provision of, and reimbursement for, home care could tap the potential demand for the alternative forms of care.

The requirement in the 1981 Reconciliation Act for waiver requests clearly distinguishes between persons who under existing conditions are institutionalized and those who live in the community. The provision of home care to the former group is based on the premise that it may reduce public expenditures per resident. Home and community-based care provided to persons already in the community, however, would either substitute for care now provided by family or friends or would add to care now provided. Reimbursement for such care, though perhaps desirable, would increase public expenditures. The waiver requests submitted by the states are required to provide community-based services only for those persons who would otherwise be institutionalized, thereby not tapping the population currently using home or community-based services. Inevitably, however, some states may define more broadly than others those individuals who would "otherwise be institutionalized."

Oregon. Oregon was one of the first states to submit and receive a waiver to offer alternatives for those who qualify for institutional care provided under Medicaid. The waiver was requested in response to escalating nursing home costs and the limited varieties of care that are reimbursed under Medicaid. Residential care and homemaker services are among the alternative services now available to the elderly and disabled as well as to the mentally and emotionally disturbed and the mentally retarded and developmentally disabled. The alternative forms of care will be provided only to those individuals who qualify for a skilled nursing facility (SNF) or intermediate care facility (ICF). Even with the favorable ratio of unit costs for home versus institutional care, the state does not expect substantial savings in the first few years of the program. Start-up costs, including appropriate placement of patients, will be incurred. Moreover, start-up time for the projects will be required since community-based facilities and home services will need to be expanded to meet the anticipated increase in demand.

Wisconsin. Wisconsin is considering several options to address its particular problems with escalating long-term care costs. Over the past five years, the institutional care portion of Medicaid has been growing at an average annual rate of 24.5 percent. Moreover, 70 percent of the nearly $1 billion budget is allocated for institutional care. Additionally, the use of nursing homes by recipients in Wisconsin is considerably higher than the national average; the elderly in Wisconsin between the ages of seventy-five and eighty-four use nursing homes 36.9 percent more than in the nation as a whole.

The state has developed several initiatives that offer viable options to institutional care. The Department of Health and Social Services, for example, has applied for a federal long-term care research and demonstration project to test an HMO concept for Medicaid recipients over age sixty-five in several parts of the state. The department also is exploring the feasibility of a strategy incorporating competitive bidding by private providers for long-term care services. The department would identify and select county or multicounty areas for pilot purposes. It would then determine a specific target population and initial bidding procedures whereby private providers, including nursing homes and home health agencies, would contract to provide services to Medicaid recipients.

These initiatives complement the ongoing, mostly state-funded, Community Options Program, which provides limited funding for alternatives to nursing home services. The state is also considering submitting a Medicaid waiver request to place institutionally based recipients in community-based services, as is being done in Oregon. The key difference in the Wisconsin proposal is that the nursing beds that would become available would be closed, in attempts to mitigate the institutional bias that characterizes the state's program.

Kentucky. Kentucky has submitted a waiver request for home and community-based care which emphasizes deregulation in Medicaid. For example, the existing standard under the Medicaid program requires a supervisory visit by a registered nurse or appropriate professional staff member for home health aides every two weeks. The state is requesting HHS to relax this regulation, requiring supervisory visits every sixty days when the aide services are the only services ordered by the physician. Existing requirements also stipulate that reimbursable home health services must be provided at the patient's place of residence. The state is requesting a waiver to allow professional staff of the home health

99

agency to be reimbursed for a visit to the patient before discharge from the hospital or nursing home to assist the patient in choosing alternatives to institutional care.

Conclusion

The development of primary care networks and case management, the increased use of cost sharing, and the provision of community-based alternatives to institutional care represent incremental yet long-term changes in the way medical care is provided and financed under Medicaid. These changes parallel some of the trends in health care markets where preferred provider organizations and alternative health plans are emerging and employees are increasingly purchasing low-option insurance plans. Public policy needs to be cognizant of these market changes, especially in health care where federal, state, and local governments bear 42 percent of all health expenditures. The health care market alternatives in delivery and financing may be applicable to public sector programs, although the programs may need to respond to the particular needs of their beneficiaries. Indeed, public policy can be a follower as well as a leader in the changing health care markets.

Except for the Gephardt bill, however, the proposed market-oriented federal legislation makes little, if any, reference to the Medicaid program. Proposed changes appear as an afterthought to the private insurance and Medicare systems.

In spite of the lack of explicit legislative changes in the Medicaid program, incremental changes have been made in the 1981 and 1982 budget acts and in the Health Care Financing Administration (HCFA) regulations. Indeed, a number of states have cut back eligibility and scope of services, thereby limiting access to care and causing greater cost shifting to private paying patients. These short-term changes are palliative measures that meet immediate budget crises but do not address ways in which Medicaid can be structured to incorporate long-term cost-effective measures. These shortcomings in the political process should not, however, deflect attention from the creative initiatives in the states and counties to provide not only more cost-effective care but also better access to care for those who are eligible for the program.

By spreading the financial risk to include providers and recipients, and the states themselves, states perceive that program cost increases can be controlled rather than eliminated through restrictions on eligibility and services. Moreover, by eliminating the duplication and lack of coordination in health care delivery, which is fostered by the existing unlimited fee-for-service system, the states envision savings through coordination of the Medicaid recipient's care.

100

A second objective of these state initiatives is to offer providers and the states themselves some predictability in Medicaid costs and reimbursements. Currently, as bill payer, the states have little control over expenditures, whereas under case management the state will be able to anticipate more readily the magnitude of Medicaid expenditures.

The prospects for the Medicaid program and these emerging state initiatives must take into account several critical considerations. Any progress toward more incentives for greater consumer and provider cost consciousness will clearly be neither rapid nor smooth. Indeed, the growing activity in the states documented above still represents exceptions rather than the rule in state Medicaid administration. Moreover, an overhaul of the existing cost-based reimbursement system is not likely to result in substantial savings in the largest and fastest growing expenditure category in Medicaid—long-term care.

Even with these cautionary notes, however, the initiatives outlined in the discussion are the first major efforts by the states to think decidedly differently about how to provide and finance medical services for the indigent—with both cost and quality as primary considerations. These structural reforms have been developed in spite of and because of budgetary concerns. It is these initiatives that offer the possibility of maintaining access and existing levels of benefits in the Medicaid program.

Notes

1. Robert M. Gibson and Daniel R. Waldo, "National Health Expenditures," *Health Care Financing Review* (September 1981), p. 19.
2. Ibid., p. 18.
3. Gary Clark, "The Role of the States in the Delivery of Health Services," *American Journal of Public Health,* vol. 2 (January 1981), p. 61.
4. Kathleen Brennan, *Medicaid* (Washington, D.C.: The Intergovernmental Health Policy Project, 1981), p. 1.
5. Ibid.
6. Commonwealth of Virginia, Department of Health, "Proposed Amendments to Medical Assistance (Medicaid) Plan Regarding Recipient Eligibility and Covered Services," 1981.
7. California State Legislature, Assembly Bill No. 799, and Assembly Bill No. 3480, passed June 24 and 25, 1982, respectively.
8. General Accounting Office, *Impediments to State Cost Saving Initiatives under Medicaid* (Washington, D.C., July 1981), pp. 8–17.
9. Health Insurance Association of America, "Hospital Cost Shifting: The Hidden Tax" (Washington, D.C., 1982), p. 2.
10. See Linda Ellweth and David Gregg, "Inter Study Researchers Trace PPOs, Provide Insight into Future Growth," *Review* (July/August 1982),

pp. 20–25. Also, "Competition Seen as Key to Lower Medical Costs," *New York Times,* April 1, 1982, p. D23.

11. National Governors Association, "Alternative Medicaid Cost Containment Recommendations" (Washington, D.C., 1980).

12. Ibid.

13. Mancur Olson, "Introduction," in Mancur Olson, ed., *A New Approach to the Economics of Health Care* (Washington, D.C.: American Enterprise Institute, 1981), p. 6.

14. Ibid.

15. Massachusetts Department of Public Welfare, *Budget Request: FY 1983.*

16. Olson, "Introduction," p. 25.

17. Ibid.

18. Becky E. Belangy, "Multicare of Multnomah County, Oregon," in *Medicaid and Primary Case Networks* (Washington, D.C.: National Governors Association, March 1982), p. 98.

19. U.S. General Accounting Office, Letter to Richard Schweiker, Secretary, U.S. Department of Health and Human Services, July 20, 1982.

20. Bruce Spitz, "Primary Care Networks and Medicaid: A Background Paper," in *Medicaid and Primary Care Networks,* p. 6.

21. Harold S. Luft, "How Do Health Maintenance Organizations Achieve Their Savings?" *New England Journal of Medicine* (June 15, 1978), p. 1337.

22. William Pollak, "Long Term Care," in Judith Feder, John Holohan, and Theodore Marmor, eds., *National Health Insurance* (Washington, D.C.: The Urban Institute, 1980), p. 482.

6
Market-Oriented Options in Medicare and Medicaid

Paul B. Ginsburg

Medicare and Medicaid finance medical services for the aged and disabled and for the poor, respectively. Because these population groups have high rates of use of medical services, the programs account for an important proportion of the medical care market. Medicare and Medicaid patients are responsible for 45 percent of gross revenues in community hospitals, for instance. Given the importance of these programs in the financing of medical care, changing their provisions would be an important component of a policy to encourage greater use of market forces to contain costs.

This paper reviews Medicare and Medicaid options that are market oriented. It begins with a discussion of mechanisms by which market forces can play a role in medical care delivery. Since the potential for such mechanisms is much greater in Medicare, more attention is devoted to options specific to that program. After a brief description of the Medicare program, aspects that impede the use of market forces are identified. Then three groups of options are discussed:

- benefit redesign options
- reimbursement options
- voucher options

In a final section, the applicability of these options to the Medicaid program is discussed.

Market Mechanisms

Widespread use of a passive form of third-party payment for medical care has suppressed much of the potential of market forces to allocate re-

NOTE: This paper was written in a private capacity. It is not a statement by the Congressional Budget Office.

sources in the United States. Most persons have health insurance to provide financial protection against large medical bills. Instead of the patient paying the provider for services, the insurer pays. But insurers pay in a very passive manner. In the case of hospital care, some simply pay whatever the charges are, while others calculate incurred costs and reimburse them. In the case of physician services, charges are paid in full (less any deductible or coinsurance that the patient is responsible for) as long as they are not outside the range of what comparable physicians in the area charge.

When such payment is widespread, incentives to economize are seriously diluted. For the patient, services cost only a small fraction of their prices, and going to a less expensive provider yields minimal financial returns. For the provider, patient insensitivity to charges lessens the incentive to keep them down.

Two basic mechanisms are available that would increase incentives to contain costs. One would make the insurance coverage less complete so that the patient would pay a share of the cost. The insured, for example, could be made responsible for the first $500 per year in covered medical expenses, or for 20 percent of the charges. An extensive research literature indicates that cost sharing reduces rates of service use and medical care prices.[1] Cost sharing is controversial, nevertheless, because some feel that it could lead to the forgoing of important medical care, especially among low-income persons.

The second mechanism would continue relatively complete insurance coverage, but would give a more aggressive role to the insurer. Rather than simply paying bills that are reasonable, the insurer would negotiate with the provider about fees and patterns of service use. Examples of this mechanism range from the health maintenance organization (HMO) at one end of a spectrum to the preferred provider organization (PPO) at the other.

In the health maintenance organization, the insurer and the provider are the same organization. This is clearest in the prepaid group practice type of HMO, where a medical group contracts with consumers to provide a year's medical services for a set fee. By combining the insurance function with the delivery of medical care, physicians' incentives are shifted away from overprescribing of services toward economizing on them.

In preferred provider organizations, the insurer limits choice to those providers believed to be relatively low cost. (Low-cost providers either have low fees or practice in a conservative style.) In some cases, the provider may offer the insurer a discount in order to get on the preferred provider list. Since most states do not permit insurers to limit the insured's freedom of choice of providers, PPOs do not deny reimbursement to other providers but require more cost sharing by the consumer.

104

Somewhere between HMOs and PPOs are primary care networks (PCNs). In this arrangement, the insurer contracts with physicians to provide primary care to the policyholder and to manage referral care and hospitalization. The contract requires the primary physician to accept some risk for the total covered medical care costs of the policyholder.

Of these arrangements, we have the most experience with the HMO. More than 10 million persons are now enrolled, with the number growing at 13 percent per year. HMOs have been studied extensively, with the consensus of analysts being that persons enrolled in group-practice HMOs experience lower costs than those with traditional health insurance.[2] Whether those enrolled in individual practice associations (IPAs) —another type of HMO—experience lower costs is still an open question.

Experience with other forms of organizations such as PPOs or PCNs is limited, however. Whether they are economically viable under either current policies or policies more conducive to competition in the health care field is not yet known.

The Present Medicare Program

Medicare provides hospital insurance (Part A) for about 29 million persons eligible for Social Security and railroad retirement who are sixty-five and older or who are disabled, and for chronic renal disease patients who have Social Security coverage either as workers, spouses, or dependents. The Supplementary Medical Insurance program (Part B) is an optional supplement available to this same population and to all those sixty-five and over. It covers primarily physician services. Part A is financed exclusively by a payroll tax, whereas Part B is financed roughly one-quarter by premiums paid by beneficiaries and the rest through appropriations from general revenues. In fiscal year 1981, Medicare outlays totaled $42 billion.

The present program has a number of features that impede the working of market forces. Its hospital coverage is quite extensive. After the payment of a deductible for the first day in the hospital for an episode of illness ($260 for calendar year 1982), no payments by the patient are required for the next fifty-nine days in the hospital. While the deductible probably discourages hospital admissions to a degree, there is no incentive to shorten lengths of stay.[3] Nor has the patient an incentive to use a hospital with lower prices, because the deductible is based on costs averaged over all hospitals rather than costs in the particular hospital used.

Medicare pays hospitals on the basis of incurred costs, so that the reimbursement policy does little to offset the insulation of patients from costs in the particular hospitals used. Two exceptions are limits on reim-

105

bursements for routine costs and the formula for reimbursement of capital costs. The first, known as "Section 223 limits," is based on comparisons of hospitals with their peers. While yielding some budget savings (roughly 1 percent of hospital reimbursements), this approach is unlikely to have done much to affect costs. It focuses on deviant hospitals only (about 25 percent of hospitals will be affected in 1982 under recently tightened limits) and thus far has been limited to routine costs (essentially room and board and nursing services), whereas much of the cost problem involves ancillary services, such as diagnostic laboratory and X-ray tests.[4] Capital costs are reimbursed by paying interest costs and depreciation on a historical cost basis. During periods of inflation, reimbursement of only historical costs probably diminishes incentives to invest somewhat.

Physician service coverage is not as extensive as hospital coverage. Beneficiaries pay a $75 annual deductible and 20 percent coinsurance. Furthermore, reasonable charge criteria, or screens, are not particularly generous, and physicians may bill patients for the difference between charges and what Medicare reimburses.

An important part of Medicare cost sharing is offset by extensive purchasing of private supplemental coverage. More than half of Medicare beneficiaries either purchase or obtain through employment private coverage that supplements Medicare. (An additional sixth receive Medicaid benefits, which act as a supplement to Medicare.)

An implicit subsidy from Medicare to the purchasers of supplemental plans may explain why supplementation is so extensive. The reduction in cost sharing that results from purchasing such plans induces higher rates of use of medical services, but Medicare pays a large portion of the costs of the additional use.[5] As a result, the private plan is underpriced and Medicare outlays are higher than they otherwise would be—by more than $3 billion per year.

Finally, Medicare presently offers no encouragement of lower-cost delivery of services that involves an active role by the insurer because Medicare retains the insurance function. Medicare beneficiaries may enroll in HMOs, for example, but Medicare reimburses the HMOs on a fee-for-service basis. Since most of HMOs' favorable cost experience comes from lower rates of hospitalization and of surgery, the savings accrue directly to Medicare. As a result, potential financial incentives to beneficiaries to enroll in HMOs are reduced substantially.

This disincentive may be removed by a provision of the Tax Equity and Fiscal Responsibility Act of 1982 (Public Law 97-248), which authorizes HMO reimbursement on a capitation basis. Prior to implementation, however, the Secretary of Health and Human Services must certify that the actuarial problems associated with setting capitation rates have been resolved, an endeavor likely to be difficult.

Benefit Redesign Options

Medicare could continue its role as a passive insurer, but encourage market forces by increasing incentives for patients to use medical care more judiciously. This section begins by examining an option to discourage supplemental insurance. Only if supplementation is reduced can benefit redesign options contain medical care costs as opposed to simply reducing federal outlays. Next, two hospital cost-sharing options are discussed—coinsurance and indemnity benefits.

Discourage Supplementation. The mechanism by which the purchase of private insurance to supplement Medicare increases federal outlays and reduces cost sharing was described above. A tax equal to the amount of additional costs to Medicare—about 35 percent of the private plan's premium—could alleviate this problem.

Such a tax would have two major effects. First, it would increase the amount of cost sharing. Because the tax would offset the implicit subsidy from Medicare to purchasers of supplemental plans, some participants would decide that such coverage was not worth the price and would instead pay deductibles and coinsurance out of pocket at the time services were used. Second, it would reduce federal costs for Medicare. Some of the savings would come from surcharge receipts, while the remainder would come from lower rates of Medicare claims by those deciding to discontinue their supplemental policies. (Predicting the proportion of beneficiaries who would drop their supplemental coverage—the key consideration for a market-oriented policy—is very difficult, however.)

This option would lead to more equal government aid for all participants by requiring those with private supplemental coverage to bear the additional costs they impose on the Medicare system. Elderly and disabled persons with the lowest incomes would not be affected because their deductibles and coinsurance are paid by Medicaid. But some who would otherwise have purchased supplemental coverage would face difficulties in meeting out-of-pocket costs during a year of unusually high medical expenditures. Supplemental plans that provide only catastrophic coverage could be excluded from such a tax.

Restructure Hospital Coinsurance. In addition to the first-day deductible, beneficiaries could be required to pay 10 percent of the amount of the deductible for each of the next thirty days of a hospital stay in each calendar year—$26 per day in 1982. Medicare would cover all charges in excess of any stay beyond thirty-one days, or of separate stays totaling more than thirty-one days in a year, thus improving coverage for participants with unusual hospitalization needs.[6] Enrollees would pay only one $260 deductible, no matter how many times hospitalized in a year.

107

This option would implicitly set a maximum yearly out-of-pocket individual liability for hospital costs of about $1,040 in 1982. The Medicaid program would continue to pay the coinsurance costs for those elderly and disabled persons enrolled in both programs.

In addition to limiting federal expenditures, coinsurance would induce patients to make less use of hospital care. The impact would be reduced significantly to the extent that private supplemental plans were revised to cover the new coinsurance charges, however. Also, coinsurance in itself does not give the patient an incentive to choose low-cost hospitals.[7]

Under this option, out-of-pocket costs would rise substantially for the majority of elderly and disabled who are hospitalized. Only a small number of Medicare participants would benefit from the improved catastrophic coverage in any one year, whereas the potential $1,040 in cost sharing represents about 15 percent of average per capita income for the elderly. In addition, since physicians' fees are currently subject to co-insurance under Part B of Medicare, the burden of an illness requiring hospitalization could rise to well over $1,040.

This conflict between the need to economize on the use of medical services and the burden that cost sharing would place on low-income beneficiaries might be resolved by varying coinsurance rates with income. Low-income persons, for example, could be assessed 5 percent of the amount of the deductible while all others could pay 15 percent.

The administrative difficulty of varying coinsurance rates by income would depend on how refined were the criteria used to determine who was entitled to the lower rates. The simplest would be based on the level of Social Security benefits. Beneficiaries who were hospitalized and whose monthly benefit was below a certain amount could apply to their Social Security office to obtain the lower coinsurance rate.

Some might consider such a criterion to be inequitable, since among persons with low Social Security benefits some might have high incomes from other sources. A second criterion might be added—for example, that both low Social Security benefits and low adjusted gross income be required to get the low coinsurance rate. This would be feasible, though more complicated than the first.

Restricting income testing to hospital benefits, as in this option, would keep the administrative workload down. Only 22 percent of Medicare beneficiaries have a hospital stay during a calendar year.

Restructure Indemnity Benefits. Under current law, the deductible and coinsurance amounts due from the beneficiary do not vary with the institution used. Under this option, the benefits paid by Medicare would not vary from hospital to hospital, so that cost sharing would. The higher the hospital's charges, the more the cost sharing. Such a restructuring of benefits would introduce significant incentives to use hospitals with lower charges and thereby increase competition among hospitals. If indemnity benefits were based upon the average paid by Medicare under current law (or under the coinsurance option discussed above) and if provision was made for patients to retain Medicare's discount (the difference between charges and the amount reimbursed by Medicare), the additional competitive pressures would be felt without increasing the burden of cost sharing by the patient.[8]

Indemnity benefits would have some technical difficulties—indeed, difficulties quite similar to prospective payment of hospitals (discussed below). Specifically, Medicare payments would have to vary according to the beneficiary's diagnosis, age, and local medical costs. For reasons of both administrative feasibility and equity among beneficiaries, the variation might be made in hospital reimbursement rather than in the benefit structure itself. Thus, Medicare reimbursement would be based upon a hospital's case mix and other factors, and hospitals would be permitted to charge patients the difference between allowable costs and the reimbursement rate.

Reimbursement Options

The manner in which Medicare pays hospitals and HMOs could be changed in order to make greater use of the market.

Prospective Payment of Hospitals. As discussed above, Medicare pays hospitals on the basis of incurred costs, a method that fails to combat the cost-increasing incentives associated with extensive third-party payment. Setting payment rates prospectively, or in advance, would give hospitals incentives to contain costs.

Prospective payment of hospitals is a complex topic that requires more space than is available in this chapter.[9] Consequently, the discussion here is limited to whether the prospective payment option is in fact consistent with a policy of using the market.

Prospective payment has aspects of both competition and regulation. It is competitive in the sense that it gives hospitals a broad economic constraint that has been lacking under current policies. It gives hospitals incentives to reduce costs, and flexibility in doing so. Indeed, where rates are set on the basis of costs in peer hospitals, competition among hospitals, though indirect, is fostered.

On the other hand, prospective payment is not market oriented, in that consumers do not play a role since their incentives are not changed. Prospective payment leaves a tension between the consumer, who continues to demand the best, and the government, which prevents hospitals from delivering it. Since prospective payment applies only to hospitals, it establishes an incentive to shift services into that part of the medical system not covered—ambulatory care. It concentrates a great deal of power in the agency that sets the rates, but—unlike the market—includes no automatic mechanism to correct errors.

Prospective payment is more market oriented when hospitals are allowed to make extra charges to patients. In this case, errors made by the rate-setting agency can be corrected through the market process, and consumer demands can be satisfied. When charges are permitted under a prospective payment system, the result is similar to making the benefit into an indemnity.

But making prospective payment more market oriented would not necessarily make it better. Some are concerned that Medicare beneficiaries might not have sufficient economic power as consumers to restrain hospitals from raising charges, and that hospitals would not feel powerful incentives to contain costs. Coverage of extra charges by private supplemental plans would make effective consumer control even less likely.

Per Enrollee Reimbursement for HMOs. Medicare could reimburse HMOs on a per enrollee basis instead of the present fee-for-service basis. Under Public Law 97-248, Medicare will be permitted to pay HMOs an amount equal to 95 percent of what Medicare spends on similar persons in the area who obtain care through the fee-for-service sector. If the HMOs' costs were lower, consumers would benefit. This would significantly increase financial incentives for Medicare beneficiaries to enroll in HMOs, which in turn would lower aggregate spending on medical care.

A near-term problem with this option is its potential for an initial small increase in Medicare outlays. First, for those already enrolled in efficient HMOs, Medicare would pay out more benefits. If an HMO's costs were 20 percent lower than the fee-for-service sector, for example, its Medicare claims would be 80 percent of the average in the area; under this legislation, Medicare would increase its payments to 95 percent of the average. The legislation deals with this problem by limiting conversions of existing enrollees to risk contracts. Public Law 97-248 requires two new enrollees for each existing enrollee converted.

Second, demonstrations of this option have indicated that those beneficiaries opting for HMO enrollment had a lower than average rate of claims in the four years preceding their opting for an HMO during the demonstration.[10] This may reflect a possible negative correlation between a person's rate of service use and his willingness to entertain the change of physicians that is often required to enroll in an HMO; this correlation would probably erode over time. If HMOs were reimbursed on the basis of the average experience in the fee-for-service sector, but persons with lower than average claims were more likely to join, federal outlays would increase. Refinements in the method for setting per enrollee reimbursements—required of the Secretary of Health and Human Services under the legislation—may mitigate this problem, however.[11]

The Voucher Option

In contrast to the benefit redesign and reimbursement options, under which Medicare would continue as the insurer, beneficiaries could be given vouchers to be used to purchase any qualified private health plan operating in their locality. (Plans would qualify by providing minimum benefit packages and meeting other requirements such as annual open enrollment periods.) Those choosing plans with premiums lower than the voucher amount would receive the difference in cash from Medicare, whereas those choosing plans with higher premiums would pay the extra amounts from their own funds. Voucher amounts could vary according to the age and sex of the enrollee and relative medical spending in the locality.

Medicare vouchers could be either voluntary (an alternative to Medicare) or mandatory, in which case Medicare would be transformed from an entitlement to services to an entitlement to a voucher. Only the former has been discussed by elected officials, although the latter is considered by some analysts to be more workable.

The attraction of the voucher idea is that it would permit the Medicare population to participate in new types of health plans in which insurers play a more aggressive role than at present, such as HMOs, PPOs, and PCNs. It would be necessary, however, to overcome certain obstacles: the disadvantages of private insurers in competing with Medicare, and adverse and preferred-risk selection (the process by which individuals choose health plans on the basis of their expected rates of use of services). Vouchers could also increase cost sharing, but they are not a particularly attractive option with which to pursue this goal since cost sharing could be increased directly by redesigning Medicare benefits. Increased HMO enrollment would not require a voucher, since it could be encouraged by per-enrollee reimbursement. Given the lack of experience to date with delivery systems in which the insurer plays an active role, Medicare vouchers may be premature at this time.

111

The Potential of Voluntary Vouchers. Vouchers would encourage HMO enrollment by establishing incentives to join HMOs having lower costs than fee-for-service medicine. Under current law, since HMOs are reimbursed by Medicare on a fee-for-service basis, much of the savings from lower rates of hospital use accrues directly to Medicare, not to the beneficiary. Under a voucher system, the Medicare payment would not be based on the experience of the particular HMO, but on Medicare's experience in the fee-for-service system in the same locality. To the extent that an HMO's premium was lower than the voucher amount, the beneficiary would keep the difference. Other alternative delivery systems such as PPOs and PCNs would have an opportunity to attract Medicare beneficiaries for the first time.

Vouchers would encourage enrollment in HMOs and other systems by easing their marketing problems as well. In any locality, an annual listing of the HMOs that qualify for vouchers, their benefits, and their premiums would reduce their costs of marketing to the Medicare population in that area—costs that might otherwise preclude substantial efforts to enroll this population.

Cost sharing might be increased if enrollees were given a cash refund in return for accepting additional cost sharing. Under current law, Medicare beneficiaries willing to pay additional premiums to reduce their cost sharing can do so by purchasing private health insurance that supplements Medicare—but those wanting to convert some of their Medicare benefits to cash cannot do so. The voucher proposal would provide such an outlet.[12]

Problems with Voluntary Vouchers. Medicare vouchers would have some serious problems. Private plans might have difficulty in competing with Medicare. Vouchers might also stimulate adverse and preferred-risk selection. These problems would be more severe in the case of traditional insurance plans with greater cost sharing than in the case of HMOs or other alternative delivery systems.

Some of these problems would be significantly reduced by having Medicare play an active role in structuring the system. Alain Enthoven, one of the major proponents of the voucher concept, has long envisioned such an active role.[13] Both of the legislators who have developed bills have favored an open system, however.[14] The remainder of this section discusses a relatively unstructured voucher system, like the one envisioned in H.R. 850. A later section discusses the potential of a more structured system.

Competitive problems. Private insurers might have cost disadvantages in competing with Medicare. First, private insurers have selling costs whereas Medicare does not, and the costs of selling insurance to individual aged and disabled persons could be very high. Administrative costs (other than claims processing) for individual health insurance policies average about one-third of their premiums today.

The costs of private insurers would also be higher for another reason: they must often pay providers at higher rates than Medicare. The problem is most serious for hospital care, where Medicare, with few exceptions, does not permit additional charges to the patient. Data from the Health Care Financing Administration indicate that Medicare determinations of allowable hospital costs average 19 percent less than charges in 1978.[15]

These competitive problems would affect HMOs, but to a lesser degree than traditional health insurers. First, many HMOs either have their own hospitals or obtain discounts through bulk purchasing of hospital care, reducing Medicare's advantage. Second, HMOs offer more than just a different benefit structure than Medicare. Their alternative delivery systems emphasize comprehensiveness of benefits and coordination of services that might be attractive to some Medicare enrollees on other than financial grounds.

Adverse and preferred-risk selection. Vouchers could lead to substantial adverse and preferred-risk selection to the disadvantage of Medicare, and thus increase rather than reduce federal outlays. Again, this would be less serious for HMOs than for traditional private plans.

Persons choosing to use vouchers to purchase traditional private health insurance policies would likely be lower users than those remaining in Medicare, for two reasons. First, private plans would be more attractive to those interested in less extensive benefits than to those seeking more extensive benefits. Second, insurers would have strong incentives to market selectively in order to obtain the best risks.

Vouchers would be quite unattractive to persons seeking traditional plans with more comprehensive benefits than Medicare because private supplements are already available—implicitly subsidized by Medicare. In most cases, Medicare plus the supplemental plan would have a lower price than a private plan obtainable with a voucher.

Since some persons seeking less extensive coverage might find vouchers attractive, while few seeking more extensive coverage would, the adverse selection would tend to be to the disadvantage of Medicare. In other words, the costs to the federal government of the vouchers for persons opting out of Medicare would exceed what their Medicare benefits would have cost had they remained, so federal spending on the program would increase.

In the case of HMOs, adverse selection would be a very different phenomenon, but the direction, at least initially, would be the same. Since HMO benefits would tend to be similar to those in Medicare, there would be no chance for low users to gravitate toward less comprehensive plans. But the persons switching to group-practice HMOs would tend to be low users. Even if the difference eroded over time, federal outlays consistently could be higher than under current policies, especially if large numbers of beneficiaries switched to HMOs each year.

Finally, preferred-risk selection could also be a serious problem. It would pay insurers to enroll persons likely to be low users. Preventing this by regulation would not be feasible because of the difficulty of proving intent.[16] The net result would be a transfer from Medicare to those insurers who succeeded in such endeavors.

Mandatory Vouchers. Some of these problems might be dealt with by making vouchers mandatory, at least for those newly eligible for Medicare. Medicare would provide only a set amount of funds toward the purchase of a qualified health plan, not reimbursements for covered medical care services.

Mandatory vouchers would eliminate the problems that private health plans would have in competing with Medicare. They would also avoid an increase in federal outlays caused by adverse and preferred-risk selection, since voucher amounts would not be affected by such developments.

On the other hand, mandatory vouchers would have several negative features. They might channel a significant amount of resources into the process of choosing among plans. The selling costs discussed above would be included in the premiums paid by all of those eligible for Medicare. The voucher amount would either reflect the selling costs directly—thereby raising federal costs for the same coverage—or enable beneficiaries to buy less coverage for the same federal cost. Moreover, adverse and preferred-risk selection might result in a significant transfer of resources from the high users to the low users. In addition, Medicare would lose its ability to use its purchasing power to drive a hard bargain with providers on behalf of taxpayers.[17]

Perhaps more important than the pros and cons outlined above is the change in the nature of the Medicare entitlement that would be associated with mandatory vouchers. Under current law, persons eligible for Medicare are entitled to reimbursement for a defined set of medical services when needed. As the cost of purchasing these services has soared, federal reimbursements have increased automatically. Under a mandatory voucher, the entitlement would be not to reimbursement for services but to a certain amount of money to be applied toward the premiums of qualified private health plans.

The entitlement might be set equivalent to the current cost of the service entitlement, but it could be set lower. Some, for example, have proposed basing the voucher on current spending in Medicare and indexing it by the GNP implicit price deflator. If the GNP deflator increased by six percentage points per year less than per capita spending in Medicare, as is projected, the voucher amount would soon be substantially less than the cost of the services included in Medicare today. To the extent that beneficiaries enrolled in plans whose premiums grew more slowly than Medicare spending, the problem would be reduced. On the other hand, the voucher amount could be indexed by a more generous factor so as not to affect the level of federal support for health services for Medicare beneficiaries, or a compromise might be found between the need to reduce the budget deficit and the needs of the elderly.

A Structured Voucher System. The problems of adverse and preferred-risk selection and high administrative costs associated with vouchers could be reduced if Medicare played an active role in structuring the competition. Such a role might include standardizing benefit packages, performing the marketing function, and limiting the number of plans. Many of these functions are already performed by the federal government in the Federal Employees Health Benefits Program and are performed by the company or the union in most employment-based health plans. The disadvantage of such an approach is that it raises barriers to new plans. Also, some advocates of competition might object to such an active role for Medicare as involving too much regulation.

Standardizing benefit packages would increase competition among plans by making comparisons easier for consumers. Among traditional plans, for example, the benefit structure might vary only by the size of the deductible or by the coinsurance rate. The consumer could then easily choose the preferred degree of cost sharing and compare plans with the same cost sharing on the basis of price.

Having Medicare do the marketing of plans by informing beneficiaries of what plans were available in their area, and their prices, would reduce administrative costs substantially and avoid much preferred-risk selection. With Medicare marketing the plans, opportunities for approaching only low-risk persons would be eliminated. Medicare could also handle the differences between premiums and the voucher amount through the Social Security system, which sends monthly checks to most Medicare beneficiaries.

Limiting the number of plans would be useful, especially among traditional plans, to make choices easier and to help police compliance with open-enrollment requirements and marketing practices. But the procedure used to choose participants would be critical. A bidding system would have to be established to maintain competitive pressure on insurers. Medicare actuaries might choose those plans offering the best value to consumers; or plans might pay Medicare for the privilege of participating (with Medicare using the proceeds to increase the voucher amounts). The process of limiting the number of plans, which is an easy one for employers sponsoring plans, might be quite difficult for government, however.

Applicability to Medicaid

The Medicaid program finances medical care for the needy.[18] State agencies administer Medicaid under federal guidelines, while financial responsibility is shared by federal and state and sometimes by local governments. The states vary substantially both in the categories of persons covered and in the benefits to which they are entitled.

All recipients of Aid to Families with Dependent Children (AFDC) and virtually all Supplemental Security Income (SSI) recipients are eligible for Medicaid. About thirty states also cover the medically indigent: persons with large medical bills who would have qualified for AFDC or SSI except for their incomes and whose incomes less medical payments fall below state-established levels. About half of Medicaid recipients are under age twenty-one; one-sixth are over sixty-five, in which case Medicaid generally acts as supplemental coverage to Medicare. Large segments of the poor population—poor childless couples, single persons under age sixty-five, the working poor, and intact families—generally do not qualify for Medicaid, however, because they do not qualify for AFDC or SSI. In fiscal year 1981, Medicaid financed medical services to more than 22 million persons at a cost of $30 billion, of which 56 percent was paid by the federal government and the rest by state and local governments.

Because the recipient population is so poor, the options for using the market in Medicaid are more limited. For example, although some cost sharing may be appropriate in this program, the amounts would have to be nominal, lest the primary objective of the program—increased access to care by the poor—be sacrificed. But nominal amounts of cost sharing might have little deterrent effect if providers did not make much effort to collect them. Providers might find it more economical to treat the cost-sharing requirement as a reduction in program reimbursement.

The low incomes of Medicaid recipients would also hinder the use of vouchers. Behind the voucher concept is the notion of persons choosing either a plan with a premium lower than the voucher amount and getting a rebate, or one with a higher premium that requires an extra payment. But Medicaid recipients have very limited resources to pay extra premiums, and the concept of some of them receiving rebates might generate a great deal of political opposition.

Although cost sharing and vouchers have serious limitations, Medicaid programs can do a lot as large purchasers of care. Bulk purchasing of HMO enrollments on behalf of Medicaid recipients is permitted under current law, for example, and is being pursued in a number of states. Such arrangements are also being pursued with PCNs. Alternative delivery systems such as HMOs and PCNs are particularly attractive for providing services to the Medicaid population because they emphasize provider incentives rather than consumer incentives.

A recent change in federal law has made such prudent purchasing arrangements easier to pursue. Section 2175 of the Omnibus Budget Reconciliation Act of 1981 (Public Law 97-35) authorizes waivers of the freedom-of-choice requirement in Medicaid. This change will permit states to enroll groups of recipients in HMOs or PCNs without the need to set up a multiple-choice mechanism. In this way, Medicaid can avoid the risk of predominantly low users being selected by HMOs and thus increasing program expenditures. The law also specifically permits the bulk purchase of laboratory services.

Guarding against low-quality services could be a major problem, however, to the extent that Medicaid recipients were denied the opportunity to "vote with their feet." Perhaps the most effective way to avoid this problem would be to insist that the proportion of Medicaid recipients among an HMO's enrollees be small. Since practicing two classes of medicine within an organization is often impractical, competition for private patients would tend to ensure that Medicaid recipients received services of reasonable quality.

Notes

1. This literature is reviewed in Congressional Budget Office, *Containing Medical Care Costs through Market Forces* (Washington, D.C., May 1982), chapter II.

2. For a comprehensive review of this literature, see Harold Luft, *Health Maintenance Organizations* (New York: Wiley-Interscience, 1981).

3. The Professional Standards Review Organization (PSRO) program, enacted in 1972 but recently scaled down, attempts to deal with this problem through utilization review.

4. At the time of this writing, both the Senate Finance Committee and the House Ways and Means Committee have reported bills that would expand the coverage of Section 223 limits to ancillary services and place limits on the rate of increase of reimbursements for inpatient costs per admission.

5. The supplemental plan, for example, may pay the 20 percent coinsurance for physician services. But if physician visits increase by 20 percent because of the extra insurance, Medicare pays 80 percent of reasonable charges for the additional visits—or, in this case, 40 percent of the full costs of the additional coverage.

6. Under current law, Medicare beneficiaries pay coinsurance charges (generally 25 percent) for days after the sixtieth day.

7. Under this option, the coinsurance would not vary at all between hospitals. If, instead, coinsurance was 10 percent of each hospital's charges, it would vary, but the incentives to choose the low-cost hospital would still be weak.

8. The Medicare discount could be retained by permitting hospitals to charge patients only the difference between their allowable costs and the indemnity benefit.

9. For a discussion, see my "Issues in Medicare Hospital Reimbursement," *National Journal,* vol. 14 (May 21, 1982), pp. 934–37.

10. Paul W. Eggers and Ronald Prihoda, "Pre-Enrollment Reimbursement Patterns of Medicare Beneficiaries Enrolled in 'At-Risk' HMOs," *Health Care Financing Review,* vol. 4 (September 1982), pp. 55–74.

11. Prior claims experience might be taken into account in setting the reimbursement rate during the first few years of a beneficiary's enrollment in an HMO.

12. Some voucher proposals, such as H.R. 4666, introduced by Congressman Willis D. Gradison, Jr. (Republican, Ohio) and Richard A. Gephardt (Democrat, Missouri), would permit vouchers to be used to purchase only those health plans with benefits at least equivalent to Medicare's. Proposals such as these would work only through alternative delivery systems.

13. See Alain C. Enthoven, *Health Plan* (Reading, Mass.: Addison-Wesley, 1980).

14. H.R. 850, introduced by Congressman Richard A. Gephardt and now Office of Management and Budget Director David Stockman, and H.R. 4666, introduced by Congressmen Gradison and Gephardt, would limit structuring to an open-enrollment requirement and a minimum benefit package. The current antiregulatory mood in Washington may preclude a system as structured as the one discussed below. Indeed, H.R. 850 has been (probably unjustly) criticized as excessively regulatory.

15. A few Blue Cross plans may not face this problem of paying hospitals at higher rates than Medicare. They sometimes have discounts comparable to those of Medicare.

16. Insurers could, for example, target marketing campaigns to areas having populations that are relatively young and well-off.

17. As discussed earlier, Medicare pays hospitals considerably less than their charges. To the extent that charge-paying insurers replaced Medicare under a mandatory voucher system, these gains to taxpayers would be lost.

18. For a more detailed description of Medicaid, see Congressional Budget Office, *Medicaid: Choices for 1982 and Beyond* (Washington, D.C., June 1981).

7
Economic Incentives in the Provision of Long-Term Care

Lynn Paringer

Over the past decade, spending on nursing home and other long-term care services has risen faster than spending on any other component of health care, including hospital care. In 1980, more than 40 percent of each Medicaid dollar was consumed by nursing home services.[1] Given projected increases in the size of the population over sixty-five, long-term care can be expected to expand further its share of health expenditures. If current trends continue, it is estimated that by 1990 spending on nursing home care will account for 11.2 percent of personal health spending, up substantially from the 8.8 percent share in 1980.[2]

National debate on appropriate strategies to control health care costs has focused primarily on the acute care sector of the health market. A principal concern is that a lack of incentives for cost-conscious behavior by consumers and providers of services has in part fueled the rapid rate of increase in health spending. A suggested method of reducing the rapid rate of expenditure increase is to provide economic incentives to consumers and providers for efficient behavior. Assuming that economic incentives can be successfully used to curtail spending increases for acute care services, the question remains whether the same strategies can be used to similar effect for long-term care services. The structure of the long-term care market may be sufficiently different to warrant a separate analytical framework for assessing it and developing viable solutions to the rapid increase in costs.

The major characteristics of the long-term care marketplace that serve to differentiate it from the acute care sector are the following: (1) virtually no insurance coverage is available through the private sector; (2) the public sector finances over 50 percent of the care pro-

NOTE: The author wishes to thank William Scanlon, Richard Scheffler, Margaret Stassen, and Jack Meyer for their comments on earlier versions of this paper.

119

vided in nursing homes, but public support for alternatives is fragmentary; (3) individuals use the whole spectrum of outputs provided by nursing homes to consume the services actually desired; (4) the majority of care is currently provided not in the market but informally by family and friends; and (5) the long time dimension of use and the structure of the Medicaid program distort the price of services faced by both public and private consumers leading to overconsumption of some types of long-term care and possible underconsumption of others. In the first section of this chapter, I will assess the impact of each of these characteristics on the functioning of the long-term care market. Much of the discussion will center on comparing the hospital market with the nursing home market, which is where the bulk of spending occurs.

In the second section, I will discuss the current regulatory environment within which the long-term care market operates. Government has attempted to curtail the rate of spending growth and maintain quality by imposing regulations that limit the supply of services and the price of care and that define the mix of inputs used in producing a nursing home day. I will assess the impact that these different types of regulations have had on efficiency in the long-term care market.

The following section will consider alternatives to direct regulation as a means of improving the functioning of the long-term care market. Increased cost sharing by consumers, the use of vouchers for direct service purchase, and efficiency incentives for providers will be examined along with methods of improving regulation. The conclusion presents some implications of the current debate on the merits of competition versus regulation.

Is Long-Term Care Unique?

Economists generally agree that the market has failed substantially in the provision of health care. Pervasive health insurance coverage and the tax deductibility of insurance, which encourage even more expansive coverage, have resulted in providers and consumers of care being insensitive to real resource costs. It is now well understood that insurance reduces the out-of-pocket costs that consumers pay when they purchase care and results in the use of more medical services than would occur if individuals faced the full resource cost at the time care is consumed. Consumers have little incentive to search out low-cost providers of care since the monetary gains are small and the time costs associated with search may be substantial. The presence of comprehensive insurance coverage leads to a phenomenon known as "moral hazard"—the tendency of the insured to spend the insurer's money more readily than he would spend his own money. The tax system, by allowing employers to deduct health insurance costs from wages paid to employees, further encourages the purchase of health insurance. The extra insurance in turn leads to even more moral hazard. When consumers are not motivated to search out low-cost providers, providers are not forced to compete for patients. Furthermore, if consumers are ignorant of the medical appropriateness of different health care strategies, they may contract with a physician to act as their agent and to make medical care decisions on their behalf. Since the physician has a financial stake in the outcome and the consumer is likely to put up little resistance to increased amounts of care (both because the consumer's financial stake is small and because the consumer may not be able to make intelligent medical care decisions), physicians may increase service provision beyond a level that is economically efficient. Proponents of increased competition argue that, by making both sides of the market face costs that better reflect the true resource costs, consumers will be encouraged to shop around for the most cost-effective mix of services and providers will be motivated to compete on the basis of cost for the consumer's health care dollar.

The large divergence between consumer out-of-pocket price and marginal cost is a principal cause of inefficiency. Proposed remedies are directed toward increasing the price of care both at the time care is consumed and when insurance is purchased through the employer. Expanded consumer choice of different health insurance packages combined with financial incentives to choose low-cost packages is expected to foster competition among providers and induce efficiency. Increased efficiency means that a larger amount of output can be provided for the same dollar outlay. The strategies considered may be effective in the acute care market where first-dollar insurance coverage is extensive, consumers are often unable to judge the efficacy of certain services, and providers' incomes rise with the amount of output they provide. The market for long-term care services is substantially different from the market for acute care services, however, and consequently the same remedies may not be appropriate in this setting. A comparison of the nursing home and hospital industries will serve to illustrate the similarities and differences between long-term and acute care services.

Like hospital care, the majority of nursing home care is financed by the public sector, primarily through the Medicare and Medicaid programs. In 1980, the public sector financed 57 percent of nursing home expenditures and 54 percent of hospital spending.[3] Unlike hospital care, however, for which there is virtually no cost sharing on the part of Medicaid beneficiaries and only a small amount of cost sharing on the part of Medicare recipients, there is substantial cost sharing by public beneficiaries for nursing home services. Persons eligible for nursing home care under Medicaid must forfeit all of their income minus a small personal needs allowance when they are admitted to a nursing home. On the private (nongovernmental) side of the market, the differences between hospital and nursing home care are even more apparent. Although 46 percent of hospital spending is done through the private sector, less than 25 percent of this represents consumer out-of-pocket payments. Three-fourths of private spending is financed through insurance companies. In contrast, less than 5 percent of all private spending on nursing home care is financed by private insurers. Persons not eligible for public nursing home subsidies face the full cost of care when they enter the home. This is in contrast to private consumers of hospital care whose out-of-pocket costs are small relative to the cost of care.

The time dimension of care use is also significantly different. Although many people receive nursing home care after recovering from a spell of hospitalization and will subsequently be discharged to their homes, a sizable minority of nursing home residents will live out the remainder of their lives in the facility. Nursing home care for them is a catastrophic expense, and many who enter the facility as private pay patients will exhaust their resources and become public beneficiaries.

The most basic distinction, however, between long-term and acute care services lies in the nature of the service. Unlike acute care which has a curative or rehabilitative goal, long-term care services focus on assisting the chronically disabled to function in activities of daily living. Services range from aid in meal preparation and shopping to traditional medical services. This is reflected in the financing of some long-term care services. Before 1972, for example, care provided in intermediate care facilities was generally considered a welfare expenditure rather than a medical care expenditure and was covered under state welfare programs.[4] Nursing homes, whether skilled or intermediate care facilities, provide a myriad of goods and services in addition to health care—food, housing, recreation, and social services—and thus they can appropriately be regarded as alternatives to independent living. Consequently, decisions to enter nursing homes are not solely related to health status and a need for medical attention. (In 1969, fewer than than one-third of nursing home residents received intensive nursing care.)[5]

Because of differences in the nature of the service and the type of care provided in the long-term care sector, most of the decisions to seek care rest primarily with the patient. The assumption of consumer ignorance and the use of the physician as agent for the patient in the decision-making process is not as prevalent in long-term care. Even when the physician acts as the patient's agent, the physician generally has no financial incentive to prescribe care because he or she receives no gain from placing a patient in a nursing home.

The usual reasons for market failure in the acute care sector—extensive health insurance coverage for both private and public beneficiaries with little consumer cost sharing, subsidies for the purchase of insurance, and consumer ignorance—are not as prevalent in the long-term care sector. Yet, costs for long-term care services are rising even more rapidly than costs for acute services. Although rapidly rising costs are not prima facie evidence of market failure, they do suggest that we need to identify the reasons for the rapidly increased amount and share of resources devoted to long-term care.

Market Basket Moral Hazard. Some long-term services such as meals programs or homemaker services provide only one output. Others, however, like nursing homes may appropriately be viewed as providing a range of outputs that are all consumed together. To characterize the market for long-term care services, it is reasonable to define the different services in terms of the outputs or the characteristics they provide. Using an analytical framework following that of Kelvin Lancaster, we can posit that people desire characteristics that they obtain by purchasing goods and services.[6] Their objective is to maximize their well-being subject to the amount of resources they have available to spend. Their preferences for medical care are conditioned by, among other things, their health status. Characteristics such as meals, medicine, and nursing care are consumed when they purchase nursing home services. The price a consumer pays for a good or service is determined in the market and is influenced by the level of subsidy made available by the public sector for the purchase of the good or service. Higher subsidies encourage more use of a particular good or service.

Consider the problem facing an avid skier planning a trip to Aspen for five days. She is trying to determine which of several ski packages to use. One package offers one week in a high-quality hotel, three meals a day, six days of lift tickets, tennis and swimming privileges, and round trip airfare on a given airline. The person, however, only has five days available, generally eats two meals a day, and cannot play tennis. She finds another package that includes only airfare and a motel for five days, and she must purchase meals and lift tickets separately. The skier chooses the second package. Suppose the supplier of the first package offers a 50 percent discount. The person now switches to the first package even though it contains some characteristics that convey little, if any, satisfaction.

The range of output provided by a nursing home makes it something like a bundle of service characteristics. When a day of nursing home care is purchased in the market, it consists of medical services, housing, recreation, and social interactions. Many of these characteristics can be purchased independently in the marketplace as well. When purchased in the form of a nursing home day, however, they are all consumed simultaneously. The quantity and quality of each characteristic varies from home to home, but all facilities provide some amount of each. The individual thus is confronted with the problem of selecting the optimal bundle of characteristics. He or she can purchase each characteristic either separately, or in some other combination (congregate living facilities and retirement communities are examples of some of these characteristics being provided in combination), or in the combination that is given by what constitutes a nursing home day. The optimal resource allocation would be one in which the marginal satisfaction per dollar spent on each good or service is equal across the entire range of goods and services.

In Lancaster's world, people must trade off characteristics of goods to come to a decision regarding the quantity of different goods to purchase. Among the characteristics of a nursing home are some—provision of food, shelter, and medical care—that may yield satisfaction; others, however, such as isolation from family and friends and loss of independence, reduce satisfaction. People weigh the pluses and minuses, come to a decision regarding the net increment in satisfaction relative to cost, and compare it with other possible long-term care market baskets. The bundle of characteristics that yields the greatest increment in satisfaction relative to the individual's cost is the one chosen.

Public sector financing alters the prices that people face for different goods. By lowering the cost of long-term care to the recipient, public subsidies have an impact similar to the moral hazard caused by insurance coverage. However, the moral hazard associated with long-term care is more complex. Long-term care includes services well outside the health field. Hence, changes in public policy outside the range of traditional health policy can exert an important effect on the use of certain long-term care services, particularly nursing home services. People who reside in nursing homes have the majority of their living needs provided by the facility. Changes in any public policy that alters the price of food or shelter or any other basic living need will affect the desirability of choosing nursing home care over alternative living arrangements. Cutbacks in food stamps or housing subsidies, for example, will increase the cost of maintaining oneself in an independent living arrangement and may encourage individuals to seek institutional care. In addition, the provision of adequate police protection in predominantly elderly areas and the availability of transportation will also affect the desirability of residing in a nursing home vis-á-vis an independent living arrangement. In general, policy interventions that alter either the cost or the satisfaction derived from purchasing these goods will alter the consumption bundle chosen and affect the utilization of nursing home care.

The moral hazard that occurs with nursing home care results from individuals consuming a good or service that they may not desire (or that they might acquire at lower cost elsewhere) in order to obtain a good that they do desire. Thus, individuals who need help with meal preparation and housekeeping and who, because of rapidly rising utility and housing costs, might be unable to continue to live independently, may choose nursing home care even though they may not require the level of medical care provided in the facilities. If housing and meal subsidies alone were available, the individual could maximize satisfaction by maintaining an independent living arrangement. Because of this multiple characteristic aspect of the nursing home, it is imperative to view the market in terms much broader than as a segment of the medical care market. For some people, nursing home care is a substitute for independent living necessitated by the lack of public subsidies for certain components of their overall needs. When prices of goods and services such as meals or home heating rise or fall, it affects the decisions of people in independent living arrangements about whether to switch to nursing home care.

The fact that nursing homes provide a wide range of services in addition to health services suggests that we should broaden our idea of what services may be used as alternatives to nursing home care. Medicare was introduced in 1965 as a program designed to pay for the medical services for elderly who had acute health problems. A minimal amount of nursing home care following a hospital stay is covered under the program. The motivation for such coverage was the perception that some individuals, following a hospital episode, would require skilled nursing care during the recuperative process, but that the service intensity needed was not of the magnitude of that provided by the hospital. Nursing homes were viewed as a lower-cost alternative to hospitalization.

In addition to this type of immediate post-hospitalization care, long-term care services also provide for the needs of the chronically ill and functionally disabled. The overwhelming majority of publicly financed long-term care services are nursing home services. Several studies of home health services and adult day care indicate, however, that some fraction of the nursing home population may be cared for at a lower cost in these alternative settings.[7] There may be a sizable fraction of the institutionalized population that, although they require institutionalization, do not need the intensive amount of medical care being provided to them in their current setting. Available data indicate that 10 to 20 percent of people in skilled nursing facilities and 20 to 40 percent of the residents in intermediate care facilities are receiving levels of health care that exceed their needs.[8] Other data indicate that for every person in a nursing home there are as many as two equally disabled persons living in noninstitutional settings.[9] The weak relationship

125

between health status and nursing home use suggests that numerous other factors affect demand for and utilization of care, including the availability and price of services that serve as alternatives to nursing home care. It is important, therefore, to identify the range of goods and services that can be viewed as alternatives to nursing home care and to determine the impact of changes in their availability and prices on the demand for nursing home care.

Another aspect of the moral hazard problem results not from differential subsidies that encourage the use of some services over potentially lower-cost alternatives but from the size and nature of the subsidy for nursing home care itself. The level of public subsidy provided is higher if individuals are in high-cost facilities than if they are in low-cost facilities. While out-of-pocket costs by public beneficiaries may be large, their expenditures are not related to the cost of the facility.* Therefore, the public subsidy takes up the slack in cost. As a Medicaid eligible's income rises, the amount of nursing home care that can be purchased does not rise, while the amount of other goods and services that can be purchased does rise. Thus, once the decision has been made to enter a nursing home, public beneficiaries have no incentive to search out the lowest-cost provider of care and, in effect, the government scales the subsidy directly to providers' costs. This is a built-in cost-generating feature of the market. Since many beneficiaries can expect to be nursing home residents for a long time, the total cost of this feature of reimbursement is quite significant. Use of high-cost nursing home facilities has enormous cost implications for states' Medicaid programs, yet the mandate of consumer freedom of choice precludes the state from stepping in and assigning beneficiaries to particular facilities. The extensive state subsidy available for nursing homes compared with little financial assistance for noninstitutional services encourages consumers to use institutional care. In addition, the fact that subsidy levels are higher as the facility's cost is higher further encourages the use of high-cost facilities.

The Real Resource Cost of Long-Term Care. In estimating the amount of spending devoted to long-term care, we enter into our calculations only the cost of market-provided services. The large majority of long-term care services are not, however, purchased in the market but are provided informally by family and friends. The Congressional Budget Office estimates that between 3.0 million and 6.7 million disabled per-

* Individuals who are eligible for state support of nursing home care by either being recipients of Old Age Assistance or falling into a state's medically needy category pay a price for care equal to their income less a small personal needs allowance.

sons receive long-term care services from family and friends or take care of themselves.[10] In comparison, fewer than 2 million persons reside in long-term care institutions. A principal determinant of nursing home use and use of other long-term care services is the availability of family support networks.

By not considering the cost of this informal care in determining long-term care expenditures, we seriously underestimate the amount of economic resources society devotes to long-term care. Individuals give up labor market alternatives and other uses of their time to provide services to family members and friends. The choices are made given existing prices for market-provided services, existing labor market alternatives, the value of alternative uses of time, as well as any utility one receives from providing care to the chronically disabled. If the out-of-pocket price of market alternatives falls or if market opportunities rise, individuals will be motivated to substitute more of the market-provided care for their own time. Alternatively, if the price of market-provided alternatives falls because of public subsidies for meal programs or home health or other programs, demand for these services will rise. Economic efficiency dictates that we be concerned about the amount of non-market-provided care, which represents a use of scarce resources, even though the value of those resources is not included in traditional gross national product (GNP) accounts.

Much current debate about expanding public support for alternatives to nursing home care centers on the effect such subsidies will have on the volume of non-market-provided care. On the one hand, if service coverage is expanded, alternative care may be substituted for nursing home care for patients currently in homes but who could be cared for at lower cost in an alternative setting. On the other hand, if the costs of alternative services are lowered, individuals currently receiving care informally may choose to substitute this newly subsidized care for some of the informal care. Government policy makers, concerned primarily with the level of government spending, desire to limit the extent to which the latter occurs. One way to do this is to define as a resource the presence of potential care givers in the household. Government might attempt to draw first on the resources of other family members before subsidizing the costs of care. A question thus arises about when a resource drawn on to provide services is also a resource to be counted in determining Medicaid eligibility. Should family members be held financially responsible for long-term care services when they are not held responsible for other types of health services? How can one enforce such responsibilities? Should people be given financial incentives to encourage them to provide care for disabled and functionally impaired family members? To do so would result in economic rents to those who have already decided to act as care givers. These questions revolve around the potential trade-off of private for public long-term spending.

The Time Path of Long-Term Care Service Use and Uncertainty. The long-term nature of the services rendered creates an additional problem for public programs. Although use of acute care services may extend over a number of periods, the episode of illness is generally short and, except for those persons who approach exhaustion of the deductible or are about to reach the point of a major change in coinsurance, the time dimension of service is not likely to be as important as it is for the use of long-term care services. Many nursing home residents expect to remain in an institutional setting for a long time, possibly until death. Uncertainty about the period of use means that the costs of services cannot be easily predicted. For those who enter a facility as private pay patients, the duration may affect both the total costs as well as the distribution of those costs between the private and the public sectors. Individuals who enter nursing homes as private pay patients face the full costs of care while they remain as private pay patients. (Indeed, if there is cross-subsidization occurring, they may pay more than the marginal cost of services.) Should these individuals become eligible for Medicaid during their stay, however, their price for services changes dramatically. Individuals eligible for Medicaid nursing home coverage fall essentially into two categories. In the first category are those whose incomes are below the state's cash assistance standard. They would receive a public assistance payment if they were not in a nursing home. In the second category are the medically needy. Many of them have exhausted private assets and income and have become eligible for Medicaid.

Because of the different out-of-pocket payment amounts for the private versus Medicaid-eligible patients, an important determinant of total care costs is the probability that a private patient, once admitted, will become eligible for Medicaid. This will alter both the total cost of care to the patient and the costs of the state's Medicaid program. The probability of such an event occurring is not insignificant. A study of the nursing home population in South Dakota found that 30 percent of the Medicaid patients in the homes had been private pay at the time of admission.[11] Of those who converted from private pay to Medicaid, 40 percent did so within the first year of admission. Studies in other parts of the country have yielded similar findings. The ability to convert to Medicaid eligibility means that the discounted value of the out-of-pocket amount paid to the facility for private pay patients could be well below the discounted value of costs incurred by the facility in providing care. The result is that private pay patients as well as public beneficiaries have an incentive to overconsume nursing home care.

An additional distinction between private and public pay patients is that entry to a nursing facility for private pay patients is at the discretion of the patient, whereas Medicaid beneficiaries require state approval before entering a facility. It is difficult to deny Medicaid payment to patients who are already residing in a long-term care facility or to move patients to another facility. Thus, once a private pay patient exhausts his resources and becomes eligible for Medicaid, the state is unlikely to move the patient even if it determines that the level of care provided to the patient in the current facility is excessive relative to the patient's medical needs. The result is that some patients may not be receiving services that are determined to be commensurate with need.

The distinctions between the market for long-term care services and that for acute care services are numerous and suggest that some of the remedies advocated to enhance market functioning in the latter may not be so readily applied to the former. In the following section, I will discuss the current role of regulation in long-term care and the impact it has had on the amount, price, and distribution of services.

Regulation: The Rules of the Game

Government involvement in regulating medical care has a long history, although the nature of the intervention and thus the climate within which the health industry operates have changed markedly over time. Before 1965, much government involvement was of the indirect type, such as income tax subsidies for insurance purchases. Although restrictions on supply have a long history, they traditionally were applied to medical manpower rather than facilities. Indeed, after World War II we witnessed efforts to expand the number of facilities via the Hill-Burton program.

Concern with inefficiencies in the medical marketplace became prevalent after Medicare and Medicaid were introduced, largely in response to the rising costs of those programs. Once the public sector expanded its role as a financier of care, it became very sensitive to the costs of care. The implementation of Medicare and Medicaid rep-presented an expansion in insurance coverage for large numbers of elderly and indigent Americans.

In making decisions on the financing of nursing home and other long-term care services, states must balance demand for other public services against the demand for long-term care services. Because of its large role as a financier of care, the state has strong incentive to use its regulatory powers to limit the costs of care services that it will reimburse. States attempt to constrain spending either by limiting demand for services or by limiting supply. To limit demand for publicly financed care, states may tighten eligibility standards or refuse to pay for or subsidize certain services. Tightening eligibility standards is feasible only in states that maintain broader standards than those mandated by the federal government. Also, it is politically difficult to cut back substantially on the number of eligible recipients. In addition, cutbacks in Medicaid eligibility may simply shift the cost burden of care to local governments, many of which are already in worse financial shape than the states.

An alternative to limiting eligibility or the range of services provided is to restrict supply, set the price of services, and attempt to control quality by defining certain minimum levels of input usage. In pursuing their cost-containment objectives, governments impose two types of regulations on providers of care. This first type pertains only to services provided to public beneficiaries—for example, rate setting. The second type is imposed on all providers of a service—for example, licensing.

When the public sector finances only a small fraction of care provided and when the market is competitive with nursing homes attempting to maximize profits, it is relatively easy to determine the cost of competitively provided services. One looks to the private market and observes what noninsured consumers pay for a service. When government subsidizes more than 50 percent of the consumers' medical care consumption, however, it is not possible to observe what the price of a service would be in the absence of insurance.

Before the introduction of Medicaid, many states reimbursed facilities by using a flat rate. Nursing homes were paid a daily rate that was not a function of the costs they incurred in providing the service. Homes were encouraged to keep costs down because they could keep the difference between the daily rate paid by the state and their costs. With the advent of Medicaid, a number of states switched to cost-based reimbursement. Under this system, facilities are paid the cost of providing services. Since there is no financial reward for being a low-cost facility, there is no incentive to hold down costs. The movement toward cost-based reimbursement was further encouraged by the 1972 Social Security Amendments, which required that payment rates be reasonably related to the cost of providing care in an efficiently and economically operated facility.

As costs for long-term services continued their rapid rise, governments as payers looked for methods to limit the outflow of funds for these services. Their financial role in the market and the increasing demands on their pocketbooks from this and other public services

TABLE 7–1
NURSING HOME EXPENDITURES AS A PERCENTAGE OF
TOTAL MEDICAID EXPENDITURES, BY STATE, FISCAL YEAR 1978

State	Percent	State	Percent
South Dakota	67.8	Alabama	45.8
Minnesota	64.2	Vermont	45.2
Alaska	63.2	Georgia	44.7
New Hampshire	62.2	South Carolina	44.6
Colorado	60.5	New York	44.3
Wyoming	60.5	Kansas	44.2
Iowa	58.1	Hawaii	43.8
Texas	58.1	Rhode Island	43.3
Nebraska	57.8	Kentucky	41.7
Wisconsin	56.9	Mississippi	41.1
Idaho	56.7	Florida	40.3
Arkansas	55.5	Ohio	40.0
Montana	54.0	North Carolina	39.8
North Dakota	53.8	Delaware	39.7
Connecticut	53.1	Michigan	39.3
Indiana	53.1	Missouri	38.8
Oklahoma	52.8	Massachusetts	38.7
Utah	52.5	Washington	38.4
Nevada	51.0	New Jersey	36.4
Oregon	48.9	Maryland	34.3
Maine	48.4	New Mexico	31.3
Pennsylvania	47.6	Illinois	29.5
Louisiana	47.0	California	23.9
Virginia	46.3	West Virginia	22.5
Tennessee	46.0	District of Columbia	13.1

NOTE: Arizona does not have a Medicaid program. Guam, Puerto Rico, and the Virgin Islands are not included.

SOURCE: Health Care Financing Administration, *Medicaid Statistics Fiscal Year 1978,* DHEW Publication No. (HCFA) 78-03154, Research Report B-5 (FY 78) (Preliminary), June 1979, table E.

gave them a strong incentive to use their abilities as regulators to hold down the rate of increase in costs. They began to consider options to limit supply (certificate of need), limit demand (restrictions in Medicaid eligibility), and limit prices on long-term care services.

By 1978, many states devoted over one-half of their Medicaid budgets to financing long-term care services (see table 7–1). In response, they have adopted three types of regulatory mechanisms to control rising long-term care costs and yet try to maintain quality standards:

(1) setting prices, (2) limiting the quantity of services supplied, and (3) regulating the use of inputs.

Price Rules. The first tool used to control costs is rate setting, which generally applies only to services provided to public beneficiaries. Although required by law to set payment rates that are related to reasonable costs, states nevertheless exercise substantial control over payment levels for nursing home care. By altering rates, states alter the rate of return to entering the industry. They can also alter the mix of facilities by varying the differential between their payment for skilled nursing home facilities and intermediate care facilities. The rates that states pay facilities for services rendered to Medicaid beneficiaries are generally well below the rates that facilities receive for treating private patients. The incentive for the facility is to treat first those patients for whom it can receive the highest fees—that is, the private patients. Once demand by the private sector has been exhausted, facilities may drop down and provide services to public beneficiaries. This situation is depicted in figure 7-1.[12]

Because of imperfect information and product differentiation, one would expect nursing homes to face downward-sloping demand curves. Marginal revenue in the private market lies below the demand curve. The rate that the state sets for treating public beneficiaries is M. The marginal revenue curve is therefore kinked at the point where the private marginal revenue curve intersects the Medicaid reimbursement level. For-profit facilities will provide output to the point where the incremental revenue (MR) they receive from treating a patient just equals the incremental cost. If the incremental cost of providing an additional nursing home day is less than the rate that a home can receive from treating a Medicaid eligibile, some output will be provided to Medicaid beneficiaries. Nonprofit facilities may behave somewhat differently depending on their service goals. Nevertheless, one would not expect them to provide services unless they obtain some positive return. Higher Medicaid payment levels will encourage greater provision of services to public beneficiaries for both types of facilities. Depending on the rate that is set, facilities may either exhaust demand for services by public beneficiaries or provide fewer services than are demanded. With rate setting and free entry, one would expect firms to enter the industry and bid away any excess profits. A reduction in the Medicaid payment rate would discourage firms from treating Medicaid beneficiaries and could lead to an exodus of the less efficient firms from the industry. A possible effect of low rates is to encourage firms to provide a lower quality of care.

FIGURE 7-1

DEMAND AND COST CURVES OF A NURSING HOME

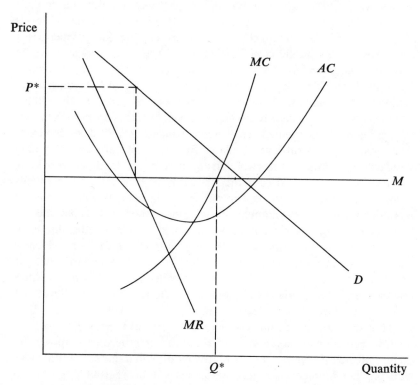

Q^* = profit-maximizing level of output	M = Medicaid reimbursement level
P^* = profit-maximizing private price	AC = average cost
D = demand in the private sector	MC = marginal cost
MR = marginal revenue	

Quality Rules. To counter industry incentives to reduce quality of care to public beneficiaries and to protect private consumers who are generally frail, elderly, and very vulnerable, states have attempted to set their own quality standards. The heterogeneity of the product, however, makes it extremely difficult to set output standards. The states have thus responded by setting input requirements. They have defined certification standards that providers must meet to be eligible for state payments. The introduction of Life Safety Codes in the 1970s represented a major effort at quality control. The result of such standard setting was to raise the costs of providing care and consequently to alter the character of the industry. The costs of meeting the new standards was likely to have a more significant impact on small homes than on large ones. In 1969, 40 percent of nursing homes had less than twenty-five beds.[13] Burton Dunlop reported that many of these small homes were forced to close because of the new quality standards.[14]

Another effort at quality control is to mandate the input levels of certain types of personnel. Thus, to be eligible for payments for care provided to public beneficiaries, long-term care providers would have to be certified. In general, one set of certification standards exists for skilled nursing facilities and another set for intermediate care facilities. Medicare will only pay for services rendered in the skilled facilities and states generally set higher payment rates for these facilities. Depending on the mandated certification standards, the costs of achieving them, and the payment level available from the state, the use of quality standards and rate setting will affect the type of facilities providing services in the state. Also, if the standards require certain increments in inputs for a given increment in patient load, facilities will congregate around certain sizes to minimize costs. Since labor costs constitute the large majority of costs incurred by facilities, regulating the inputs of labor resources can enormously affect the costs of the facilities. Homes that cannot meet the costs imposed by the quality standards will be driven out of the market. Whether they will be replaced by facilities that can meet the standards will depend on the reimbursement level and whether the state heavily restricts entry to the market.

Nursing homes are not the only long-term care providers to have quality regulation or some type of certification procedure imposed on them. Medicare regulations currently require that home health aides who provide Medicare services be supervised by registered nurses to qualify for payment. In addition, to qualify for Medicare payments, home health agencies must provide skilled nursing care and at least one other therapeutic service. In the past, proprietary agencies had to be certified by the state in order to be eligible for reimbursement under Medicare. Since numerous states did not have licensing requirements for home health agencies, this requirement effectively excluded all for-profit facilities in the state from participating in the program.

Whether input restrictions and certification standards have raised the quality of long-term care services above what they otherwise would have been is not known. If they have served to maintain a higher quality of care, it may only have been accomplished through a trade-off for quantity and an increase in costs.

Quantity Rules. The third regulatory tool available to the government in its efforts to cut costs is to impose direct controls on the supply of services. In 1974, Congress passed the National Health Planning and Resource Development Act. The act required that, before a state could receive grants from the Public Health Service, it had to implement certificate-of-need legislation. By 1979, virtually all states had enacted such laws.

The available evidence indicates that certificate-of-need legislation has had little, if any, significant impact on reducing hospital costs. The question of possible cost savings is now being extended to the long-term care sector. Most available evidence points to an existing excess demand for nursing home care.[15] Occupancy rates in nursing homes are well above those for hospitals. Numerous states have difficulty finding placement for public beneficiaries in nursing homes. Whether this is due solely to certificate-of-need legislation or to a combination of measures is difficult to sort out. Depending on which tool is used most heavily to achieve a given end has important implications for the structure and performance of the industry. If its objectives are to stay within some budgetary amount, a state can attempt to do so using rate regulation, certificate-of-need legislation, or a combination of both. If the state relies primarily on rate regulation to achieve its ends, firms will be encouraged to enter the market or expand output so long as there are profits to be made in the industry. Nursing homes that are inefficient will be driven out of the market by the lower-cost facilities. As long as demand exceeds supply, facilities will have an incentive to discriminate against the heavy-care, high-cost patients. Unless states can queue up those most in need of services, it is likely that those requiring the most intensive level of services will not have access to care. Existing freedom-of-choice constraints on the Medicaid program further inhibit the ability of states to care for the sickest persons first. If payment rates are set low enough to meet budgetary objectives, and firms only earn a normal return, enforcement of certificate of need is unnecessary because no firm would desire to enter the industry.

If, however, states rely primarily on certificate of need to control supply, and firms still desire to enter the industry, one may consider such attempted entry as evidence that firms in the industry are earning abnormally high returns. States may set rates above those needed to maintain a given bed supply for political reasons, or they may believe that higher rates will result in a higher quality of care. If higher quality comes at a higher cost when quality standards are being enforced, returns to the facility will fall. The current presence of a queue for entry and expansion suggests that higher-than-average returns are being earned. States could finance more services to more people if they lowered payment rates. As long as there is excess demand for services, facilities continue to have incentives to skim the "light care" or least costly patients first. If nursing homes in the industry are earning above-average returns, it may certainly be in their interest to maintain, or even make more rigorous, the existing certificate-of-need laws. Eliminating the laws would permit existing nursing homes to expand via building new facilities or expanding existing facilities. Allowing entry would also eventually lower the return to nursing home investment. Existing facilities currently expand primarily by purchasing existing facilities. It should come as no surprise, therefore, that some of the most vociferous proponents of certificate of need may come from within the industry. (The desire of an industry to protect itself from outside competition is certainly not unique to the health care industry. Occupational licensing and tariffs or import restrictions represent efforts by other industries to use regulation as a means of protecting their economic interests.) If entry restrictions result in rates of return that are above the competitive levels, it is reasonable to expect continuing concentration of firms within the industry. The possibility of earning monopoly rents creates incentives for firms that already own a number of firms to expand further. In the longer run, the larger firms may anticipate an eventual capture of the regulators by the industry. This is more likely to occur with only a few firms in the industry.

The Regulator's Dilemma. Each of the states is in the position both of being the major purchaser of long-term care services and of having the authority to regulate providers of care. In theory, states would like to pay facilities the cost of efficiently provided services of a given quality. Because the state is such a large purchaser of care, however, facility costs will tend to reflect state payment rates. Unless a state can accurately estimate the costs of efficiently provided care, there is no assurance that reimbursement levels will reflect such costs. When states rely on cost-based reimbursement, facilities have no incentive to hold costs down. To meet budgetary targets, states often respond by setting payment rates and limiting the supply of services. Usually, the resulting output of services is not efficiently produced, nor is the distribution of services optimal. The inability to define effectively what is meant by a nursing home day has produced efforts to regulate quality by defining the quantity and quality of inputs to be used in the production process. By designating the quantity and types of inputs used, the state confines facilities to the use of only a limited number of production processes. Nursing homes may be unable to respond to changes in input prices. Unless the state is able to estimate precisely the most efficient production process and to alter that as prices change, production inefficiencies will occur. Inefficiencies in production mean that the same output could be produced at a lower cost.

Which Way Is Out?

Regulation, combined with large government subsidies for institutional care, has distorted prices for services and led to excess demand for institutional care. The public sector has sought to limit spending through a series of regulations that directly control prices, quantities, and the use of inputs. One could debate whether this approach has resulted in any savings to the public sector. It seems more fruitful to ask whether, with the same dollar outlays, more long-term care resources can be provided to the functionally impaired. An alternative to direct regulation of the market is to create economic incentives for firms to provide quality care at minimal cost.

Many of the incentives that have been proposed in the acute care sector relate primarily to raising the price faced by consumers at the time of purchasing care, limiting the tax deductibility of health insurance plans, encouraging the formation of prepaid group plans, and granting vouchers to the elderly and medically indigent that can be used to purchase insurance plans. Whether these incentives will improve the functioning of the long-term care market is difficult to predict. Given the numerous differences between the long-term and the acute care markets, remedies that might improve resource allocation and reduce costs in one market might have no discernible effect in the other market. In this section, I will discuss some of the proposals for encouraging efficiency and their potential impact on long-term care services.

Consumer Cost Sharing. Consumers already share a substantial amount of the costs for nursing home services. Private pay patients face the full costs of care, and public beneficiaries devote nearly their entire income to purchasing nursing home care. However, public beneficiaries—the majority of consumers—face out-of-pocket costs for care that are independent of the cost of the facility. They have no incentive to choose low-cost providers of care. Private consumers who expect to exhaust their resources and convert to Medicare also have reduced incentives to select low-cost providers. This suggests that there might be some efficiency gains in the long-term care market if the out-of-pocket costs borne by the patient were scaled to reflect facility costs. Consumers would pay more out of pocket if they selected high-cost facilities for a given level of care. The use of economic incentives to encourage consumer behavior has some potential problems, however, when applied to the market for long-term care.

First, restructuring consumer out-of-pocket payments so that they increase with the cost of the nursing home would be more expensive for the public programs than the existing structure. Public beneficiaries currently devote virtually all of their income to nursing home care. Thus, if one were to structure consumer cost sharing so that consumers who selected low-cost providers would pay less, the result would be lower out-of-pocket costs for some consumers. Those who selected high-cost providers would continue to devote nearly all of their income to nursing home care. The result would be greater public subsidies than occur under the existing system.

Second, the implementation of graduated cost sharing requires the ability to group facilities by level of care. Cost differences resulting from improved efficiency in producing output of a given quality need to be distinguished from cost differences resulting from a difference in quality of care. Since the level of service intensity varies substantially across facilities, and since input levels provide only a crude method of distinguishing among facilities, it would be necessary to develop a new approach to facility classification.

Third, given the long-term nature of the consumption package, it is unlikely that many consumers will reap any of the savings from choosing a low-cost facility. For those who use the facility to recover from a hospital episode, incentive payments may result in the selection of lower-cost providers. Many consumers, however, can expect to remain in the facility for long periods of time. For these people, response to economic incentives will be based on the strength of a person's desire to distribute income to family members since the family will be the principal beneficiary of a patient's decision to select a lower-cost provider.

A second approach that might be used to increase consumer cost-consciousness and to improve efficiency in the delivery of health care is the use of vouchers. In the broadest sense, vouchers become very nearly an income transfer program based on ability to pay and level of health impairment. At the narrow end, they become block grants to individuals that can be used to purchase a set of specific health services, possibly covering only one service such as nursing home care. Vouchers do have the advantage of allowing budgeting authorities to plan ahead more easily.

The use of vouchers in the acute care market has been advocated as a means of encouraging individuals to purchase low-cost insurance plans. Insurance is generally unavailable for long-term care so that a voucher system in this market would more likely be used for the direct purchase of services. If individuals are granted an allocation of funds that they can use to purchase a basket of services, it is in their own interest or in the interest of their families to make cost-effective decisions since they must pay the full cost for the good or service. For this reason, a voucher program should also cover the widest range of services possible. Rather than viewing publicly financed long-term care services only as health services, one may wish to broaden the view and include housing, utilities, and meals as items that can be purchased with the voucher. This will cut down on the "market basket moral hazard" problem. Theoretically, a voucher system preserves many of the incentives available in a market system while allowing better targeting of program costs.

Probably the most important problem with a voucher system is its potential cost. The overwhelming majority of long-term care services are currently provided informally by family and friends. A voucher system, if structured to include most low-income disabled persons, would probably result in an unacceptably high level of taxpayer spending for long-term care services. Even if one were willing to commit that level of resources, many tough questions would still need to be addressed: Should the value of the voucher be determined by a means test and an evaluation of health status? If so, what factors are to be considered in determining ability to pay, and how well does health status predict need for services? Regional variations in service prices would ideally need to be taken into account in setting the voucher limit. Also, given the current financing of Medicaid, a voucher system with a broad focus could result in states shifting other services such as housing subsidies and meals programs to Medicaid in order to receive federal financial participation. Still, the voucher system is one approach that could result in minimal price distortions for long-term care services.

Improving Provider Incentives. Besides consumer incentives to increase efficiency in the provision of long-term care services, incentives can also be implemented on the supply side of the market. Efficiency in the delivery of long-term care, particularly nursing home services, could be improved by eliminating certificate-of-need requirements. If nursing homes desire to enter the industry, it is because, under the current market conditions, they expect long-run profits. Monopoly rents are accruing to those already in the industry, and it is in their interest to prevent other nursing homes from entering. If nursing homes desire entry, states could reduce their reimbursement rates and maintain the same level of output to public beneficiaries at a lower cost. Certificate of need results in inefficient firms remaining in the industry; free entry would permit efficient firms to survive and would help to drive out the inefficient ones. States could control the number of nursing homes and the level of public expenditures for care by altering reimbursement rates and would not need to use certificate of need to limit bed supply.

Under conditions of excess demand, nursing homes have incentives

139

to skim the light care patients first. States can counter these incentives to some extent by structuring payment rates to reflect the costs of providing care to different types of patients. However, how these payment rates are structured is critical to the performance of the homes. If rates for heavy care patients are high relative to those for light care patients, facilities will have little incentive to improve a patient's functioning level, because doing so would result in a reduced reimbursement. If the nursing home was allowed to keep some of the gains resulting from improving patient functioning, it would be in the firm's financial interest to improve patient outcome. Thus, a system of payment based on the costs of caring for different patients and the provision of economic incentives for improved outcomes may be a useful alternative to existing payment policies. Nursing homes might be further encouraged to maintain quality if they provided a range of services to patients besides the traditional institutional services. By putting nursing homes in charge of providing services to discharged patients and by financially encouraging them to improve the functioning level of their patients, providers would have greater incentive to behave efficiently.

Subsidizing the provision of more noninstitutional services would also increase competition among providers. Current policies encourage the use of institutional care by providing little government support for alternative services. In addition, Medicaid eligibility policies are often less stringent for nursing home care than for other services so that patients have little option but to use nursing home care. The result is a distortion of relative prices for nursing home and other services, resulting in a bias toward institutional care.

Proponents of expanding noninstitutional alternatives point to studies which show that some fraction of the nursing home population can be cared for at lower cost in an alternative setting. The costs generally referred to are total public program costs rather than total social costs. While Medicaid may reduce program costs by transferring some persons from institutional to community care settings, once the additional housing, utility, and transportation costs are included, the total social cost of community care might be higher than the cost associated with institutional care. As a result, reducing program costs might be accomplished only at the expense of reduced aggregate output. Opponents of expanding noninstitutional services may also base their arguments on total program costs. They point to the amount of informal care that is now being provided by family and friends and the potential for substituting formal for informal services. This substitution could drive up public program costs substantially.

By subsidizing alternatives to nursing home care, states can remove the bias toward the use of institutional services. Subsidizing alternatives does not, however, eliminate moral hazard and the resulting tendency to overutilize services. Consumers will always be more willing to spend someone else's money than to spend their own resources.

Improving Regulation. A third approach to the problems of long-term care is to improve existing regulation. One proposed method is to eliminate the consumer's freedom of choice. This approach would permit states to develop a priority system for allowing patients to use long-term care services. Currently, any public beneficiary who has been approved by the state is eligible for nursing home care. As long as demand for services exceeds the existing supply, homes have the incentive to treat light care patients and ignore the more costly ones. If freedom of choice was eliminated, states could directly place heavy care patients. Patients could be queued on the basis of need, and the budgetary constraints of the public sector would determine how far down the queue the states could go in placing patients. Institutional services could be precluded for the lightest care patients. By eliminating consumer freedom of choice, states could better control and direct resources and could counter efforts of profit-maximizing nursing homes to skim the light care patients.

Conclusion

The long-term care sector of the health market poses problems for cost control that are quite different from those posed by the acute care sector. The reasons for market failure in acute care—extensive private and public insurance coverage, limited consumer cost sharing, tax deductions for employers' contributions to health insurance plans, and consumer ignorance—are not as prevalent in long-term care. Long-term care is essentially different from acute care, and the current structure of public programs that finance the majority of long-term care creates a different set of problems. The current public financing available for long-term care has a strong institutional bias leading to a "market basket moral hazard." People are encouraged to consume services that they may not need in order to acquire some that they do need. In addition, because consumer cost sharing is not related to the costs of care, there is little incentive to search out low-cost providers. This is true for public beneficiaries and to some extent for private beneficiaries as well, since a sizable fraction of private consumers will eventually spend down their assets and become eligible for publicly financed long-term care.

The existing approach to controlling health care costs has focused on regulation. States have used certificate of need to limit institutional bed supply, set rates for nursing homes, and restricted Medicaid coverage for noninstitutional alternatives. To counter the nursing homes' incentives to reduce the quality of care, states have regulated the use of inputs. The result has been an excess demand for institutional care and incentives for nursing homes to skim the light care patients in lieu of more costly patients. In instances where state-set payment rates are high and certificate of need is restricting entry, nursing homes can earn monopoly profits and inefficient homes will not be driven out of the market. To induce efficiency in the provision of long-term care services, states have three policy options: (1) increase the incentives for consumers to choose cost-effective methods of care; (2) improve competition among providers of care; and (3) reform regulatory constraints so that regulation can be more effective.

For short-term users of nursing homes, consumer incentives could motivate the choice of low-cost providers of care. Graduating consumer payments to reflect facility costs could encourage consumers to search for the most cost-effective methods of care. Many individuals in long-term care facilities can, however, be expected to use the services for long periods. They are not likely to exhibit a strong response to monetary incentives that encourage the use of low-cost providers.

Instituting a voucher system for long-term care represents another means of inducing consumers to behave efficiently in their selection of providers. The major problem with a voucher system is the potentially high cost associated with such a program. Even if it were limited to a small number of severely disabled persons, program costs might increase. The cost associated with purchasing care through the market currently encourages the provision of large amounts of informal care. If the voucher limit were set at the rate states currently pay for nursing home care, Medicaid costs would increase substantially. To remain within current budgetary limits, states would need to put strict limits on the size of the vouchers and on eligibility. Still, such a solution does have substantial merit on economic-efficiency grounds and research should further pursue this as a possibility.

Another method of encouraging efficiency is to create economic incentives for providers of long-term care. Eliminating certificate of need would open up greater competition among institutional providers and could force many inefficient homes out of the market. States could set rates to maintain a targeted bed supply. Although this would result in greater efficiency, nursing homes would still desire to skim the light care patients as long as rates were set so that excess demand existed in the market. One way to counter this is by restricting consumer freedom of choice. Such restrictions on consumer freedoms may be socially unacceptable, however. Alternatively, the states could set payment rates that reflect the cost of caring for patients with different impairment levels. In addition, incentives could be created so that nursing homes would be encouraged to improve patient outcomes. Improving the method for determining the costs of care applicable to specific impairments and adding incentives for improved patient outcomes are areas of research that may produce significant improvement in the ability of the public sector to finance long-term care services at a reasonable cost to taxpayers.

Notes

1. Robert M. Gibson and Daniel R. Waldo, "National Health Expenditures, 1980," *Health Care Financing Review*, vol. 2 (September 1981), p. 20.

2. Mark Freeland, George Calat, and Carol Ellen Schendler, "Projections of National Health Expenditures, 1980, 1985 and 1990," *Health Care Financing Review* (Winter 1980), p. 11.

3. Gibson and Waldo, "National Health Expenditures, 1980," p. 20.

4. William Scanlon, "Public Policies and the Nursing Home Industry's Growth: Findings and Gaps," Urban Institute Working Paper 1095–2 (Washington, D.C., April 1981), p. 9.

5. William Scanlon, "Aspects of the Nursing Home Market: Private Demand, Total Utilization and Investment," Urban Institute Working Paper 1218–1 (Washington, D.C., February 1978), p. g.

6. Kelvin Lancaster, "A New Approach to Consumer Theory," *Journal of Political Economy*, vol. 74 (April 1966), pp. 132–57.

7. See for example, U.S. Congress, Senate, Special Committee on Aging, hearing on *Health Care for Older Americans: The "Alternatives" Issue*, Part 5, 95th Congress, 1st session, September 21, 1977, pp. 499–515.

8. Congressional Budget Office, *Long Term Care for the Elderly and Disabled* (Washington, D.C., February 1977), p. x.

9. James Callahan, Lawrence Diamond, Janet Giele, and Robert Morris, "Responsibility of Families for Their Severely Disabled Elderly," *Health Care Financing Review*, vol. 1, no. 3 (Winter 1980), pp. 29–48.

10. Congressional Budget Office, *Long Term Care*, p. 17.

11. General Accounting Office, *Entering a Nursing Home—Costly Implications for Medicaid and the Elderly* (Washington, D.C., November 26, 1979), pp. 29–43.

12. Frank A. Sloan and Bruce Steinwald, "The Role of Health Insurance in the Physicians' Services Market," *Inquiry*, vol. 12 (1975), pp. 275–299; Scanlon, "Aspects of the Nursing Home Market."

13. Scanlon, "Public Policies," p. 13.

14. Burton Dunlop, *The Growth of Nursing Home Care* (Lexington, Mass.: Lexington Books, 1979), pp. 80–81.

15. Ibid., pp. 81–83; Scanlon, "Aspects of the Nursing Home Market," p. 81.

8

Health Care Cost Containment through Private Sector Initiatives

Patricia W. Samors and Sean Sullivan

The sharp increase in health care costs in recent years has led to new public policy initiatives designed to contain these costs. Many new government regulations pertaining to reimbursement of doctors and hospitals, expansion of facilities, and utilization of services have been established, and a variety of comprehensive national health plans have been proposed. Congress is considering several "procompetition" plans, emphasizing incentives for consumers and providers to lower costs. The numerous private sector initiatives developed to reduce the rate of increase in health care costs are often overlooked in the debate over regulatory versus market-oriented approaches to public policy. Frequently, these initiatives are taken by employers whose soaring costs of providing employee health benefits correspond to the steep rise in the national health bill. Ford Motor Company's health costs, for instance, rose from $68 million in 1965 to $650 million in 1981, doubling roughly every five years. Health costs for Caterpillar Tractor Company grew from $65 million in 1975 to $146 million in 1981. This growth does not reflect an increase in the number of employees covered nor in benefits offered.

Private sector activities in health care span a wide range; some are sponsored by individual employers, some by unions, and some by insurers and providers. Other efforts involve coalitions of interested parties in a given community.

Some of these initiatives correspond closely with the thrust of the current procompetition legislative proposals by trying to change consumer or provider incentives.[1] Others, however, attempt to improve the existing system without altering the basic incentives.

Flexible Benefits

A prime example of the incentives approach is the cafeteria or flexible benefit plan that allows employees to shape their benefits to meet their

144

individual needs while giving them incentives to alter their health care consumption patterns. Several companies offer these plans. TRW Corporation originated the concept in 1974 at its California branch, where 18,000 employees now have a choice of four company-sponsored health plan options as well as six health maintenance organizations (HMOs). Employees who choose either of the two low-option plans are given credits that can be used to "purchase" other specified benefits or—under limited conditions—can be converted to taxable cash payments. Only 5 percent of employees have chosen this option, although 40 percent have selected the standard health plan under which the employee is neither charged extra nor eligible for credits.

American Can Company offers each employee a choice of four options in addition to the core medical plan. Credits are determined by subtracting the value of the core benefits from the value of the company's old major medical plan. These credits can be applied to the four other plans (one of which is the original major medical policy) or to other specified benefits. The four plans have various deductibles, copayment shares, and stop-loss catastrophic limits. Fewer than 10 percent of the employees select the old plan; about 50 percent are in the next most expensive plan; 10 percent choose only the core benefits; and the remaining 30 percent are in the other two lower-option plans. The company expects more employees to choose the least expensive plans as other benefits are offered to make those options more attractive.

Educational Testing Service (ETS) has a plan under which its employees are offered essential coverage in medical care, life insurance, and disability income replacement as well as vacation, education, and retirement benefits. ETS pays the entire cost of these basic benefits. Every year each employee is allotted flexible credits based on calendar years of service with ETS and determined by a percentage of the employee's salary. Employees can use their flexible credits to buy optional benefits to supplement the traditional benefit program or they can receive these credits in cash.

Incentive Plans

A few plans incorporating cost-saving incentives are especially intriguing. Mobil Oil Company has a bonus plan that may be unique in U.S. industry. Rather than providing their employees with specified health benefits, oil companies contribute a flat monthly amount toward health insurance. Mobil self-insures and compares its total monthly cost per employee with the flat-rate monthly contribution. For each month that the cost is below the contribution, employees are credited with the difference; there is no offset for months in which costs exceed contributions. As of December 1981, the plan covered 29,000 active Mobil employees (80 percent of the total domestic work force), who were grouped into nine geographical "experience" units. Calculations are made separately for each unit; bonuses vary among units but are uniform within a unit. The plan was introduced in 1977, and bonuses have been paid to nearly all eligibles each year. The average bonus in 1981 was $115, and the largest was $197. This plan has two of the principal elements of the procompetition bills—fixed employer contributions and cash rebates.

Another interesting plan is offered to employees of the Mendocino County Schools Office north of San Francisco. Although not strictly a private sector initiative, it merits attention because of its originality. For the past two years, the schools office has administered a stay-well self-insurance plan instead of purchasing full first-dollar coverage from an outside insurer. It now deposits $500 for each employee in a local account, to be used for the first $500 of medical expenses during the year. At the same time, it purchases a $500 deductible group major medical policy from Blue Cross to cover employees after the first $500 of expenses. Any portion of the $500 deposit not used by an employee is carried over to the following year, when another $500 is deposited. Any unused portion of this second $500 is also carried over; if the employee's expenses in the second year exceed $500, the excess is paid under the group major medical policy and not out of his first-year carryover. When the employee leaves the schools office, he may take any unspent amounts that have accrued as severance pay, or use them to purchase continuing coverage. The plan encourages employees to stay well and to use discretion in incurring future medical expenses. Some choose to pay part of their medical costs themselves rather than spend their allowances, thereby gaining tax benefits. The schools office retains any interest accruing on unspent balances. The record so far shows a quarter of the employees with no medical expenses at all, a quarter with expenses exceeding $500, and half with expenses less than $500.

Interest in plans similar to the Mendocino plan can be found across the country in both the private sector and the public sector. Berol Corporation's new program pays each employee at the end of the year $500 less any reimbursement made by the insurance plan, which pays 80 percent of covered expenses after a $150 deductible.

In Pennsylvania, the Lehigh County Medical Society has encouraged the state medical society to develop a prototype plan based on the Mendocino concept. Once formulated it will be offered to doctors in the state and will serve as a model to be recommended to industries in the area. In Delaware, Blue Cross/Blue Shield has developed an innovative concept, corresponding closely to the Mendocino plan, for members of the

Medical Society of Delaware and their employees. For those who elect to participate in the new Stay Well Program (which is available only to those who choose the comprehensive 100 percent policy), Blue Cross/ Blue Shield will set aside $500 of the annual premium to serve as a "good health" incentive. The first $500 of expenses incurred for medical services will be paid out of this fund. If the full $500 is not depleted over the course of the year, the remainder will be refunded at the close of the contract year.

Bank of America, the California state legislature, and the state of Florida are trying plans similar to Mendocino's, on a test basis. In June 1981, the Florida state legislature passed a law that called for the implementation in January 1982 of a pilot cost-containment health insurance plan for state employees working in Dade County. The success or failure of this project will determine whether or not it is extended to all state employees. Dade County was chosen as the test site because its health care costs are high and a change in its health care expenditures can be measured. Under this Health Incentive Program, premium payments are deposited in a special trust fund. Any money remaining after payment of claims and administrative expenses for a calendar year will be distributed from the fund to plan participants based on a system of points. The points are awarded according to the dollar amount of claims paid by the state. Individuals with $1 to $150 in claims, for example, will receive four points; $151 to $300, three points; and over $500, no points. The value of each point is determined by dividing the total number of points into the remainder in the fund. Participants will then receive an incentive payment equal to the number of points times the value of each point.

Eight hospitals in southern California are offering their employees a multiple deductible plan that includes incentive bonuses to elect higher deductibles. Under this Optional Multiple Deductible Program, the hospital workers have a choice of three health plans including the original major medical plan with a $100 deductible and plans with $250 and $400 deductibles. An employee choosing either of the two higher deductible policies will receive a rebate at the end of 1982 equal to $226 or $366, respectively. Because the hospitals self-insure they are able to set the amount of the deductibles and the rebates. Although the bonus is not directly linked to service use, it does act as an incentive for the employee to choose the higher deductible, which in turn causes him to be more selective in service use because of his potentially greater out-of-pocket expenses. The lower utilization of medical services and the higher deductibles reduce the hospitals' cost of providing health benefits to their workers. Orthopaedic Hospital of

Los Angeles, the first hospital to opt for the program, estimated that in 1981 it saved $380,000 in costs predicted for that year under the previous major medical program.

Sun Company offers its employees several health care alternatives. Sun pays a portion of the premium for a traditional health insurance package, but absorbs the entire cost of the premium for a second fee-for-service option. This latter plan contains specific cost-containment features. For instance, in order to induce the employee to obtain care outside the hospital, only 90 percent of semiprivate hospitalization costs are covered—compared with 100 percent of costs for ambulatory surgery. Also, to eliminate unnecessary Friday and Saturday hospital admissions, only 80 percent of such costs are covered except for emergencies.

There are also employer- and union-sponsored plans, such as wellness programs and direct provision of care that attempt to curb the rate of growth in health care costs within the existing financial and service delivery structure.

Health Management

Several companies have initiated large-scale wellness or health management programs. Their objective is to promote employees' health, thereby reducing absenteeism, increasing productivity, and slowing the rate of growth of health care costs. Kimberly-Clark Corporation established a health maintenance effort in 1977 called the Health Management Program. Through the program, employees, their spouses, and retirees are helped to recognize their health risks and to control them. The company encourages lifestyle changes and provides an exercise facility and health education classes for this purpose. This program, which is offered in two locations, is expected to achieve significant annual savings within ten years.

Control Data offers a Staywell Program to nearly one-third of its 60,000 U.S. employees. Each employee fills out a questionnaire on family health history and personal lifestyle. Computers process the results to appraise the ten greatest risks to the employee's health, and steps are suggested for reducing them. This program also offers courses in stress reduction, smoking cessation, nutrition, weight control, and fitness.

IBM offers the Plan for Life program of health promotion for its employees and their dependents. In addition to exercise facilities at some of its locations, IBM has a national contract with the YMCA/YWCA that enables employees and their families to use local facilities at no charge. An interesting feature of IBM's health management program is tuition reimbursement for local college adult education courses that fit into the Plan for Life program.

New York Telephone's Health Care Management program saved the company an estimated $16 million in 1981 (expressed in 1980 dollars). Despite this apparent success, one criticism of these programs is that, while they may reduce the demand for health care services, they do not alter consumer incentives and, therefore, will have limited impact on health care costs.

Employer as Provider

Several companies have recently begun to provide direct care for their employees as a way of controlling costs. The Gillette Company, a forerunner in this regard, provides primary care and some specialty care to more than 90 percent of its work force at three clinics in the Boston area staffed by fourteen physicians and ten nurses and technicians. Some of the physicians are on salary and others are reimbursed on a fee-for-service basis, while most maintain outside office practices as well. By providing peer review, monitoring utilization, and stressing preventive and primary care, Gillette provides its employees with quality comprehensive care while saving an estimated $1 million or more annually.

R. J. Reynolds developed a staff model HMO (the physicians are employees of the HMO, rather than independent contractors) that serves only its employees and their dependents The company's Winston-Salem Health Care Plan provides regular HMO services and refers patients to outside specialists and hospitals as needed. Again, utilization—including decisions on surgery—is monitored. With 85 percent of its employees enrolled, Reynolds has saved money on the plan because of the emphasis on preventive care and the lower hospitalization rate commonly found among HMOs.

Unions have historically been involved in the delivery of health care through HMOs and union-sponsored delivery systems. This approach to cost containment has declined, however, as a result of the demand for free choice of physicians and location of care, residential shifts away from the urban areas where the centers were located, and the geographic service limitations of the centers. Many of the centers did exhibit a high degree of efficiency—the United Mine Workers Association's program cost $360 per beneficiary in 1976 compared with a national average of $551.[2]

In addition to providing direct care, labor unions and management have negotiated cost-containment provisions in collective bargaining agreements. United Auto Workers' contracts establish pilot programs for hospital, professional, and drug utilization reviews, for second surgical opinions, and for hospital preadmission testing. Labor-management committees have been established to oversee these programs. The United Department Store Workers Union mandates that its members receive a second opinion for surgery. In the ten years since this program was initiated, the incidence of surgery has dropped by 18 percent.

Self-Insurance

A growing number of employers have been developing self-insurance programs, so that by the end of 1981 such programs accounted for nearly 20 percent of the health insurance market—an increase from 5 percent in 1975. Since self-insurance does not attempt to contain costs by altering consumer or provider incentives, it is not clear whether procompetition legislation would help or hinder this trend. Self-insurance does reduce employers' administrative and financial costs.

Some employers insure against and administer all claims themselves; some self-insure but contract with insurance companies or claims administrators for administrative services only (ASO); and others self-insure against some but not all claims. The Health Insurance Association of America, the trade association of large commercial insurers, estimates that more than 25 percent of all group health benefits are self-insured. A survey by Hay Associates of more than 500 companies shows that nearly 40 percent either are self-insured or combine self-insurance with some degree of commercial coverage. (Hay surveys mostly large firms, which are more likely to self-insure.) Examples of the trend are Caterpillar Tractor, Deere and Company, and Mobil Oil, which are fully self-insured and self-administered. Honeywell is self-insured but contracts with Blue Cross/Blue Shield and commercial insurers for administrative services. Citicorp self-insures against medical claims while taking advantage of Blue Cross's negotiated discount with hospitals in New York.

The Employee Retirement Income Security Act (ERISA) exempts self-insurance from all state regulation of insurance plans, letting the companies avoid premium taxes and reserve requirements. As a result, employers avoid the "tax costs" of insurance and the loss of earnings on funds held in reserve.

Another benefit to firms that self-administer the medical claims of their employees is the data they collect that enable them to determine how and where their money is being spent. Using this data, an employer can negotiate with providers, such as hospitals serving the firm's employees, for price discounts, and it can identify providers that are overusing procedures. Control Data, after being self-administered for two years, is just beginning to use its data for this purpose.

Coalitions

The private sector initiatives already surveyed help contain employer health care costs, but they are primarily individual company or union efforts. A number of activities, however, bring the major participants together to work jointly toward a reduction in the cost of health care. The most visible of these joint cost-containment activities has been the formation of health care coalitions. Of the fifty to sixty coalitions in existence, about thirty-five are actually carrying out their programs. The remainder are still forming their agendas.

Membership in the coalitions always includes business and sometimes government, labor, providers, and insurers. Blue Cross/Blue Shield plans are involved in fifty area coalitions, and many plans have played a key role in sponsoring or helping coalitions get started. While many of the coalitions consist only of business, leaders of the American Medical Association and the American Hospital Association are encouraging their members to join. In this way, the medical profession's views will be heard and health policy decisions will not be made only by business people. Coalitions work on several fronts: promoting and developing HMO alternatives; collecting cost and utilization data for employers using different providers; working with insurers to redesign health benefit plans to encourage less costly utilization practices; participating in local health-planning activities through involvement with Health Systems Agencies (HSAs); educating companies, employees, and local hospital board members on health care cost-containment programs; and negotiating with providers and suppliers to contain costs. In addition to their involvement in coalition activities, business and labor often work independently on similar fronts to contain costs.

HMO Development. The Twin City Health Care Development Project was initiated by major Minneapolis–St. Paul employers such as General Mills, Honeywell, Control Data, and Cargill even before the federal HMO act was passed in 1973. This project put up seed money and helped to get HMOs operating. A Group Health Plan already existed with 36,000 enrollees, but the project has now helped to produce seven HMOs with total enrollment of more than 25 percent of the metropolitan population. Honeywell has about two-thirds of its 18,000 local employees enrolled in six HMOs, and General Mills has approximately 80 percent of its headquarters' employees in three plans. After five HMOs were formed, many of the remaining physicians signed up with Physicians Health Plan, an individual practice association (IPA) HMO established by the Hennepin County Medical Association in response to the growth of the prepaid group practices.

151

Individual companies have occasionally supported the establishment of HMOs in their localities. Ford Motor Company was active in launching an HMO in Detroit (Health Alliance Plan of Michigan) and tries to offer new plans each year at various locations. Sun Company helped finance the Greater Delaware Valley HMO in Philadelphia. Deere and Company provided money to start an HMO in its home office Quad City area in Illinois and worked to gain support from a major segment of the community's two medical societies. As of June 1982, the plan had enrolled nearly one-third of Deere's work force living in the market area (12,000 employees) and half of the community's physicians. Deere is working with the business and medical communities to set up similar prepaid plans at its two major locations in Iowa. Caterpillar Tractor financed a feasibility study for an HMO in York, Pennsylvania, but decided against it because of provider opposition. After a similar study, it is going ahead with an IPA-type HMO at its headquarters in Peoria. As mentioned earlier, in 1976 R. J. Reynolds developed a staff model HMO for its employees and their dependents. As of mid-1982, 85 percent of its employees were enrolled in the plan. IBM Corporation has also worked diligently at offering employees choice of alternative plans; it has 147 HMOs available at its various facilities across the country.

Digital Corporation has taken an innovative approach to providing its employees with information on health plans by identifying the HMO options available to each worker according to ZIP code. In 1981, after that information was made available to its employees, the portion of Digital's work force enrolled in HMOs increased by two percentage points, bringing the total to 15 percent.

Labor unions have also actively promoted HMO alternatives. In the early 1960s, the United Auto Workers organized a prepaid group practice in Detroit, which has since merged with the Health Alliance Plan of Michigan that Ford helped to start. The Rhode Island AFL-CIO initiated the Rhode Island Group Health Association in 1968 to enroll members of the United Steelworkers, the International Association of Machinists, and the American Federation of State, County, and Municipal Employees in that state. The Communications Workers negotiated a nationwide HMO dual-choice option with the Bell System in 1971. The International Union of Electrical, Radio, and Machine Workers had negotiated a similar provision with General Electric in 1970. The International Longshoremen's and Warehousemen's Union on the West Coast encourages its members to join HMOs by not negotiating for more expensive benefits in non-HMO plans; consequently, a majority choose Kaiser or other prepaid group plans.

Insurer involvement in HMO development deserves particular

notice. At the end of 1981, Blue Cross/Blue Shield plans were sponsoring fifty-four HMOs with about 1,039,000 members, an enrollment increase of 21 percent over 1980. Wisconsin Physicians Service's HMO with 183,100 enrollees is the largest of the Blue plans. The HMO of Minnesota, with 63,000 enrollees, is the second largest plan in the Twin Cities. Eight new plans were put into operation in 1981, and four started in 1982 with additional HMOs planned at least through 1984.

Among the commercial insurance companies sponsoring HMOs are Prudential, John Hancock, and CIGNA (which was formed through a merger of the Insurance Company of North America and Connecticut General). Through its PRUCARE subsidiary, Prudential operates six HMOs with an enrollment of about 170,000. The company has two additional plans in the development stage, which are scheduled to open in January 1983. Forty percent of current enrollees are in Houston, where Prudential opened its first HMO in 1975. Its Chicago HMO, acquired in June 1981, has 36,000 members; the remaining 66,000 are enrolled in Austin, Nashville, Atlanta, and Oklahoma City HMOs—all opened within the last few years. PRUCARE took from 1975 to 1979 to reach a total enrollment of 50,000, but it expects to add another 75,000 to 100,000 enrollees annually over the next several years. The company also plans to add two new HMOs a year for the next two years.

John Hancock recently became involved in operating HMOs by purchasing the Dikewood Corporation of Albuquerque, New Mexico. Hancock/Dikewood Services, Inc., the wholly owned subsidiary of John Hancock, currently operates three HMOs. In Hartford, Connecticut, the HMO works in partnership with the Hartford Hospital; in Atlanta the HMO is set up as an IPA model; and in Philadelphia the company acquired a group practice plan.

Through INA Healthplan, Inc., a subsidiary of the newly formed CIGNA Corporation, CIGNA has the largest share of the commercial insurers in the HMO market. Working principally through acquisitions, INA Healthplan has 600,000 enrollees in nine HMOs—300,000 of them in Los Angeles, where it acquired the well-established Ross-Loos Plan. Other acquisitions include those in Phoenix, Spokane, Miami, and St. Petersburg. The company started its own HMOs in Dallas, Tucson, and Tampa and expects that an additional plan will be operating in Houston in 1982.

Although Prudential and CIGNA see profitable opportunities in the HMO market, SAFECO—an innovator among commercial insurers—incurred losses at its United Healthcare subsidiary (formerly Northwest Healthcare). United was structured as a primary care network whereby each primary care physician had a separate account into which money was deposited each month as payment for his participating patients—payment for inpatient and outpatient services rendered by himself, specialists, or the emergency room. At the end of the year, the doctor shared in any surplus or paid part of any deficit. In 1979, roughly 52 percent of the participating primary care physicians had a surplus; in 1980, that number fell to 25 percent with a loss to United of $1.6 million. In 1981, total losses were running between $3 million and $4 million, and United was finding it difficult to compete in the marketplace because its premiums were rising. Thus, in November 1981, SAFECO began to phase out the program.

United Healthcare failed for several reasons: the low limit on the primary care physician's liability did not contain an incentive to keep expenses low; the physicians were unable to control specialists' costs; and patient benefits were too open-ended. In Seattle, however, a new program, Network Management, has picked up where United left off. The new plan is based on the SAFECO program but with several modifications that are expected to control specialists' fees, benefit design, and primary care services.

Aetna Life and Casualty has taken a different step toward creating competition in the delivery of health care by developing a program, Choice, that tries to combine the strengths of both traditional health insurance and HMOs. The freedom to choose one's own primary care physician is incorporated into Choice by allowing the patient, at the time of enrollment, to select physicians and hospitals for referral and specialty services from a list of those chosen for their quality, efficiency, and cost effectiveness. This component of the program combines the freedom to choose referral physicians with the HMO's ability to control the costs of specialty care by restricting the choice of providers. Aetna seeks out specialty physicians and associated hospitals known for their high standards and appropriate utilization of tests and surgery, because at least three-fourths of claims costs are for these services. Choice will be available in the Chicago area in late 1982. The company expects to extend the program to several additional areas within the year as well.

Alternative Avenues. While some coalitions, individual companies, labor unions, and commercial insurers have worked to promote HMO development and enrollment, others have focused on containing costs through utilization review, planning activities, and Professional Standards Review Organizations (PSROs). The Joint Health Cost Containment Program of the Greater Philadelphia Chamber of Commerce/ Penjerdel Council, for example, has developed a data base on hospital utilization for its forty member companies, enabling them to reshape benefit packages to encourage lower utilization and to make providers more conscious of the high cost of hospitalization. Penjerdel also

154

educates hospital trustees to exercise more cost-conscious leadership and to develop better local health-planning mechanisms as alternatives to HSAs.

Another coalition is the Fairfield/Westchester Business Group on Health, with twenty-five member companies including IBM, Mobil, and American Can. The Fairfield/Westchester Business Group seeks to emulate Penjerdel in gathering data on utilization and in improving areawide hospital planning in Fairfield County, Connecticut, and Westchester County, New York.

The Michigan Cost Containment Coalition consists of representatives from the Big Three auto companies, the United Auto Workers union, and Blue Cross. It worked with state legislators to develop and secure passage of a bill that makes HSAs responsible for planning and implementing bed reduction in Michigan hospitals.

The Boston University Health Policy Institute has helped establish a process for using hospital data to highlight utilization and cost problems. The institute is currently working with ALCOA in Blunt County, Tennessee, and with Du Pont in Wilmington, Delaware— where these companies are the dominant employers. The purpose of the project is to bring health care cost and utilization problems to the attention of the local hospitals. The institute meets with providers, presents the findings from its analyses, and discusses actions that can be taken to clear up the problems. The project emphasizes a cooperative effort between payers and providers. In contrast to PSROs, the project seeks, not to have physicians reviewed by their peers or singled out for how they practice, but to influence the way all providers practice and to provide information on how to do so more efficiently. Although it is too early to determine the effect of the project, the Health Policy Institute has gained the attention and support of local physicians.

The PSROs were originally started to review health care provided under Medicare, Medicaid, and the Maternal and Child Health Programs. They attempt to ensure quality care and to contain costs through a peer review system funded by the federal government. Interest in this form of utilization review has recently grown in the private sector.

The Midwest Business Group on Health, based in Chicago, has encouraged some of its eighty-three member companies to sign contracts with PSROs to review the quality and volume of services provided to the companies—but not the price. Projects are under way in Minnesota, where fifteen major companies including Honeywell, Control Data, and the 3M Corporation have signed with the Twin Cities Foundation for Health Care Evaluation. Plans covering approximately 170,000 individuals will be reviewed under this contract.

PSROs also perform review for individual companies not affiliated with coalitions. For the past three years, Deere and Company has contracted with the Midstate Foundation for Medical Care in Illinois and with its Iowa counterpart to conduct both admission and concurrent stay review. The results have been significant: within the Midstate Foundation's area of responsibility, in-patient days per 1,000 Deere workers declined by 26.8 percent, the average length of stay declined by nearly one full day, and admissions per 1,000 workers declined by 14.0 percent; within the Iowa Foundation's area, in-patient days declined by 21.4 percent, admissions declined by 14.6 percent, and average length of stay declined by one-half day. The company is now looking for a PSRO in Wisconsin.

PSROs are subject to some criticism. The effectiveness of having providers review their own peers is questioned. In addition, there are virtually no incentives to save money. A recent study by the Congressional Budget Office (CBO) found that PSROs reduce hospital days for Medicare patients only slightly (saving little more than the cost of the review itself) and that much of the small reduction in government outlays involves transferring costs to private patients whose charges rise in proportion. When these cost-shifting effects are accounted for, the CBO concludes, the costs outweigh the benefits.[3]

U.S. Administrators (USA), a California-based claims-processing firm, does provide utilization review with an incentive to reduce costs. If costs are not consistent with industry norms, the physicians are not paid the excess. This firm works on an administrative-services-only basis and has gained attention for its rigorous review of all claims for both appropriateness and cost. Using a set of model-treatment screens (MTSs) developed from a computerized data base by physician panels, USA identifies providers who overutilize, underutilize, overcharge, or whose services fail to meet practice standards determined by the physician panels. USA has also been willing to assume the role of advocate for the patient against providers whose claims have been rejected by the insurer. In addition to the MTSs, USA uses screens to check hospital length of stay, hospital ancillary charges, and utilization in prepaid group practices. USA's procedures can identify and bring pressure on outliers, but they are unlikely to change the prevailing style of medical practice significantly.

Negotiating to Reduce Costs. A different experiment in cost containment has been initiated in Rochester, New York, by the business community together with hospitals, local government officials, Blue Cross, the New York State Health Department, and the federal Health Care Financing Administration (HCFA). The major insurers—Blue Cross, and the federal and state governments—guaranteed area hospitals a specified total revenue for five years. This community revenue ceiling was based on 1978 costs adjusted annually for inflation. State and federal regulators agreed to waive many regulations governing reimbursement for the same period, and the hospitals formed the Rochester Area Hospitals Corporation (RAHC), which agreed to share any savings below the revenue cap with the insurers. This Hospitals Experimental Payment (HEP) Program became effective in 1980. Although Rochester-area hospital costs had risen more slowly than the national average for the past few years because of tight state reimbursement regulations, RAHC members managed to improve their financial condition in 1981 while keeping cost increases at about half the national average. This suggests that HEP may have had some impact.

In areas of increasing competition for patients, preferred provider organizations (PPOs) are springing up. There are three in Denver and a number in California. A PPO is a physician association or a hospital that negotiates a lower schedule of fees with a self-insured employer or a union trust fund in exchange for referral of patients and quick payment of bills. Employees or members of the union may then use a doctor who is a member of the PPO and be fully covered for their health care expenses or use a physician or hospital that is not on the "preferred provider" list and pay a percentage of the bill. For hospitals and doctors operating in areas that have an excess of beds or providers, a PPO offers an expanded patient market. Mountain Medical Associates (MMA) in Denver has 320 member physicians providing health care to roughly twelve groups. The doctors contracting with MMA accept discounts of between 5 and 20 percent below the usual and customary rate. In return, they are reimbursed within ten working days. Under the PPO arrangement, claims and utilization of services are reviewed by physician panels. In 1981, the peer review committees for MMA reduced the cost of claims by roughly 30 percent for the employer and union funds it serves. While medical costs grew by 12 to 15 percent in the Denver area in 1981, payments by union trust funds participating in the program rose by only 5 percent.

Pratt & Whitney Aircraft developed the equivalent of a PPO at its West Palm Beach, Florida, location. In response to complaints from employees about high medical fees that were not fully covered by the company health insurance plan, Pratt & Whitney negotiated a reduced fee schedule with certain local physicians. Employees are given the fee schedule and are directed to participating physicians; if they go to other physicians, they pay any additional charges themselves. Started as a program to save money for employees, it saves money for Pratt & Whitney because employees use health care services in less costly ways and thereby stimulate competition among providers. PPOs prevent

157

reimbursement for inefficient services and thus reward more efficient providers.

Several attempts by labor unions to lower medical costs for their members are worth noting. The United Federation of Teachers Welfare Fund in New York contracts with retail pharmacies to pay the wholesale price plus a fixed service fee for prescription drugs. This example has been copied by other unions in New York and other cities and has been incorporated in national agreements covering auto and steel workers. The International Ladies Garment Workers Union offers a mail-order prescription service under its nationwide Health Services Plan. By having members send prescriptions to one of four large pharmacies where they are filled in a semi-automated manner, the union achieves economies of scale that reduce prices.

Conclusions

This survey reflects the variety of programs that have been established in response to the rise in health care costs. It does not mention all of the private sector initiatives in the health care field. In spite of all the voluntary activity, however, it is difficult to say whether these efforts will have the desired impact on costs.

Most of the initiatives lack incentives for consumers to change their use of health care and for providers to alter their fee schedules or practice patterns. Outside of Minneapolis–St. Paul, Hawaii, and perhaps California and Seattle, there are no significant competitive markets offering multiple choices to consumers in the private sector or in which contributions to the plan of choice are made on a fixed-dollar basis. Such markets are available only to employees of individual employers offering multiple plans. As a result of the Federal HMO Act, most major companies offer two choices in some locations. Many companies, however, have not found or cannot find qualified HMOs to offer their employees. The efforts of coalitions to promote HMOs and other alternative delivery systems have generally fallen short of what employers in the Twin Cities did years ago. Most coalitions are concentrating on more restricted ways of trying to contain costs. Some work to limit supply—serving on health systems agencies to improve area planning. Some seek to limit demand—developing data on local practice patterns to identify outliers or contracting with PSROs for utilization review. These activities are burgeoning and will have some impact at the margin, but they will not change the incentives for either the consumer or the provider. Interestingly, insurers like John Hancock, CIGNA, Prudential, and the Blues are doing more to change the marketplace by establishing new lines of business—developing their own alternative delivery systems.

The initiatives of individual companies are more intriguing than those of business coalitions, and some even provide those needed incentives. Employers like American Can, Educational Testing Service, TRW, and Sun are offering employees a choice of plans and are providing incentives to choose plans with more cost sharing. Others—Mobil and the Mendocino County Schools Office and its imitators—are encouraging employees to utilize their plans carefully by offering financial rewards. These experiments—if proven successful, as some have been—may spread and eventually cause some change in the system.

Although private sector initiatives are important and worth studying, changes in government policies may be needed to alter the health care system and reduce the escalating costs that are a by-product of that system. Unless accompanied by changes in federal and state tax and regulatory reimbursement policies, private efforts to reduce costs might be futile.

Notes

1. Examples of procompetition proposals include the Health Incentives Reform Act, S. 433, introduced by Senator David Durenberger (Republican, Minnesota); the National Health Care Reform Act, H.R. 850, introduced by Congressman Richard A. Gephardt (Democrat, Missouri); and the Comprehensive Health Care Reform Act, S. 139, introduced by Senator Orrin G. Hatch (Republican, Utah).

2. Stephen C. Caulfield and Pamela L. Haynes, *Health Care Costs: Private Initiatives for Containment* (Washington, D.C.: Government Research Corporation, 1981), p. 88.

3. Congressional Budget Office, *The Effect of PSROs on Health Care Costs: Current Findings and Future Evaluations* (Washington, D.C., June 1979).

Part Three
Federal Policy Reform:
Fiscal and Administrative Issues

9

The Effect of Tax Policies on Expenditures for Private Health Insurance

Amy K. Taylor and Gail R. Wilensky

Current efforts aimed at controlling costs in the health care sector have focused on strategies for making consumers and providers more cost conscious in their use of health services. Many of these strategies have included provisions that limit or eliminate the tax exclusion of employer contributions to employee health insurance. Under current law, such contributions are excluded from employees' taxable income and from the earnings to which payroll taxes are applied. The reason for focusing on employment-related health insurance is that it constitutes the bulk of private health insurance. Recent estimates indicate, for example, that almost 85 percent of private health insurance is employment related.[1]

Two concerns have been raised about the treatment of employer contributions for employee insurance. The first concern, and the one that has received the most attention lately, is that it has resulted in large revenue losses to federal and state governments. These revenue losses have been mostly to the U.S. Treasury in terms of forgone federal income tax revenues and liabilities. To a lesser extent, they represent losses to state and local governments as a result of lower state and local income tax revenues. Second and more important, the exclusion effectively reduces the price of insurance to consumers and thereby provides an incentive for employees to purchase more insurance than they would if they were using taxable income. The resulting increased level of insur-

The authors are grateful to Allen Kendal, of Social and Scientific Systems, Inc., and Amy Bernstein for programming assistance, to Pamela Farley for assistance in the analysis, and to John Carrick and Barbara Bottazzi for typing the manuscript. The views expressed in this paper are those of the authors, and no official endorsement by the National Center for Health Services Research is intended or should be inferred.

ance is thought to exacerbate the rate of inflation occurring in the health care sector.

Much of the work to date on this subject has been concerned either with estimating the revenue losses associated with the current tax treatment or with describing at a theoretical level the effect of the tax subsidy on the demand for insurance. In the 1970s, federal income tax losses were estimated by Feldstein and Allison and by Steurle and Hoffman.[2] More recently, Wilensky and Taylor and the Congressional Budget Office have estimated federal income tax and payroll tax (FICA) losses under existing law as well as selected limits on the exclusion.[3] These studies, however, ignore any behavioral changes that would result from changing the tax laws. Conceptual and/or theoretical discussions of the tax effects have been presented by Ginsburg and Vogel.[4] Theoretical effects of tax subsidies on coinsurance rates, given various assumptions about the price elasticity of the demand for health care, have been specified by Feldstein and Friedman and by Greenspan and Vogel.[5] What has been missing is an empirically based estimate of the effects of the tax laws on the amount of insurance purchased. Because much of the concern has been on the incentives current tax law provides for the purchase of excessive amounts of insurance, this has been a serious omission.

This chapter focuses on the changes in expenditures for health insurance that would result from specified changes in the tax treatment of employer-provided health insurance. Several legislative proposals have been introduced that place limits on the amounts of health insurance employers can provide on a tax-free basis. Examples include S. 433, introduced by Senator David Durenberger (Republican, Minnesota), and H.R. 850, introduced by Congressman Richard A. Gephardt (Democrat, Missouri). These bills typically include other provisions designed to increase cost-conscious behavior in the health insurance market, such as requiring a fixed contribution for all policies. The effects of requirements other than changing the tax subsidy are ignored here, although a recent study indicated that these changes would require a major restructuring of the health insurance industry.[6]

Predicted changes in expenditures on health insurance are shown in the aggregate and for subscribers at various income levels. Estimates of changes are based on the observed responsiveness to price changes and on variations around the observed estimate that we regard as plausible alternatives. These variations are presented in part to demonstrate the sensitivity of the results to the responsiveness assumed or observed and in part because we believe that the observed responsiveness represents a conservative estimate of the changes that would result if employer contributions were taxed. Basing estimates of change on behavior observed in the current environment is likely to be conservative because consumers do not now have much knowledge about their employment-related health insurance. We think that this is because they have little reason to be knowledgeable; only 18 percent of subscribers are offered options regarding their coverage and employers pay 100 percent of the premium for almost half of the subscribers. Even so, the tax subsidies are large and the tax effects on behavior are expected to be significant.

Data Sources

The data used in this analysis come from the 1977 National Medical Care Expenditure Survey (NMCES), which provided detailed national estimates of the use of health services, health expenditures, and health insurance coverage. The survey was undertaken to provide data for a major research effort in the National Center for Health Services Research and was cosponsored by the National Center for Health Statistics.[7]

The characteristics of the subscribers, including their income and tax filing status, were derived from the household survey, the primary source of data for the study. The household survey included 14,000 randomly selected households chosen to be representative of the civilian noninstitutionalized population. These households were interviewed six times over an eighteen-month period during 1977 and 1978. Information reported by households regarding tax status, filing relationships, and the use and amount of medical and other itemized deductions were edited so as to be consistent with tax laws in effect in 1977.

Data on employer contributions and the presence of employment-related insurance and type of coverage were derived from the employer and insurance carrier reports in the Health Insurance/Employer Survey.

NMCES data for 1977 have been updated to provide 1983 estimates using a variety of procedures and sources of information. Population data have been updated using U.S. Census Bureau projections; income has been updated using Data Resources, Inc. (DRI), long-term projections; insurance premiums and employer contributions have been updated using projections provided by the Actuarial Research Corporation. Major federal tax law changes that will be in effect for 1983 have been incorporated into the tax model used to calculate the subscribers' marginal tax rates.

Employment-Related Health Insurance

Employer contributions to health insurance premiums in 1983 are predicted to be about $77 billion, amounting to 77 percent of total employment-related group insurance premiums of $100.6 billion. These premiums cover 68 million subscribers, including about 6 million with zero employer contributions.[8]

TABLE 9-1

AVERAGE EMPLOYER CONTRIBUTIONS, EMPLOYEE CONTRIBUTIONS,
AND TOTAL PREMIUMS FOR GROUP SUBSCRIBERS,
BY FAMILY INCOME, 1983
(dollars)

Family Income	Total Number of Subscribers (thousands)	Average Contribution by Employer[a]	Average Contribution by Employee	Average Total Premium[b]
1 to 9,999	4,263	763	295	1,071
10,000 to 14,999	5,665	855	304	1,170
15,000 to 19,999	7,499	1,025	330	1,371
20,000 to 29,999	17,045	1,098	343	1,466
30,000 to 49,999	23,076	1,287	315	1,626
50,000 or more	10,979	1,188	288	1,443
Total[c]	68,627	1,126	317	1,466

a. Includes those with zero employer contributions.
b. Employer and employee contributions do not add to total because of "other" contributions.
c. Includes persons with income less than $1.00.
SOURCE: National Center for Health Services Research, National Medical Care Expenditure Survey, unpublished data.

Overall, the average employer contribution is expected to be $1,126 (see table 9-1). Although this contribution increased with subscriber family income, the highest income class being the exception, the relationship between employer contribution and family income is not very strong. The average total premium for subscribers with employment-related insurance is $1,466. Total premiums exhibit the same relationship to income as employer contributions. The distribution of employer contributions by family income is shown in appendix table 9-A, and the percentage of subscribers potentially affected by a change in tax laws is shown in appendix table 9-B.

The figures shown in table 9-1 represent projections for 1983 assuming that tax laws and other incentives regarding the purchase of health insurance remain unchanged. In the next section, we specify an econometric model of the determinants of employment-related health insurance premiums and use this to estimate subscriber behavior with respect to tax rates and income. This will enable us to predict changes in expenditures for health insurance that would result from specified changes in the tax laws.

Model Specification and Data Description

As explained earlier, the current income tax system makes the "price" of health insurance less than the price of other goods and services. Because employer contributions to health insurance premiums are excluded from employees' taxable income, an individual with a marginal tax rate of 40 percent who receives $100 in wages actually has only $60 remaining after taxes for the purchase of insurance or other personal consumption. If the employee is given $100 in the form of tax-free benefits, however, as is the case for employer-provided health insurance, he or she gets a full $100 worth of health insurance. Thus, the opportunity cost of one dollar of employer-provided health insurance is only sixty cents. More generally, for an individual whose marginal tax rate is mtr, the price of one dollar of employer-provided health insurance is $P = 1 - mtr$.

The specification of the behavioral equation relating health insurance premiums ($PREM$) to income (INC) and price (P) is the constant elasticity relation:

$$\log PREM_i = b_0 + b_1 \log P_i + b_2 \log INC_i + b_3 SEX_i + \sum_{j=1}^{9} a_j IND_{ij}$$
$$+ \sum_{k=1}^{3} c_k REG_{ik} + b_4 \log GRPSIZ_i + b_5 HSTAT_i$$
$$+ b_6 ICFFAM + b_7 \log AGE \qquad (1)$$

where

SEX	= dummy variable indicating that the subscriber is female
IND	= dummy variable for the industry in which the subscriber works
REG	= dummy variable for the region of the country
$GRPSIZ$	= size of the firm in which the subscribed is employed
$HSTAT$	= dummy variable indicating good or excellent health
$ICFFAM$	= dummy variable indicating family insurance policy
AGE	= age of the subscriber

In this equation, the measure of the dependent variable, expenditures on health insurance, should be interpreted as reflecting the level of health insurance benefits rather than the cost or loading charges of insurance. The definition of income used in the regressions is adjusted gross income minus total taxes paid, which approximates the disposable income of the appropriate family unit. Marginal tax rate is calculated for each tax filing unit by adding one dollar to taxable income and measuring the increase in taxes that would have to be paid. Thus, this measure

167

is independent from the amount of health insurance benefits actually received.

Regression Estimates

The estimate of the basic equation relating total insurance to income and price, for all individuals in the sample with employment-related group insurance, is given in table 9–2. The price elasticity is —0.21 and the income elasticity is 0.02. These results proved to be very stable across different specifications and data subsets used. In spite of the potential problem of collinearity between price and income, the standard errors on these coefficients are very small. The coefficient of the variable for sex of subscriber (—0.10) indicates that expenditures on health insurance are 10 percent less for women than for men, which probably reflects the tendency of women to be in occupations with lower wages and benefit structures. The industry variables are not statistically significant, although region of the country appears to be an important determinant of premiums. Compared with those in the Northeast, health insurance premiums were significantly higher in the North Central region (11 percent) and the West (7 percent), whereas they were almost 9 percent lower in the South. As expected, premiums for family plans were nearly twice as expensive as individual insurance policies. The effect of age on expenditures for health insurance also shows the expected sign, with premiums rising slightly as age increases. On the other hand, health status does not have a significant independent effect on total premiums, holding age and other variables constant. Group size also is not statistically significant, reflecting the fact that increasing size is related both to increased benefits of larger groups and decreased loading charges, which might tend to cancel each other out. When employer contributions are held constant, the coefficient of the group size variable is negative.

The basic equation was also estimated including separate price variables for various income groups. The results indicate that price elasticity does not appear to differ significantly across income classes.

Simulation Results

This section uses the parameter estimates from the basic equation relating health insurance premiums to tax rates and income to calculate the effects of changes in the income tax treatment of employer-provided health insurance. The simulations show, for various ceilings on tax-free employer contributions, changes in average total premiums and average employee contributions by income class, as well as changes in aggregate health insurance premiums for 1983. We also present estimates of the

TABLE 9–2

ESTIMATES OF THE EFFECTS OF TAX RATES AND INCOME ON
EXPENDITURES FOR HEALTH INSURANCE
(dependent variable: log of health insurance premiums)

Independent[a] Variables	b_1 Coefficient	t-value[b]
Constant	5.40	39.15
1 − marginal tax rate (= P)	−0.21	3.35
Income	0.02	2.67
Sex[c]	−0.10	3.33
Industry[d]		
Mining	0.13	1.52
Construction	−0.01	0.30
Transportation and utilities	0.06	1.61
Wholesale and retail trade	−0.07	1.83
Finance	−0.07	1.40
Services and miscellaneous	−0.03	1.12
Public administration	0.07	1.31
Military	−0.16	0.26
Unknown	−0.06	2.10
Region[e]		
North Central	0.11	3.37
South	−0.09	2.59
West	0.07	1.98
Group size	0.003	0.47
Health status[f]	0.002	0.17
Family policy	0.90	28.61
Age	0.05	2.02

a. All variables except the dummy variables are in logarithms.
b. Adjusted for sample design.
c. Omitted variable is male.
d. Omitted variable is manufacturing.
e. Omitted variable is Northeast.
f. Omitted variable is fair or poor health.
SOURCE: National Center for Health Services Research, National Medical Care Expenditure Survey, 1977.

number of subscribers affected, average increased tax liability by type of tax, and total increases in tax revenues.

For the purpose of comparison, four hypothetical plans with different ceilings on tax-free employer contributions to health insurance premiums are analyzed. In the first plan, all employer contributions to health plans would be fully taxable. Plan II would place a tax-free ceiling of $1,125 per year on family plans and $450 per year on individual plans. Under Plan III, tax-free employer contributions would be limited to $1,800 for family coverage and $720 for individual coverage. The limitations for Plan IV would be $2,400 and $975. The dollar limits in these plans all refer to projected estimates for 1983.

Any change in the tax treatment of employer-provided health insurance will affect the price of health insurance to a subscriber. Let P_i be the current price faced by individual i, and P_i' the price after a proposed change in the tax law. Similarly, let $PREM_i$ be the current health insurance premium of that individual, and $PREM_i'$ the premium after the change in tax law. We assume that employer contributions after the changes in the law will be no greater than the tax-free ceiling and that compensation received previously in the form of tax-free benefits will go to employees as additional wages.[9] This means that income (INC_i), as well as price, will be affected by the tax law change. The change in net income included in the simulation equation is measured by any additional monetary compensation minus the new taxes that would be required. The following formula, based on equation (1), is used to calculate the predicted change in subscribers' premiums:

$$\log PREM_i' - \log PREM_i = -0.21(\log P_i' - \log P_i)$$
$$+ 0.02(\log INC_i' - \log INC_i)$$
$$(2)$$

Results are also derived based on two alternative values of the price elasticity. This is done to test the sensitivity of the results to various parameter estimates. At the lower end, we have used a price elasticity of zero, which corresponds to no behavioral response in reaction to changes in the tax laws. Results based on an elasticity of -0.5 will also be included and can be interpreted as a measure of a long-run response. Because employees currently have so little choice among health insurance plans, the initial estimate of -0.21 should be viewed as a short-run elasticity, much smaller than the response that might occur over a long period, when employees would be better able to adjust to new conditions. The initial value of -0.2 compared with a long-run elasticity of -0.5 indicates that 40 percent of the long-run response would occur in the short run. If, in fact, movement toward the long run does not occur so

TABLE 9–3

CHANGES IN TOTAL HEALTH INSURANCE PREMIUMS FOR SPECIFIC
LIMITATIONS ON TAX-FREE EMPLOYER CONTRIBUTIONS, 1983
(billions of dollars)

Tax Status of Insurance Premiums	No Behavioral Response $b_1 = 0.0$	Change When $b_1 = -0.2$	Change When $b_1 = -0.5$
I. No exemptions	100.6	−7.5	−16.7
II. $1,125 for family, $450 for individual policies exemption	100.6	−6.0	−13.3
III. $1,800 for family, $720 for individual policies exemption	100.6	−3.6	7.3
IV. $2,400 for family, $975 for individual policies exemption	100.6	−1.8	−3.6

SOURCE: National Center for Health Services Research, National Medical Care Expenditure Survey, unpublished data.

quickly, 0.5 is probably an underestimate of the value of the true long-run response parameter.

Table 9–3 shows the changes in total expenditures for health insurance in 1983 that would result from various limitations on tax-free employer contributions. For the price elasticity value of −0.2, estimates of the decrease in total premiums range from $7.5 billion to $1.8 billion, from a base of $100 billion in premiums that would occur in 1983 if the tax law is not changed. Using an elasticity of −0.5 indicates a larger response to changes in the price of insurance, and the resulting predicted decrease in total premiums ranges from $16.7 billion to $3.6 billion.

Changes in average total premiums and employee contributions by income class are shown in table 9–4. The pattern of changes in total premiums is stable across all plans and elasticities. Average premiums decrease monotonically as income increases. The change is almost four times greater for those with incomes above $50,000 than for those with incomes below $10,000. The reason is that, with a progressive income tax structure, marginal tax rates go up as income increases. For those with employer contributions above the tax-free limit, the price of one dollar of health insurance increases from 1 − mtr to 1. This means that the change in price is much greater for those with high marginal

171

TABLE 9-4

CHANGES IN AVERAGE TOTAL HEALTH INSURANCE PREMIUMS AND AVERAGE EMPLOYEE CONTRIBUTIONS FOR SPECIFIC LIMITATIONS ON TAX-FREE EMPLOYER CONTRIBUTIONS, BY INCOME CLASS, 1983
(dollars)

Family Income (dollars)	Average Premiums			Average Employee Contributions		
	No behavioral response $b_1 = 0.0$	Change when $b_1 = -0.2$	Change when $b_1 = -0.5$	No behavioral response $b_1 = 0.0$	Change when $b_1 = -0.2$	Change when $b_1 = -0.5$
I. No Exemptions						
1 to 9,999	1,071	−44	−100	971	+929	+874
10,000 to 14,999	1,170	−65	−149	1,001	+937	+853
15,000 to 19,999	1,371	−84	−192	1,161	+1,078	+970
20,000 to 29,999	1,437	−109	−246	1,223	+1,115	+977
30,000 to 49,999	1,495	−149	−332	1,415	+1,268	+1,084
50,000 or more	1,599	−171	−377	1,335	+1,164	+958
Total	1,466	−123	−275	1,269	+1,147	+995
II. $1,125 for Family, $450 for Individual Policies Exemption						
1 to 9,999	1,071	−52	−118	576	+525	+459
10,000 to 14,999	1,170	−74	−168	564	+490	+396
15,000 to 19,999	1,371	−98	−221	628	+531	+407

20,000 to 29,999	1,437	−128	−286	665	+538	+380
30,000 to 49,999	1,495	−169	−374	801	+632	+428
50,000 or more	1,599	−230	−438	636	+407	+198
Total	1,466	−144	−317	710	+567	+394

III. $1,800 for Family, $720 for Individual Policies Exemption

1 to 9,999	1,071	−61	−135	502	+442	+368
10,000 to 14,999	1,170	−89	−189	558	+470	+370
15,000 to 19,999	1,371	−112	−233	506	+394	+273
20,000 to 29,999	1,437	−149	−310	547	+399	+237
30,000 to 49,999	1,495	−198	−402	668	+470	+266
50,000 or more	1,599	−230	−438	636	+407	+198
Total	1,466	−170	−344	604	+434	+260

IV. $2,400 for Family, $975 for Individual Policies Exemption

1 to 9,999	1,071	−76	−162	556	+480	+394
10,000 to 14,999	1,170	−101	−214	687	+588	+415
15,000 to 19,999	1,371	−122	−250	548	+426	+299
20,000 to 29,999	1,437	−166	−333	497	+332	+164
30,000 to 49,999	1,495	−217	−424	629	+413	+206
50,000 or more	1,599	−265	−505	730	+466	+226
Total	1,466	−190	−375	607	+418	+234

SOURCE: National Center for Health Services Research, National Medical Care Expenditure Survey, unpublished data.

TABLE 9-5

NUMBER OF SUBSCRIBERS AFFECTED AND THE AVERAGE INCREASED
TAX LIABILITY FOR SPECIFIC LIMITATIONS ON TAX-FREE
EMPLOYER CONTRIBUTIONS, 1983

Tax Status of Insurance Premiums	Number of Subscribers Affected (thousands)	Average Tax Increases (dollars)			
		Federal income taxes[a]	FICA[a,b]	State income taxes[a]	All taxes[a,b]
I. No exemptions	61,575	332	105	62	499
II. $1,125 for family, $450 for individual policies exemption	44,431	180	56	34	270
III. $1,800 for family, $720 for individual policies exemption	23,497	147	45	28	220
IV. $2,400 for family, $975 for individual policies exemption	10,786	145	43	28	216

a. Excludes subscribers not affected by any tax changes.
b. Includes employers' share of FICA.
SOURCE: National Center for Health Services Research, National Medical Care Expenditure Survey, unpublished data.

tax rates than for others. For example, for an individual whose marginal tax rate is 0.6, the price of insurance would increase 2.5 times, from 0.4 to 1.0 under the proposed law. For someone with a tax rate of 0.2, however, it would only change by 25 percent, from 0.8 to 1.0.

The effects derived for different elasticities also show the expected variations. The decrease in average premiums is greater for an elasticity of −0.5 than for an elasticity of −0.2, reflecting the greater responsiveness associated with the higher value of the parameter. The changes in average employee contributions to health insurance also reflect these patterns. Expenditures on health insurance by employees increased less for higher elasticities, since the decrease in total premiums was greater in these cases.[10]

The various exclusion limits show that the change in average premiums increases as the tax-free limit increases. Although this may seem counterintuitive at first, it must be remembered that when all or most employer contributions are subject to tax, many small changes in premiums may be included in calculating the average change. At

TABLE 9–6

NUMBER OF SUBSCRIBERS AFFECTED AND TOTAL INCREASE IN
TOTAL TAX LIABILITY FOR SPECIFIC LIMITATIONS ON TAX-FREE
EMPLOYER CONTRIBUTIONS, 1983

		Total Revenue Increases (millions of dollars)			
Tax Status of Insurance Premiums	Number of Subscribers Affected (thousands)	Federal income taxes	FICA[a]	State income taxes	All taxes[a]
I. No exemptions	61,575	20,443	6,465	3,818	30,726
II. $1,125 for family, $450 for individual policies exemption	44,431	7,998	2,488	1,511	11,996
III. $1,800 for family, $720 for individual policies exemption	23,497	3,454	1,057	658	5,169
IV. $2,400 for family, $975 for individual policies exemption	10,786	1,564	464	302	2,330

a. Includes employers' share of FICA.
SOURCE: National Center for Health Services Research, National Medical Care Expenditure Survey, unpublished data.

higher limits, a smaller number of subscribers are affected, but for each of them the change is larger on average.

Revenue Effects

The revenue effects of imposing these limits on tax-free employer contributions to health benefit plans are shown in tables 9–5, 9–6, and 9–7. These effects are invariant to price elasticity when all additional compensation is given in the form of taxable income.[11] This is because the tax would apply to either additional money wages or the amount of employer-provided health benefits over the limit. The number of subscribers affected and average tax increases are given in table 9–5, whereas table 9–6 shows the total tax revenues that would be raised by each of these plans.

As expected, Plan I, which would treat all employer contributions for health insurance premiums as taxable income, results in the largest

175

TABLE 9–7

NUMBER OF SUBSCRIBERS AFFECTED AND THE AVERAGE INCREASED TAX LIABILITY FOR SPECIFIC LIMITATIONS ON TAX-FREE EMPLOYER CONTRIBUTIONS, BY INCOME CLASS, 1983

Family Income (dollars)	Total Number of Subscribers (thousands)	Number of Subscribers Affected (thousands)	Percentage of Subscribers Affected	Average Increase in Federal Income Tax[a] (dollars)	Average Increase in Total Tax[a,b] (dollars)	Increased Total Tax as a Proportion of Family Income[a,b]
I. No Exemptions						
1 to 9,999	4,263	3,145	74	105	174	0.0317
10,000 to 14,999	5,665	4,788	85	161	242	0.0190
15,000 to 19,999	7,499	6,650	89	213	317	0.0180
20,000 to 29,999	17,045	15,547	91	277	394	0.0157
30,000 to 49,999	23,076	21,384	93	420	552	0.0146
50,000 or more	10,979	9,984	91	464	576	0.0085
Total[c]	68,627	61,575	90	332	467	0.0153
II. $1,125 for Family, $450 for Individual Policies Exemption						
1 to 9,999	4,263	1,907	45	62	102	0.0182
10,000 to 14,999	5,665	2,988	53	87	130	0.0103
15,000 to 19,999	7,499	4,647	62	113	168	0.0095
20,000 to 29,999	17,045	10,818	63	143	204	0.0081

30,000 to 49,999	23,076		71	225	296	0.0078
50,000 or more	10,979		70	241	301	0.0044
Total[c]	68,627		65	280	242	0.0080

III. $1,800 for Family, $720 for Individual Policies Exemption

1 to 9,999	4,263	938	22	54	86	0.0139
10,000 to 14,999	5,665	1,365	24	79	118	0.0096
15,000 to 19,999	7,499	2,306	31	91	135	0.0077
20,000 to 29,999	17,045	5,273	31	113	163	0.0064
30,000 to 49,999	23,076	9,335	40	180	235	0.0061
50,000 or more	10,979	4,261	38	194	245	0.0038
Total[c]	68,627	23,497	34	148	198	0.0063

IV. $2,400 for Family, $975 for Individual Policies Exemption

1 to 9,999	4,263	388	9	62	96	0.0166
10,000 to 14,999	5,665	632	11	88	137	0.0113
15,000 to 19,999	7,499	967	13	97	143	0.0060
20,000 to 29,999	17,045	2,301	13	105	152	0.0060
30,000 to 49,999	23,076	4,650	20	164	214	0.0055
50,000 or more	10,979	1,829	17	212	269	0.0038
Total[c]	68,627	10,786	16	145	195	0.0063

a. Excludes subscribers not affected by any tax change.
b. Excludes employers' share of FICA.
c. Includes persons with income less than $1.00.

SOURCE: National Center for Health Services Research, National Medical Care Expenditure Survey, unpublished data.

increase in taxes (by an average of $499 per subscriber) and would affect over 61 million people, or 90 percent of all subscribers with employment-related health insurance. In fact, only those with zero employer contributions or no taxable income would be unaffected. For each subscriber affected by any tax increase, federal income taxes would be raised by $322 on average, payroll taxes (both employer and employee shares) by $105, and state taxes by $62. If there were a limit of $1,125 on tax-free employer contributions for family coverage, the number of affected subscribers would be reduced to 44 million, or 65 percent of all those with employment-related health insurance. The average total tax increase per affected subscriber would be much smaller than under Plan I—only $270. Under Plans III and IV (with family limits of $1,800 and $2,400, respectively), these amounts would be reduced still further. Although the average tax increases for these two plans are quite similar, more than twice as many subscribers would be affected by Plan III as by Plan IV. The implications of these average figures for aggregate revenue increases are shown in table 9–6.

The total tax increases projected for 1983 under the proposed changes in the tax treatment of employer-provided health insurance range from $2.3 billion to $30.7 billion. Of this, roughly two-thirds is attributable to increases in federal income taxes, with the remainder almost equally divided between employee and employer contributions to payroll and state income taxes. Again, Plans III and IV, with relatively high limits on tax-free benefits, on average will affect substantial numbers of subscribers but will not produce large aggregate tax increases. For example, an $1,800 limit in 1983 would affect 23 million people but would raise only $5.2 billion in tax revenues. In contrast, taxing employer contributions to health insurance in full would affect more than twice as many subscribers, but would raise more than five times as much in tax revenues, or $30.7 billion. An intermediate limit, such as $1,125 for family coverage, would affect 44 million people but would raise less than half the taxes of Plan I ($12 billion).

Table 9–7 shows for each plan the number of subscribers affected, the average increase in federal income tax, the average increase in total tax, and the tax increase as a proportion of income by family income class. In each case, the percentage of subscribers affected is lowest for the under $10,000 class. There are two reasons for this: a higher percentage in this category report zero employer contributions, which means that they would be unaffected by these limitations, and a higher percentage have no tax liability as a result of their low incomes. The peaks at the $30,000 to $50,000 level are because this group is most often found in the high-employer-contribution categories (see appendix table 9–A).

Although the average increase in federal income tax liability for those affected varies substantially (from $332 in Plan I to $145 in Plan IV), the variation across income groups is even greater. In Plans I to III, the average federal income tax increase for the highest income group is about four times as large as the increase for the lowest group; in Plan IV, it is about three times as large.

Because the payroll tax is regressive and state income taxes tend to be proportional or only slightly progressive, the average increase in total tax shows less variation. In Plans I to III, the increase for the highest income group is about three times that of the lowest group, and in the case of Plan IV, it is about 2.5 times. This rise in the total tax, although substantial, is less than the increase in income itself, as is seen when the increase in tax is shown as a proportion of family income. As noted above, the percentage of subscribers affected in the lowest income class is much less than for other income groups. For those affected, however, the increase would represent a large proportion of their income.

Conclusion

Concern about the current tax treatment of employer contributions to employee health insurance has been twofold. First, it results in large losses of tax revenues. Second, it provides incentives for employees to purchase more health insurance than they would if they were using after-tax dollars, thereby exacerbating the rate of inflation in the health care sector.

With no change in the tax laws, employers' contributions to health insurance are predicted to increase from $34 billion in 1977 to $77 billion in 1983. The total amount of forgone tax revenues associated with the exclusion of employer-provided health benefits from employee taxable income is predicted to be $30.7 billion by 1983. Of this, roughly two-thirds represents federal income tax losses. The remainder is almost equally divided between employee and employer contributions to payroll and state income taxes. Under the present system, all subscribers whose employers contribute to their health insurance receive some saving. The average federal income tax saving for those with any type of saving is projected to be $332, varying from an average of $105 for those with incomes under $10,000 to $464 for those with incomes over $50,000. For all types of taxes, the average saving is projected to be $467 (ranging from $174 to $576).

We considered four different limitations on tax benefits. They varied from taxing all employer contributions to taxing employer contributions greater than $2,400 for family coverage or $975 for individual coverage. The number of subscribers affected varied from 90 percent (or all sub-

179

scribers with any employer contribution) to 16 percent. The total tax increases range from $30.7 billion to $2.3 billion.

The amount of revenue that would be raised by limiting tax-free employer contributions does not depend on the response of subscribers to tax law changes, given two assumptions: first, employers would continue to provide the same total compensation to their employees as they did before a tax change; second, employees are not given an option to take previously tax-free employer contributions as another type of tax-free fringe benefit or as a tax-free rebate (as is provided in some legislation). Given these assumptions, the revenue generated is not sensitive to changes in employer contributions because the tax would apply either to additional money wages or to the amount of employer-provided benefits over the limit.

The more important concern about the current tax treatment has not been the revenue loss but the incentives it provides for the purchase of an excessive amount of insurance. Given this concern, we estimated the relationship between subscriber's income, the "price" of insurance that results from the current tax treatment, and the amount spent on health insurance premiums. The findings were used to simulate changes in average total premiums, average employee contributions by income class, and aggregate health insurance premiums for 1983 that would result from various ceilings on tax-free employer contributions.

Using the estimated responsiveness to price that we interpret as the short-run change (that is, a price elasticity of -0.2), we predict a decline in total premiums ranging from $7.5 billion to $1.8 billion, relative to a base of $100 billion. Using a higher level of responsiveness that we believe is closer to the long-run response (a price elasticity of -0.5), we predict that total premiums will decline between $16.7 billion and $3.6 billion, depending on the limit chosen. As was the case for the potential tax increases, the changes in premiums were even greater across income groups than across plans, with the decline being almost four times greater for those with incomes above $50,000 than for those with incomes below $10,000. This happens because the effective price change is much greater for those with higher incomes—and therefore higher marginal tax rates—than it is for lower-income subscribers.

The different limitations clearly have different effects on the amount of revenue that would be produced and the number of subscribers affected. If the purpose of the tax law change is to raise revenue—and the amounts potentially at risk are substantial—all or most employers' contributions should be taxed. If the purpose is to reduce the amount of insurance purchased in an absolute sense, the reductions will be much greater if all or most employer contributions are taxed. However, if the purpose is to keep subscribers from purchasing additional insurance, a

180

APPENDIX TABLE 9-A
EMPLOYER INSURANCE CONTRIBUTIONS FOR FAMILY AND INDIVIDUAL GROUP INSURANCE COVERAGE, BY FAMILY INCOME, 1983 (percent)

Family Income (dollars)	Total Subscribers (thousands)	Employer Insurance Contributions						
		$0	$1– 399	$400– 799	$800– 1,199	$1,200– 1,799	$1,800– 2,399	$2,400 or more
Family Coverage								
1 to 9,999	1,672	12.4	8.7	20.0	9.3	24.2	13.4	12.1
10,000 to 14,999	2,743	9.1	11.6	18.3	15.7	26.7	12.1	6.5
15,000 to 19,999	4,650	11.6	8.2	16.7	10.1	26.5	18.3	8.7
20,000 to 29,999	11,802	9.5	6.8	15.3	13.1	28.6	15.9	10.9
30,000 to 49,999	16,708	7.9	5.5	11.3	12.3	26.7	20.2	16.3
50,000 or more	7,246	8.5	7.8	9.9	10.9	28.6	21.4	13.0
Total[a]	44,854	9.1	7.0	13.4	12.1	27.4	18.3	12.8
Individual Coverage								
1 to 9,999	2,591	27.5	22.5	32.9	11.7	3.0	2.1	0.5
10,000 to 14,999	2,922	20.0	19.1	39.3	13.9	4.2	1.8	1.6
15,000 to 19,999	2,849	12.1	14.1	47.2	16.6	6.2	2.4	1.4
20,000 to 29,999	5,242	11.9	22.5	39.5	17.4	6.7	1.5	0.6
30,000 to 49,999	6,368	12.2	16.8	42.5	16.8	8.0	2.2	1.6
50,000 or more	3,734	15.9	17.9	39.7	15.3	6.2	2.5	2.6
Total[a]	23,773	15.3	18.8	40.5	15.7	6.2	2.1	1.4

a. Includes persons with income less than $1.00.
SOURCE: National Center for Health Services Research, National Medical Care Expenditure Survey, unpublished data.

higher cap, such as $1,800 for family coverage, which affects a substantial number of subscribers at the margin without large increases in their tax burden would be appropriate.

We hypothesize that the long-run response to a change in the tax treatment is likely to be greater than the short-run response. This would occur for several reasons. One of the most important is that in order to respond to new incentives, subscribers must have choices with respect to their health insurance coverage. A recent study indicated, however, that fewer than 20 percent of subscribers with employment-related health insurance had more than one option. Legislation that mandates options in addition to limiting tax-free exclusion would facilitate this adjustment.

APPENDIX TABLE 9–B
PERCENTAGE OF SUBSCRIBERS AFFECTED BY SUBSCRIBER CHARACTERISTICS FOR SPECIFIC LIMITATIONS ON TAX-FREE EMPLOYER CONTRIBUTIONS, 1983

Personal Characteristics	Total Number of Subscribers (thousands)	Plan I	Plan II	Plan III	Plan IV
Total	68,627	90	65	34	16
Sex					
Male	43,348	89	66	36	17
Female	25,279	90	63	31	14
Age (years)					
15–24	10,219	88	59	30	15
25–34	20,245	92	68	36	15
35–44	13,629	91	65	33	15
45–54	11,850	91	69	41	19
55–64	8,767	89	67	35	17
65 and over	3,689	74	41	15	6
Race					
White	54,054	90	65	34	15
Black	6,588	91	63	31	15
Hispanic	2,434	91	72	46	25
Other	5,551	88	64	32	16
Poverty indicator					
Poor/near poor	3,005	73	43	21	6
Other low income	6,910	85	52	26	11

APPENDIX TABLE 9–B (continued)

Personal Characteristics	Total Number of Subscribers (thousands)	Plan I	Plan II	Plan III	Plan IV
Middle income	28,215	90	63	32	14
High income	30,404	92	71	39	19
Industry					
Agriculture, forestry, fishing	906	67	47	30	12
Mining	862	97	87	47	30
Construction	2,560	88	64	36	18
Manufacturing	14,019	94	71	43	21
Transportation, commerce, utilities	5,128	93	73	48	18
Sales	8,742	89	59	30	14
Finance, insurance	3,518	91	58	27	15
Repair services	2,854	89	62	31	13
Personal services	706	82	53	21	7
Entertainment/recreation	465	89	56	26	18
Professional services	7,785	91	63	30	12
Public administration	1,986	92	63	31	13
Military	158	91	58	16	16
Region					
Northeast	14,794	90	69	36	16
North Central	20,863	91	72	43	21
South	20,343	90	53	22	9
West	12,630	87	66	37	18

SOURCE: National Center for Health Services Research, National Medical Care Expenditure Survey, unpublished data.

Notes

1. Pamela Farley and Gail R. Wilensky, "Options, Incentives, and Employment Related Health Insurance Coverage," in *Advances in Health Economics and Health Services Research*, vol. 4 (Greenwich, Conn.: JAI Press, forthcoming).

2. Martin S. Feldstein and Elizabeth Allison, "Tax Subsidies of Private Health Insurance: Distribution, Revenue Loss, and Effects," *The Economics of Federal Subsidy Programs*, pt. 8, A Compendium of Papers Submitted to the Subcommittee on Priorities and Economy in Government of the Joint Economic Committee, 93rd Congress, 2nd session, (July 1974, pp. 977–94; and Eugene Steurle and Ronald Hoffman, "Tax Expenditures for Health Care," *National Tax Journal*, vol. 32 (June 1979), pp. 101–14.

3. Gail R. Wilensky and Amy K. Taylor, "Tax Expenditures and Health Insurance: Limiting Employer Paid Premiums," *Public Health Reports*, September/October 1982; and Congressional Budget Office, *Containing Medical Costs through Market Forces* (Washington, D.C., May 1982).

4. Paul B. Ginsburg, "Federal Taxes and Health Care Costs: Present Treatment and Policy Alternatives" (presented at National Tax Association—Tax Institute of America, 73rd Annual Conference on Taxation, New Orleans, Louisiana, 1980, mimeograph); and Ronald Vogel, "The Tax Treatment of Health Insurance Premiums as a Cause of Overinsurance," in Mark V. Pauly, ed., *National Health Insurance: What Now, What Later, What Never?* (Washington, D.C.: American Enterprise Institute, 1980).

5. Martin S. Feldstein and Bernard Friedman, "Tax Subsidies: The Rational Demand for Insurance and the Health Care Crisis," *Journal of Public Economics*, vol. 7 (April 1977), pp. 155–78; and Nancy Greenspan and Ronald Vogel, "Taxation and Its Effect upon Public and Private Health Insurance and Medical Demand," *Health Care Financing Review*, vol. 1 (Spring 1980), pp. 39–45.

6. Farley and Wilensky, "Options, Incentives."

7. For further descriptions see: Steven B. Cohen and William Kalsbeek, "NMCES Estimation and Sampling Variances in the Household Survey," in *Instruments and Procedures*, vol. 2 (Hyattsville, Maryland: National Center for Health Services Research, 1981); and Gordon Bonham and Larry Corder, "National Medical Care Expenditure Survey: Household Interview Instruments," in *Instruments and Procedures*, vol. 1.

8. Based on projections from 1977 data.

9. The employer's share of payroll taxes will be ignored in this part.

10. It is difficult to interpret the implications of the change in employee contributions without considering the change in monetary compensation that also took place.

11. If the law included a provision for tax-free rebates, this would not hold. This case will not be considered here.

10

Tax-Related Issues in Health Care Market Reform

Sean Sullivan and Rosemary Gibson

A major thrust of the procompetition health legislation is to alter existing tax policy, which is a significant force behind spending on health care. Total tax expenditures related to health care amounted to $25.1 billion in 1981 and are expected to reach $28.1 billion in 1983.[1] They constitute approximately one-third of the federal government's direct expenditures for health and are larger than all federal health programs except Medicare.

The largest tax expenditure results from the exclusion of employer contributions to employee health insurance plans from taxable employee income. In addition, employers deduct their payments for insurance premiums as business expenses. Total revenue losses from the employer exclusion are estimated at $19 billion in 1981 and $20.6 billion in 1982.

Many of the proposed health care bills incorporate incentives to economize on health spending by imposing various limits on this tax subsidy. Estimating the effect of the exclusion on the demand for health insurance is difficult, but the available evidence suggests that it has been substantial. The exclusion allows employees to receive employer-paid health benefits for significantly less cost than if the income in the form of employer contributions were taxed. For example, an employee receives a full dollar in income for each dollar of employer contribution for health insurance, but would receive only sixty-five cents if the payment were taxed and the employee were in a 35 percent marginal tax bracket. The effect of the tax subsidy, therefore, is to lower the cost of health insurance, which encourages the purchase of more insurance.

As coverage expands, evidence shows that consumers demand more medical services. As some health analysts have argued, providers respond to the growth in demand by increasing charges and by providing a higher level of services. The greater intensity of services enhances patient expectations, augmenting demand that fuels the rise in health care costs.

The second largest tax expenditure for health care is the medical expense deduction, which consists of two parts. Under current law, those who itemize their deductions can subtract from taxable income one-half of the cost of insurance premiums, up to $150. The second part of the deduction allows taxpayers to deduct all remaining out-of-pocket medical expenses that, in total, exceed 5 percent of adjusted gross income. The total revenue loss from the medical expense deduction is estimated at $3.6 billion in 1981 and $3.9 billion in 1982 (when the threshold was 3 percent of adjusted gross income).

The medical expense deduction has also been addressed in some of the procompetition health care legislation, although to a lesser extent than the employer exclusion. Unlike the employer exclusion, the medical expense deduction offsets part of the cost of uninsured medical services, which was intended in the original legislation establishing it. In cases in which the deduction subsidizes expenditures for elective rather than necessary procedures, however, it encourages the consumption of medical care. As with the employer exclusion, those taking the deduction have less incentive to choose cost-conscious medical providers, since each dollar of the deduction is subsidized—although only to the extent of the individual's marginal tax bracket.

The deduction for health insurance premiums offers a limited subsidy to all taxpayers who pay for all or part of their insurance premiums. The subsidy is especially useful to those who are self-employed or whose employers do not provide health insurance benefits, so that they cannot benefit from the tax subsidy provided by the employer exclusion. Like the employer exclusion, the deduction for premiums offers incentives to taxpayers to purchase more extensive coverage which, in turn, encourages the use of medical services.

Part of the impetus behind these subsidies stems from what is perceived to be the special nature or "merit good" aspect of medical care. The medical expense deduction, for example, was included in the tax code to provide relief from extraordinary medical expenditures at a time when the newly expanded income tax created an additional burden on the new tax-paying population. By their very nature, however, the subsidies distort health care expenditures by increasing the demand for care.

The legislative proposals suggest alternative means of limiting the tax subsidy for medical care, thereby changing the incentives for consumers when they purchase insurance and medical services. With consumers making more cost-conscious decisions regarding their purchase of insurance, procompetition advocates anticipate that insurers will offer more varied and innovative health benefit plans. In turn, insurers would have the incentive to bear down on providers to be more efficient so that they could offer more attractive benefit packages. Thus, the change in tax policy is considered to be a linchpin in the procompetition strategy.

186

Proposals for Changing the Tax Treatment of Health Insurance

The various procompetition proposals would alter the present tax treatment of health insurance in several important ways. All of the proposals call for a "cap" on the tax subsidy for employer-paid premiums for employees' health insurance. The different proposals would set the level of the cap differently, but all of them would change the tax consequences of premium payments above the cap. This could be done in either of two ways: (1) by taxing any excess amount as income to the employee; (2) by disallowing employers' expense deductions for excess amounts. Employers might strongly oppose the latter way because of the precedent it could set for disallowing other business expense deductions. Therefore, current proposals favor taxing the excess premiums as employee income.

Some of the proposals provide for cash payments to employees who choose plans with premiums below the cap, or below the level of their employer's contribution if it is less than the cap. These payments are taxable under some proposals but tax-free under others. They are intended to give employees additional incentives to choose less costly plans.

The more comprehensive proposals would give tax credits to individuals who are not covered by employer-provided plans, so that they might also enjoy subsidized health insurance. If the credit exceeded an individual's tax liability, he would receive the excess as a tax-free cash rebate.

Finally, at least one of the proposals would eliminate part of the present medical expense deduction for individual health insurance premiums and replace it with the individual tax credit.

Limits on Tax-Free Employer Contributions

Most of the procompetition proposals introduced in Congress would impose a ceiling on the amount of an employer's contribution to a qualified health insurance plan that will not be taxed as income to an employee (if the plan is not qualified, the entire contribution becomes taxable income to the employee). Such proposals include H.R. 850, introduced by Congressman Richard A. Gephardt (Democrat, Missouri); S. 433, sponsored by Senator David Durenberger (Republican, Minnesota); and S. 139, sponsored by Senator Orrin G. Hatch (Republican, Utah). These bills have different methods, however, of determining the "tax cap," and this raises other issues regarding equity, economic efficiency, and administrative feasibility.

The cap can be set basically in two ways: (1) make it uniform nationally for ease of administration and probably greater economic impact on total health care costs; (2) vary it by region or actuarial status or employer to give roughly equal treatment to all individuals regardless of how old they are or where they live.

187

Uniform National Cap. The most obvious argument for a single cap nationwide is its simplicity. It would be much simpler to administer, both for government as the regulator and for employers who must comply with it. The Durenberger bill, which takes this approach, would establish a first-year limit of $125 per month for family coverage ($50 for employee only and $100 for employee and spouse), effective in 1984; the limit would then be indexed for inflation in succeeding years. Such a uniform cap would obviate the need for the Department of Health and Human Services (HHS) to build a large data base and make calculations for geographical areas and actuarial groups each year. It would also simplify matters for employers with employees in various locations. A variable cap would require them to keep track of separate contribution limits for each region in which they operate and to identify any taxable amounts on employee W-2 forms. The administrative simplicity of a single national cap makes it appealing to those who must do all the paperwork.

A uniform cap might have more impact on total health care costs than a variable one. This is because a uniform cap would presumably be lower in areas with high medical costs than a cap that is adjusted to account for differences in costs among areas. It would, therefore, have more "bite" in these high-cost areas, which contain the greatest potential for cost savings within the total health care system. Of course, the objective of a tax cap is to reduce the demand for insurance coverage to a level that more truly reflects a balancing of costs and potential benefits by consumers. The current uncapped tax subsidy encourages consumers to ignore the costs and think only of the benefits, thereby stimulating demand for more insurance coverage than an efficient market would produce. Reducing the subsidy would reduce the amount of subsidized demand and thus the extent of insurance coverage. The effect of reduced demand on medical care prices would presumably be largest in the most heavily insured markets, because these are the markets with the highest and most rapidly rising medical costs.[2]

The argument most often made against a uniform national ceiling is that it would discriminate against employees in areas with high medical costs and those in high-risk actuarial categories by allowing employees in low-risk categories and those in areas with lower costs to purchase more generous tax-free benefits. This equity problem can be dealt with only by sacrificing simplicity—and perhaps efficiency—and setting caps that vary according to area medical costs or actuarial status or some other factor. The Gephardt and Hatch bills incorporate this variable cap approach.

Variable Cap. The Gephardt proposal would establish separate caps for each actuarial group in each health care area. Health care areas are defined as urbanized portions of Standard Metropolitan Statistical Areas (SMSAs) determined by the Office of Management and Budget and as areas outside SMSAs delineated by the Secretary of Health and Human Services. During the first three years after the bill takes effect, the cap would be set at the average per capita expenditure for an aged individual under Medicare in 1981, indexed for inflation as measured by the gross national product (GNP) deflator. Thereafter, it would be set at the weighted average premium of qualified plans selected during the previous general enrollment period by individuals in the same actuarial category and health care area, again adjusted similarly for inflation. This would be akin to setting the cap at whatever it costs insurers to provide the specified minimum benefits also called for by the Gephardt bill. A variable cap of this kind assumes implicitly the desirability of subsidizing some minimum "real" level of benefits for all health care consumers by varying the nominal dollar level of tax-free premiums with regional differences in medical costs as well as differences due to an individual's actuarial status.

The Hatch bill, originally proposed by HHS Secretary Richard Schweiker, would set the cap for employer contributions at the premium cost of the most expensive plan in which at least 10 percent of the employees are enrolled. The Hatch cap would thus be individual for each employer. It is not very restrictive, starting as it does at the current cost of what is probably the most expensive plan already offered, but it would prevent employers from enriching their plans because they were below a regional or national cap.

Alternatively, the cap could be set at a level that would immediately affect some target proportion of the insured population in each health care area—for example, one-third of the individuals currently covered by group plans.

A variable cap would affect the marginal behavior of more people than a uniform cap, because it would reach more of those in the lower-cost areas. As mentioned earlier, however, it would probably have less impact on total health care costs because it would not impinge as much on the behavior of individuals in high-cost areas.

A trade-off between equity and simplicity could be made by dropping one or the other of the Gephardt adjustments without going all the way to the Durenberger single cap. Alain Enthoven's Consumer-Choice Health Plan, for example, would gradually phase out regional caps but retain adjustments for actuarial status.[3] This would eventually put greater pressure on consumers in areas with high medical costs to economize on their choice of insurance plans, but would allow them time to make some adjustment while continuing to recognize cost differences based on actuarial factors.

Indexing Cap to Inflation. Whatever kind of cap was established, it would have to be adjusted for inflation. The choice of an inflation index for making this adjustment affects the real level of the tax subsidy over time. Choice of a more conservative—or less generous—index, for example, reduces the subsidy and, hence, the real level of benefits it can buy. As an extreme example, failure to index the cap at all would eventually reduce the subsidy to a small fraction of its original value. Over time, the proportion of people affected by any cap would increase to the extent that the cap was updated by an inflation index that failed to keep up with actual increases in health care costs. Politically, it would be easier to implement a conservative indexing formula the more liberal the initial value of the cap itself.

The Gephardt and Durenberger bills propose different indexes of inflation. Gephardt uses the GNP deflator, and Durenberger the medical care component of the consumer price index. Because the latter has consistently risen more rapidly than the former, Gephardt would put a tighter lid on tax-free employer contributions over time.

Adverse Selection

The tax-cap proposal raises new issues concerning adverse risk selection, which some health care analysts consider the most serious problem with the procompetition approaches. The degree of adverse selection that would result from implementing any of the bills depends on several factors. The level of minimum benefits required of all qualified plans and the frequency of open enrollment seasons for switching plans are both important, but the limit on tax-free employer contributions is perhaps the most important factor. It gives employees a choice between taxable benefits above the cap and cash payments below the cap. Employees who are higher health risks will probably continue to choose the more expensive plans, perhaps even if it means being taxed on some of the premium cost if high-option plans have premiums that exceed the tax cap. Better risks are more likely to choose the less expensive plans—to the extent that their lower premiums result from trimmer benefit packages rather than just more efficient provision of services. As this occurs, the high-cost plans—saddled with the costlier members—will become even more expensive, causing further flight of the better risks into lower-cost plans and eventually establishing, in effect, a two-tier system of health insurance.

A comprehensive set of minimum required benefits can help to reduce incentives for risk selection, because it cuts off plan shopping below that level. Enthoven makes this an important feature of his consumer-choice proposal, and the procompetition bills all specify such a set of benefits, which varies from bill to bill but generally includes Medicare-type basic services plus a provision for catastrophic coverage. The laudable effort to prevent extreme adverse selection, however, also reduces the extent of effective consumer choice and, thereby, the potential savings from choosing less comprehensive plans. The trade-off in "lost" savings would be greater the more comprehensive the minimum set of benefits.

Restrictions on plan switching during open enrollment periods would limit opportunities for "free riding" by consumers who buy minimal coverage when they are well and then change to more comprehensive coverage when they are ill—perhaps changing back to minimal coverage when they are well again. Restrictions would not keep people from making long-term choices on the basis of expected use but would cut down on annual switching based on short-term variations in expected use. Paul Ginsburg suggests that putting restrictions only on switches to plans with higher premiums would interfere least with the purpose of getting people to choose lower-cost plans.[4]

The Gephardt bill tries to protect qualified plans from adverse selection by providing for maximum limits on the number of high risks that any plan must accept. This enables high risks to be spread around proportionally, but it could probably not stem a flood of better risks out of more expensive plans. Thus, numerical limits on high risks that a plan must accept might be ineffective if the high risks all wanted to get into the same plans that the better risks were leaving. The result would still be a two-tier system, with high risks even subsidizing tax-free refunds for better risks while being taxed on part of their own benefits because of the cap on tax-free employer payments.

One way to prevent such a result would be to mandate risk pooling. However this were done, it could defeat some of the intent of the procompetition proposals to subject the health care market to more competitive forces. Assuming that all plans were required to accept a proportional number of medically high-risk people whether or not they applied, this would blunt the competitive edge of the more efficient plans somewhat and weaken the incentives for consumers to choose them. It is possible that mandated risk pooling would raise the costs of more efficient plans by more than it would lower the costs of less efficient plans, thereby increasing the total cost of health care. Of course, the requirement in most procompetition proposals that premiums be community-rated rather than experience-rated is itself a form of risk pooling, and one that Enthoven considers important as a check against preferred risk selection by insurers.

Alternatively, plans that are stuck with a disproportionate load of high risks could be subsidized, either through direct payments or through tax credits of comparable value. Either way, it would be difficult to determine the appropriate amount of the subsidy. A formula for doing so would have to relate a plan's premium to the average premium for all plans. It would have to separate the portion of the higher cost attributable to risk selection from the portion attributable to a costlier benefit package and/or costlier medical practice habits. Otherwise, the more expensive plans would be rewarded for the same costly practices that are supported by the present system of cost reimbursement. Premiums for all qualified plans would have to be risk-adjusted.

The Gephardt bill would further mitigate adverse selection by providing for actuarially adjusted employer contributions to insurance plans. These adjustments for characteristics such as age reduce incentives for preferred risk selection. It is probably preferable to make separate provisions for plans with a concentration of high risks than to weaken the general incentives for economizing on the choice of plans.

Adverse selection is not a creation of the procompetition reformers; it is a natural feature of any market for insurance. Nevertheless, all proposals calling for tax caps and refunds as incentives to choose lower-cost plans could intensify the problem and make health insurance costlier for many high-risk people. The Gephardt bill tries to alleviate the problem through its complex scheme of varying employer contribution limits by region and actuarial group, but the tax incentives could still lure enough healthy people out of higher-cost plans to leave a serious adverse selection problem.

Grandfathering

The Gephardt bill makes allowance for employees whose employer contributions already exceed the cap by "grandfathering" them. Amounts currently contributed by the employer, either under a collective bargaining agreement or not, are to remain untaxed until adjustments raise the cap to the level of such contributions. This may seem unduly deferential to the already benefit-rich, but it would probably not be politically feasible to pass a reform bill that immediately began to tax a significant portion of previously untaxed benefits. Even grandfathered workers would feel a short-term pinch as any increases in employer contributions needed to maintain or raise existing levels of coverage were taxed. Many companies already provide generous health insurance benefits to their employees, sometimes because of collective bargaining agreements reached with unions representing part of their work force. The grandfather clause may lessen unions' opposition to consumer choice proposals, but they would still oppose any scheme that would replace their present arrangement of uniform fixed-benefit packages with fixed contributions that would purchase different levels of benefits in each location.

Effect of Cap on Tax Revenues

Ginsburg has estimated the effect of the Gephardt tax cap on federal revenues. Initially, the cap would be based on the value of Medicare benefits, which according to the Congressional Budget Office would be about $154 per month in 1984, increasing in succeeding years.[5] Ginsburg estimates that at first it would affect about one-third of those with employment-based health insurance, and would increase federal tax revenues by nearly $5 billion in 1984 and almost $12 billion by 1986.[6] The Durenberger cap—at $125 per month—would be lower, and the consequent revenue gain greater. The Hatch cap is employer-specific, and the revenue effect is more difficult to anticipate; because it is based on the cost of high-option plans, however, it would probably be higher and, hence, would produce a smaller revenue gain.

Cash Rebates to Employees

The tax cap on employer contributions is designed to create incentives for employers to offer health insurance plans with premiums below the cap, so that their employees will not have to be taxed on what was previously an untaxed benefit. This is perhaps more accurately termed a disincentive to offer only plans with premiums that exceed the cap. To strengthen the incentive effect, some procompetition proponents have paired the cap with a more positive inducement for employees to choose plans with lower premiums—the offer of a cash payment equal to the difference between the premium of the plan chosen and the maximum contribution their employer is willing to make to any plan. The offer of a rebate would presumably cause employees to demand that their employers provide a choice of plans with lower premiums.

The offer of rebates could reduce political opposition to setting a lower cap that would affect more individual decisions on what insurance plan to choose. Conversely, if the cap is high, rebates are an even greater incentive.

The issues raised by the rebate are linked to those arising from the cap, because they are part of the same scheme. The refund feature of the procompetition proposals, for example, most worries those who are concerned about adverse selection. The combination of taxing employer contributions above the cap as income to the employee and offering cash refunds to those who choose plans costing less than the employer's maximum contribution may induce healthier workers to choose less expensive plans. This would leave the more expensive plans with the higher risks, which would widen the cost disparities between high- and low-cost plans. As a result, better risks—primarily younger people— would get even larger refunds, which some critics regard as "windfalls." To prevent this, they suggest computing an age factor into the rebates to determine their actuarial value, which would be lower because of the effect on costs of younger workers' switching plans. This suggestion may have merit on equity grounds, but its adoption would reduce the number of employees choosing plans with lower premiums, thereby attenuating the desired impact on health care costs.

The rebate's effect on individual choices could depend heavily on whether it is taxable. The Gephardt and Hatch bills would exempt it from income, just as are the benefits currently received under the tax exclusion for employer contributions. The Durenberger bill, however, would tax the rebate as income—although exempting it from payroll taxes. It can be argued that, given the choice between nontaxable health insurance and taxable cash, most employees would choose to keep more insurance and forgo the rebates.

The Gephardt bill would put a cap on the size of the rebate an individual could receive. It would be the lesser of $500 (indexed for inflation between 1981 and the applicable year) or the difference between the employer's maximum contribution and the tax cap itself. The purposes of such a cap on rebates would be to limit the ability of employers to provide their employees with tax-free cash by raising their maximum contributions, and to limit the potential revenue loss to the federal Treasury. Ginsburg has estimated that refunds paid to employees would be tax-free up to $49 per month in 1984, reduced by the amount —if any—by which the plan premium plus the refund exceeded the cap. He further estimates the revenue loss from this provision at more than $8 billion in 1984 and nearly $13 billion in 1986.[7] This loss would exceed the estimated revenue gain from the tax cap by about $3½ billion in 1984, but by only $1 billion in 1986. The Hatch bill would go further yet, putting no dollar limit on the rebate.

Some procompetition advocates oppose the rebate scheme. They believe that the tax cap alone would be enough incentive, because it would cause employees to prod their employers to offer plans with premiums that did not exceed the cap; otherwise, they would suffer a "tax bite." Some of these reformers are also concerned that, whatever additional incentive the rebates gave employees to choose lower-option plans, the benefits from such choices would be outweighed by the costs measured by revenue loss to the Treasury—which, as Ginsburg has estimated, would not be miniscule. Of course, considerations of budget deficits may not make for the best policy, but they could be a determining factor in a decision about whether to change the tax laws. The anticipated revenue gain from imposing a tax cap on employer contributions may be a crucial selling point for health care reform proposals, and if rebates offset that gain—and are not essential to stimulating the consumer choice process in the market place—they may entail more political risk than they are worth.

Some procompetition proponents would implement a voluntary rebate scheme under which employers could, if they wished, make cash payments to employees who chose low-option plans with lower premiums. These rebates would vary in size from one employer to another depending on the premium cost of the particular plans offered. The Hatch bill provides for just such variable rebates—although on a mandatory rather than a voluntary basis—because it sets the cap at the level of the most expensive plan in which more than 10 percent of the employees are enrolled.

A few employers already offer such voluntary rebates as part of what are called "cafeteria" or flexible benefit programs, although they are not tax-free under present law. The TRW Corporation originated the cafeteria concept at its California division. Employees have a choice of three health insurance plans as well as a health maintenance organization (HMO). Those who choose the low-option plan receive credits that can be used toward other specified benefits or, under limited conditions, can be converted to cash payments. Educational Testing Service also offers its employees flexible credits that can be either used for various optional benefits or taken in cash.

Tax Credits to Individuals

The current tax treatment of health insurance subsidizes those whose employers pay for their coverage and discriminates against those who buy insurance out of their own pockets. The first group receives a tax-free benefit in the form of employer-paid insurance premiums that are not included in taxable income; the second group must pay its own premiums with dollars of taxable income.

The procompetition proposals would try to end this unfair treatment of individuals who are not in employer-provided group insurance plans. The Gephardt bill, for example, would establish a tax credit in the amount of the premium paid to a qualified plan up to the applicable cap for excludable employer contributions for the individual's health

195

care area and actuarial category. It would also provide a credit to employees whose employer contributions were below the cap, equal to the difference between the two. If an individual's tax credit were to exceed his income tax liability, he would be eligible for the same cash rebate given to employees who choose plans with premiums that are less than their employer's maximum contribution. This tries to give all health care consumers roughly equal treatment. Such provisions would largely remove the tax shelter aspect of employer contributions to health insurance and relate the rebates more to income. Some analysts think that, because the income tax is involved, subsidies should be related to income for everyone; explicit tax credits do this best.

Ginsburg has also estimated the potential federal revenue loss from the tax credit provision of the Gephardt bill.[8] He estimates that in 1984 the credit for an individual would be about $58 per month, which is not large compared with the premiums for individually purchased insurance. Nevertheless, the projected revenue loss would be large—more than $11 billion in 1984, rising to nearly $18½ billion in 1986. These estimates include the effect of repealing the deduction for individually paid health insurance premiums. Thus, the revenue loss would exceed the gain from the cap on tax-free employer contributions.

Ginsburg's estimates for the impact of the tax cap, the tax-free rebate, and the tax credit together show net revenue losses of $14½ billion in 1984, and nearly $19½ billion in 1986.

The tax credit provision does more than just try to establish equity for people who have to buy their own health insurance. It moves the entire health insurance system away from its employment base or, as Enthoven puts it, away from a job-centered to a consumer-centered system. The Gephardt bill—the most comprehensive reform proposal in legislative form—does not go as far in that direction as Enthoven's Consumer Choice Health Plan would go, but it begins to change the focus of health insurance from individuals as employees to individuals as consumers. Employers and unions would no longer have such a dominant influence on the choice of insurance. This would be even more true if the employment link were severed entirely by separating tax credits from employer-paid insurance for all individuals.

Medical Expense Deduction

The Gephardt bill is the only procompetition proposal that would change the existing medical expense deduction along with changing the employer exclusion. The bill would continue to allow individuals to deduct up to $150 of the health insurance premiums paid out of pocket from taxable income. Therefore, the subsidy for health insurance would remain in the form of the $150 deduction, based on the taxpayer's marginal tax rate. The subsidy for health insurance is limited in the Gephardt bill, however, through means other than the cap. The bill would no longer allow any additional amount of expenditure for premiums to be included in the deduction for medical expenses in excess of 5 percent of adjusted gross income. This provision is more apt to affect individuals in higher income brackets who are more likely to take advantage of the medical expense deduction.

As discussed earlier, the Gephardt bill would add a subsidy for health insurance in the form of a tax credit. Individuals who purchase health insurance with premiums that cost more than the employer contribution but less than the cap are entitled to a tax credit equal to the difference. This provision is especially helpful to employees whose employer contributions are low and to those who are self-employed or who purchase insurance individually and are not eligible for subsidies under the existing law.

Conclusion

The scheme proposed by the Gephardt bill and—to a lesser extent—by the Durenberger and Hatch bills would constitute a major reform of the health care system. As current tax policy has been an important cause of the recognized defects in the existing system, changes in tax policy would be the moving force behind the changes in the system envisioned by the procompetition reformers.

Notes

1. Tax expenditures are revenue losses attributable to provisions of the federal income tax laws that allow a special exclusion or deduction from gross income, or that provide a special credit, preferential tax rate, or deferral of tax liability.
2. Joseph P. Newhouse, "Some Interim Results from a Randomized Controlled Trial in Health Insurance," *New England Journal of Medicine,* vol. 305 (December 17, 1981), pp. 1501-1507.
3. Alain Enthoven, *Health Plan* (Reading, Mass.: Addison-Wesley, 1980).
4. Paul B. Ginsburg, "Altering the Tax Treatment of Employment-Based Health Plans," Paper prepared for the *Milbank Memorial Fund Quarterly: Health and Society,* Spring 1981, p. 32.
5. Paul B. Ginsburg, in "An Analysis of the National Health Care Reform Act of 1981 (H.R. 850)," Staff Working Paper, Congressional Budget Office, September 30, 1981, p. iii.
6. Ibid., p. 10.
7. Ibid.
8. Ibid.

11

Tax Policy, Health Insurance, and Health Care

Charles E. Phelps

Tax policy, through a variety of ways, has provided a dominant health policy tool in the United States at least since World War II. The most readily identifiable components of the tax system affecting health care in the United States include Medicare (a payroll-tax-based, current-funded system to provide health insurance for the elderly) and the deductibility of health care expenditures on personal income tax forms. Most people in the United States probably know of these forms.

The general public sees less directly, but perhaps still knows well, the tax-exempt treatments provided for a large number of medical care providers, health insurers, and medical educators. Tax policy not only exempts these entities from paying corporate income taxes, but also provides almost automatic justification for exemption from state income and sales taxes, local property taxes, health insurance premium taxes, and other forms of tax too small to bear systematic examination. In addition, the ability to float tax-free bonds for construction, and to receive tax-deductible charitable contributions, also adds to the total government subsidy to the health sector. These tax exemptions, in concept, distort the magnitude of expenditures in health care by reducing input prices to health care providers and hence final product prices vis-à-vis other prod-

NOTE: I have had the considerable luxury of receiving the advice and attention of participants in the American Enterprise Institute's working group on health insurance and tax policy on an earlier draft of this paper, as well as benefiting from their insights from a previous session. In a sense, much of this paper is simply a reporting of their many insights. I would like to thank particularly Eugene Steuerle, Ronald Hoffman, Ronald Vogel, and Joseph Newhouse for detailed discussion of an earlier draft. Since so much of the credit for the content of this paper belongs to others, there is, perhaps, a joint responsibility for its content. Since they have not, however, had a chance to review this manuscript before publication, I hereby absolve them from responsibility for any remaining errors.

ucts. They may also distort the choice of types of providers of health care, health insurance, and health education services by taxing, in effect, industries or firms that might compete with the tax-exempt firms. In medical care, for example, physician services are generally not provided through tax-exempt organizations, whereas hospitals are typically tax-exempt.[1] Similarly, Blue Cross and Blue Shield insurance plans are typically tax-exempt, but not commercial insurance plans providing competing services of risk spreading. Understanding the consequences of the tax structure in terms of how these industries are organized (in equilibrium) may prove to be an important part of our eventual understanding of the consequences of these tax exemptions on the medical care system.

A still less obvious, and yet likely more important, tax policy within the health care sector is the prevailing tax treatment of health insurance premiums for Americans. Those who itemize deductions can claim a direct tax deduction for premiums they pay: half of the premium (up to $150 under previous tax law—$100 under the proposed revision) can be deducted routinely, and the other half contributes toward the deduction for health expenses (all expenses above 3 percent of adjusted gross income under previous tax law—5 percent under the provisions of the 1982 Tax Equity and Fiscal Responsibility Act). For individuals paying their own health insurance premiums, this deduction provides an important reduction in the relative costs of health insurance over other goods and services.

The individual deductions of health insurance premiums, however, represent only the tip of the iceberg. Approximately 85 percent of the health insurance held in the United States by those under sixty-five years of age arises through employer-group insurance, the vast majority of which employers pay in part, if not in full. The tax consequences of this form of insurance sales are considerable: the employer can deduct the insurance cost as a normal business expense, and yet the employee need not declare this compensation as taxable income, unlike most other forms of compensation.[2]

Table 11–1 sets forth crude estimates of the magnitude of tax subsidies for most of these categories of health care subsidy. These estimates are not intended to be precise but to provide the reader with a rough approximation of the magnitude of the various types of subsidy now prevailing in the economy.

Tax Subsidies for Health Care: Pro and Con

The motivation for subsidizing medical care directly and indirectly (via health insurance premium subsidies) does not seem to flow directly from

199

TABLE 11–1

APPROXIMATE MAGNITUDE OF FEDERAL TAX INTERVENTION IN
HEALTH CARE, FISCAL YEAR 1982

	Total (billions of dollars)	Per Capita (dollars)
Medicare	47	210
Medicaid	20	88
Nonprofit tax status of hospitals and certain health insurers	Not known	Not known
Income tax deductions for health care and for individuals' health insurance premiums	3	13
Tax exemption of employer group insurance premiums	23	102
Tax-exempt bonds	0.5	2
Tax-deductible charitable contributions	1	4

the usual efficiency arguments of economists for government intervention but from other issues. Consider first the efficiency arguments: medical care should be subsidized if externalities arise in consumption of care so that people purchase too little care. Immunization against contagious disease provides a classic example. Since each immunized person confers a benefit on his friends and neighbors (by reducing a possible route for contagious disease to infect them), the private incentives for innoculations are smaller than the social gain. Thus, a subsidy seems desirable. In medical care, however, infectious diseases lead to only a small fraction of all expenses and therefore do not provide a substantial argument to support government subsidy of health care.

A second argument holds that health care is a "merit good." ("I receive pleasure from knowing that you consume medical care.") This argument cannot be refuted directly, as could the previous argument. Beyond its having been posed, however, there does not appear to be any substantial empirical support for the proposition directly. Existence of charitable donations for medical charities and not-for-profit hospitals implies some sort of merit-good aspects to health care, but alternative explanations seem equally plausible.[3]

Still a third argument for providing medical care for some persons rests on the belief that those persons will not take appropriate care of themselves without the added inducement of subsidy or free care. This same logic argues for providing low-income persons with food stamps and housing subsidies rather than income subsidies. Donors—willing or unwilling—prefer their own consumption patterns to those of the recipient and, hence, offer only transfers in kind. Stated in this way, of course, it becomes apparent that this argument just restates the merit-good argument.

Other considerations about the merits of subsidizing private medical care through health insurance stem indirectly from the public provision of medical care: If the government provides free or low-cost care for some of the citizenry (for example, through county hospitals), then allowing those persons without access to such care to receive a comparable subsidy in the private sector appears appropriate. This does not, however, deal with the fundamental issue directly at hand—that is, the logic for direct governmental provision of care.

Finally, some argue for subsidizing medical care because "health care is a right," commonly asserted to flow from the Preamble to the U.S. Constitution, which establishes a goal of "promoting the general welfare." The Declaration of Independence asserts certain unalienable rights to be endowed by the Creator, including "life, liberty, and the pursuit of happiness." In contrast, for example, the Bill of Rights limits government action but does not declare duties of the government to commit resources for the benefit of individuals. (Perhaps the sole exceptions are the Sixth and the Seventh Amendments, establishing the right to speedy trial and to trial by jury.) Without broad construction of the general-welfare goal, one cannot find direct constitutional authority to support the belief that health care is a right. Indeed, only the Eighteenth Amendment speaks directly to patterns of consumption of individuals, prohibiting "the manufacture, distribution, or sale of alcoholic beverages."[4]

These direct arguments for the desirability of subsidies to medical care may enter the public policy debates about the issues, but indirect effects may also arise. Any subsidy to the consumption of medical care, housing, food, or other commodities will increase the overall demand for the product and for the factors of production associated with it. Producers of the product and its important inputs may thus become beneficiaries of medical care subsidies at least as much as the direct recipients. It therefore follows that, in a public debate over the desirability of such subsidies, providers of care will embrace at least some aspects of a health care subsidy system.

Others argue against the health subsidies and the preferred tax status of health insurance premiums. Two arguments appear commonly. The first simply denies the validity of any of the arguments in favor of the subsidies. The second accepts, at least in part, the arguments in favor but offers evidence that the costs to society of continuing this tax treatment of the health sector are increasing through time, and that (in the extreme) these costs now overwhelm any social benefits from the current policy.

The standard analysis of the effects of health insurance on demand for care suggests that increases in the level of benefits—at least as contemporary health insurance plans are structured—will increase use of health care.[5] In typical health insurance, the consumer receives insurance benefits in proportion to his medical care use or expenses. Thus, the insurance subsidizes consumption of care at the time of service, altering the decisions about consumption of health care versus other goods and services. Empirical studies show that consumption increases markedly —perhaps more than doubles in some cases—with full coverage insurance, as compared with no coverage.[6]

A randomized controlled experiment by Joseph Newhouse and others supports these results.[7] The experiment shows that, if provision of additional care to our society comes at increasing incremental costs, increasing utilization will necessarily raise the price of all medical services. Correspondingly, costs to consumers—directly and indirectly through insurance premiums—will increase and the providers of care will gain further. In such an analysis, increases in health care costs and utilization follow directly from increases in health insurance coverage. Once coverage stabilizes at some point, however, by this analysis costs should not continue to rise.

Unfortunately, this static model of industry behavior cannot explain fully the events of the past two decades. Statistical studies show that prices of care and resources used continue to climb, even when coverage does not increase.[8] This disturbing finding, if correct, suggests that health policy makers cannot necessarily rely on normal mechanisms of market equilibrium commonly praised by economists.

The argument put forth by Newhouse is quite simple in concept: Once insurance becomes nearly complete, individuals lose any incentives they might have had to shop carefully for health care. Further, and perhaps most important, business successfully introduces new procedures, techniques, and products into the medical marketplace on an unusual criterion: If the product does any good at all, it will become successful since the apparent costs to the consumer are zero. Quite in contrast, in a normal market, business successfully introduces a new product only if the benefits to consumers exceed relevant costs. With broad coverage insurance, both prices and resource use could continue to rise arbitrarily, even if the amount of health insurance coverage remained constant. Any limits to the process must come from outside: either from government regulation; or from limits on the rate at which business introduces new technologies—for example, the rate of innovation from manufacturers, universities, and the like; or from new contractual forms between providers and consumers—for example, prepaid practice plans, health maintenance organizations (HMOs), and independent practice associations (IPAs).

The Newhouse hypothesis provides the primary foundation for the argument that reductions in health insurance coverage will lead to reductions in the rate of health care price increases. Under the standard economic scenario, a once-and-for-all reduction in the level of coverage could produce only a once-and-for-all fall in the level of prices, but no effect on subsequent rates of change in health care prices. Newhouse's hypothesis suggests that eliminating full-coverage aspects of insurance could at least reduce the rate at which prices increase, and possibly also reduce the level of prices themselves.

Aside from the issues surrounding subsidies to medical care itself, there are other issues concerning subsidies to medical insurance. First, and most obvious, subsidies to medical insurance, by enhancing demand for insurance, will also enhance demand for medical care. Thus, any arguments about the desirability or undesirability of subsidies to medical care also apply to subsidies for health insurance. Similarly, increased amounts of health insurance will bestow benefits upon providers of the care.

An important argument arises in favor of subsidizing insurance because of a peculiar type of market failure. Insurance is a calculated gamble between the insurer and the insured. In a fully competitive market, the insurer would collect just enough insurance premiums, on average, to cover the costs of medical care paid out, plus any administrative expenses. But the insurer may only poorly anticipate the average of medical costs for a given person because of intrinsic differences in people's health and life style. Relatively unhealthy persons—those at relatively large risk for medical expenses—have incentives to purchase better insurance. The insurer, however, cannot easily identify such persons. This asymmetry in information between the insurer and the insured can make it difficult, or unduly expensive, for the insurance market to function fully. If so, governmental action could increase well-being, either through improvements in information or through subsidies to increase the amount of insurance in force. Taken to an extreme, this concept argues in favor of compulsory universal health insurance. (This is not to be construed that I accept such an argument.)

I will not attempt to evaluate the merits of these arguments supporting subsidies to medical care or health insurance. For whatever reasons, our political system has opted for the subsidies described at the beginning of this paper. And their magnitude grows with time, primarily because general inflation pushes the population into higher marginal tax brackets through time, and many of the subsidies are tax deductions increasing automatically with increases in the marginal tax rate. (I am not asserting here that the taxes ought not to be collected; rather, I wish to point out that relative prices, and hence patterns of consumption, are affected by the so-called bracket creep and the consequent increases in subsidies to medical care.)

Tax Subsidies to the Health Sector: Should There Be Limits to Growth?

Policy makers have considerably limited many of the tax subsidies to the health care sector, including those to health insurance; limits have been placed both on the ways in which the subsidy may be used and on the real or inflation-adjusted magnitude of the subsidies. The tax-exempt status of not-for-profit hospitals, for example, depends upon whether the hospital provides public-interest care. Section 501(c)(3) of the Internal Revenue Service (IRS) code does not automatically exempt hospitals, as it does other organizations such as colleges and churches. Typically, this has been interpreted as requiring that 5 percent of the hospitals' revenues be spent in charity care.

With the medical expense deduction for individuals, the deductibility is in large part inflation-adjusted by the condition that only expenses exceeding 3 percent of the person's adjusted gross income are deductible.

The treatment of individually purchased health insurance premiums, as noted previously, is more generous, but still limited. Similarly, life insurance premiums provided by employers become taxable income after the value of the insurance plan exceeds prescribed limits.

Employer-paid health insurance premiums, in considerable contrast, maintain a tax-exempt status as compensation to the employee essentially regardless of the magnitude or structure of the health premiums. This aspect of the "tax-based health policy" now appears open for reconsideration.[9]

The political impetus for reconsidering the tax treatment of health insurance arises from several sources. First, the long-standing increases in the relative prices of medical care continue to bother public officials. The Consumer Price Index (CPI) for medical care services has more than tripled since Medicare was introduced in 1966, increasing on average 1 percent faster per year than the general CPI, so that between 1966 and 1982 the price of medical care increased 20 percent more than the index for all other goods and services. This, of course, affects federal outlays and tax burdens. Some even argue that the increasing prices of health care help contribute to the general inflation.[10]

Next, growing budget deficits have attracted the attention of federal agencies toward alternatives for reducing the deficit in other than traditional ways. The General Accounting Office (GAO), for example, has proposed introducing or increasing user charges for federal activities such as dams, electric power, etc. Elimination of "tax expenditures" —tax revenues not collected because of definitions of income—also appears attractive.[11] Tax expenditures represent, of course, some of the most hallowed financial windfalls and subsidies of our political economy. They include the deductibility of home mortgage interest expenses, the treatment of overseas income taxes for multinational corporations, and the exclusion of employer contributions for health insurance from taxable income of employees. In 1982, the tax expenditure for employer health expenditures was estimated to be in the neighborhood of $23 billion.[12]

In part, improved information on the magnitude of the employer-exclusion tax expenditure has probably accelerated interest in tax reform. In 1973, Martin Feldstein and Elizabeth Allison first estimated the 1969 tax expenditure to be $1.63 billion.[13] Using better data and more refined methods, Bridger Mitchell and Charles Phelps in 1976 showed this to be too small by a factor of 35 percent.[14] Better data continue to accumulate to allow still more refined understanding of the extent of the tax subsidy in the future. Nevertheless, the enormous growth in employer premiums and the consequent tax expenditure over the last decade surely provide the most prominent argument for change: Employer premiums, and derivative tax expenditures, increased during the 1970s at a compound rate of 30 percent or more.

Finally, interest in limiting the tax subsidies to health care and health insurance increases as economic theories and evidence support the belief that change may be beneficial not only for controlling health care costs but also for improving consumer welfare. Most prominent among these efforts have been those of Alain Enthoven, Joseph Newhouse, and Martin Feldstein.[15] Enthoven's work on a competitive health care sector has proven particularly important in gathering public attention to the issues and to the potential importance of introducing consumer and producer competitive responses into a market now at least partly insulated from such pressures.

Alternative Mechanisms to Limit Health Insurance Tax Subsidies. The complexity of health financing allows the policy maker to approach tax subsidies for health care and health insurance from a variety of angles. The policy maker may choose between limits to subsidies for the health care market and those for the health insurance market. This choice alone seems both complex and not well illuminated by past economic studies. Elimination of tax subsidies to health care, for example, could best be interpreted as an increase in the net price of medical care to the consumer. To understand the net consequences for health care expenses, consumer welfare, and the distribution of income within the health sector (among providers, patients, institutions, insurers, etc.), one would need to know, at a minimum, how consumer purchases of health insurance would respond. Many researchers suppose that consumers respond to higher medical prices by purchasing more complete insurance.[16] Available economic theory on this issue appears ambiguous, however, and the data suggest at best that the incentives to purchase more complete insurance eventually diminish or reverse at very high levels of coverage, for high levels of medical care prices, or both.[17] One can hardly state with confidence, however, that all agree on the issue. Any policy in this area must be made, to be generous, in the face of a substantial information vacuum. This ambiguity poses an obvious embarrassment for economists attempting to advise policy makers in this area: Reduced health care subsidies may spawn more complete insurance coverage, which could drive up medical prices, possibly even more than offsetting the price-reducing consequences of eliminating the health care subsidies.[18]

Partly for these reasons, policy makers have turned to modifying the tax subsidies for health insurance: The chain of causality appears easier to understand, at least in part, and the potential for an outcome opposite to that intended seems smaller. Elimination of subsidies to health insurance would almost certainly reduce the quantity of health insurance demanded in equilibrium.[19]

To those concerned about the costs of health care markets, two potential benefits appear promising if the level of insurance coverage is reduced. First, where increases in the amount of services provided come only with increasing incremental cost, then overall reductions in the amount of medical care demanded will lead to lower prices.[20] This analysis follows from classic economic analysis, although it need not depend upon beliefs that producers of medical care are profit-maximizing entities. (The only requirement is that technology consumes increasingly more resources to produce additional amounts of care.)

In addition to this fundamental economic notion, other gains accrue if the competitiveness of the health care market increases. This notion, often not clearly defined, depends in a large part on the belief that medical markets do not function as smoothly competitive, but rather as a bunch of isolated monopolies, or perhaps as monopolistically competitive firms, each protected by geographic barriers and, more particularly, by large gaps in information among providers and consumers about appropriate prices in the market. Incentives to search for low prices, it is held, become trivially small when all, or nearly all, buyers are isolated from the effects of price, or when every buyer finds that his personal reward from an extended search for low-priced providers yields him little or no personal gain.

In this view, increased consumer payment for medical care would enhance incentives for search, leading to more information in the market and hence more competitive behavior among producers. In effect, the altered incentives to search would transform the medical market from an independent bunch of small monopolies into a more classically competitive market, with the attendant efficiencies of production and decisions about resource use.

Beyond assertions, however, I find little compelling analysis that helps to understand the actual structure of medical care markets. And the results will surely differ—for example, across medical, hospital, dental, and pharmaceutical markets.

With these considerations in mind, we can turn to the issue of how altered tax structure might modify consumer purchase of health insurance, and hence how the functions of the medical market might change. As noted previously, a consensus can be found that demand curves for health insurance (however measured) behave as for a normal good—higher insurance prices imply lower amounts of insurance demanded. Once past this general statement, however, ambiguity in detail increases with astonishing rapidity. Little, if any, evidence can be found to ascertain the dimensions of adjustment consumers would make if faced with a general change in tax structure.

Consider in turn the primary dimensions of adjustment one might expect consumers to make in health insurance: deductibles, marginal copayment rates, upper coverage limits, or scope of benefits. Each would have profoundly different effects on health care markets. In this discussion, I will emphasize the effects of changes in insurance on the price-search and competitiveness issues rather than on aggregate demand.

Modifying Deductibles. From some ways of analyzing the effects of insurance on medical markets, the most desirable consequence of a change in tax policy toward health insurance would be for people to opt for larger deductibles. This occurs because the larger the deductible, the greater the percentage of transactions that will occur at the full market price (rather than at a coinsured, reduced price rate). The distribution of expenditures for a given individual is quite skewed, as in figure 11–1, with the location and spread of the distribution affected by, among other things, the deductibles and copayment of the insurance plan. (The larger the deductible or copayment, the smaller the average expense.) Increasing the deductible not only shifts the cut-point at which the insurance begins to pay for care—thereby reducing the fraction of transactions that are insured—but also shifts the distribution itself to the left, accentuating the former effect.

FIGURE 11-1

A Prototype Distribution of Medical Expenses for Individuals

$p(x)$ = probability of expense

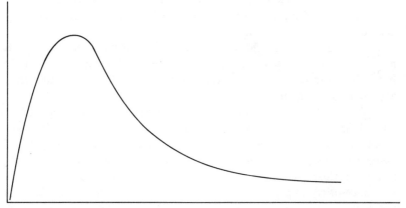

$y(\$)$ = expenditures ($)

We do not clearly understand how many "smart" buyers it takes to keep a market "honest"—either in terms of absolute numbers or as a fraction of the total buyers in a market. It seems intuitively clear that not all buyers in a market must be fully informed and have incentives for careful price shopping; at the other extreme, however, more than a small percentage of the market should be actively seeking price information in order to drive prices toward their competitive level.[21]

A promising approach to understanding the importance of incentives for comparison shopping arises from recent work by Schwartz and Wilde.[22] They rigorously develop models of market equilibrium in which only a fraction of the consumers shop comparatively, showing how the cost structure of firms and the demand elasticity of providers interact in establishing this equilibrium. In accord with Newhouse's market models, as the demand elasticity of consumers falls toward zero (as occurs with better insurance coverage), markets tend to exhibit less competitive pricing, more monopolistically competitive pricing, and a greater tendency for price dispersion (quality constant) in the market. Although their results provide a conceptual basis for understanding how health market equilibrium might be affected by comparison-shopping incentives, no direct application of their models is yet available.

Finally, deductibles would appear to affect certain medical consumption decisions only slightly. The typical hospitalization expenditure, for example, even for a short stay in the hospital, would readily exceed

208

any deductible that most families would choose for their health insurance. Thus, increasing a deductible will not affect decisions regarding length of stay, use of ancillary services, or even such decisions as whether to recuperate in a normal hospital or an extended-stay facility.

Changes in the Coinsurance Rate. If consumers, in the face of changes in the tax law, chose instead to increase the copayment rate for medical expenses, the effects on medical markets could be quite different. Consider, for example, the fictitious case in which all consumers have no deductibles but higher coinsurance rates. Each consumer would face slightly higher medical prices than previously, with corresponding reductions in the amount of medical care demanded at the market level. Correspondingly, each consumer would face somewhat enhanced incentives to search for lower prices, presumably causing lower medical prices and reduced dispersion in those prices. Missing, however, would be the strong incentive that the deductible would provide.

Modifying Upper Coverage Limits. Many health insurance policies contain upper limits of coverage, beyond which the consumer is no longer insured. Early hospital plans, for example, limited coverage to 30, 60, or 120 days of hospitalization. Major-medical insurance plans commonly include limits to payment—$25,000 to $50,000 in earlier years, now commonly $250,000 or more. Dental insurance plans commonly include upper bounds such as $1,000 per year of benefit payments.

Economic theories of consumer demand for insurance cannot explain conveniently why insurance policies contain such upper bounds of payment. Indeed, quite the contrary, economic theory suggests that the consumer would prefer a larger deductible, with the guarantee of catastrophic coverage.[23] Insurers' incentives to include the upper limits are more readily understandable, particularly if insurers do not know fully about underwriting risks. The presence of the limits suggests, however, that insurers cannot fully diversify risks. Otherwise, insurers would offer benefit plans with unlimited duration, and they would reinsure the risks. For whatever the reasons, the presence of internal limits on coverage presents another potential dimension of adjustment for the consumer faced with an increase in the cost of health insurance.

Recent evidence shows that the expenditure distribution for medical care is enormously skewed. Past beliefs that insuring the "tail" of medical expense distributions was low cost are proving erroneous. In Rand's Health Insurance Study, for example, the upper 1 percent of medical events accounts for one-quarter of all medical expenses. Similarly skewed distributions of annual expenses occur under Medicare.[24] Thus, reductions in the upper bound of coverage could potentially reduce premiums substantially.

The tax treatment of medical expenses will importantly affect the consumer's decision on the desirability of such a change in coverage. As noted, current tax law allows individuals to deduct medical expenses over 5 percent of adjusted gross income, thus saving the individual t percent of his expenses ($t =$ the marginal tax rate). Further, the "backstop" of public care—primarily county, state, and federal hospitals—and the availability of Medicaid as an ultimate insurance plan, may make reductions in the upper limits of coverage a popular choice. If tax law also prevents deduction of medical expenses, however, less consumer interest in reducing the upper bounds of coverage should be anticipated.

In terms of reducing medical costs, limitations of coverage could provide dramatic effects by implicitly substituting all of the nonprice rationing devices of government hospitals and Medicaid for the current unlimited coverage of private insurance. Further, the social benefits of many of these very large expenses may be small. Hospitalizations in the last year of life of Medicare patients, for example, account for approximately one-third of all Medicare expenses.[25]

In terms of promoting cost-conscious consumers, curtailing upper tails of coverage will not likely provide a beneficial effect, fundamentally because such a change would affect people only rarely. Thus, only a few medical encounters would have altered financial incentives, and the market would receive little additional information.

It therefore appears that reducing upper limits of insurance payment would reduce expenditures, but probably would not reduce prices very much. Even in those cases where resource use would diminish, it seems unlikely that prices would fall much, because doctors do not use such high-cost resources in many other areas of medical treatment. (Examples would include intensive care units, and other high-technology aspects of a hospital armamentarium that doctors would likely employ in those highly expensive cases that lead to unusually large total annual expenses.)

Since the current state of knowledge is so poor, one could not readily predict whether market prices would fall more in response to (1) broadly increased deductibles, or (2) broadly increased coinsurance. Reducing upper limits, as noted, will alter expenses but probably not many prices. The ambiguity arises because the effect of deductibles eventually vanishes with individuals' sufficiently large expenses, whereas copayment effects extend over a wider range—perhaps all—of possible medical expenses. In theory, both would increase the competitiveness of medical markets, lead to more search by consumers, and reduce aggregate demand. In practice, no information can predict the extent to which either would occur in reality. Policy must be made from theory, perhaps with sequential adoption of any new policy to allow learning while doing.

Changing the Scope of Benefits. A still further alternative for the consumer facing different tax treatment of his health insurance premium might be to alter the scope of benefits—for example, by eliminating certain services from the list of those covered by the health insurance, or by eliminating whole lines of health insurance completely (dental insurance, for instance). Economic theory is useful in predicting where such changes might be made, and the history of health insurance marketing substantiates this theory well.

Generally, theory views health insurance decisions as a trade-off: more complete insurance reduces risk (an economic good), but at the same time, because of the structure of the insurance, induces people to purchase more medical services than they otherwise might.[26] The loss to consumers arises because they pay, via insurance premiums, for "too large" incremental purchases of medical care made while facing the insured prices. Further, the trade-off should be less favorable for purchasing the insurance, the more consumers' purchases of medical care are sensitive to the out-of-pocket price at the time care is sought.[27]

The history of American health insurance follows this theory closely. Consumers have insured those services that are least sensitive to price—hospital care and surgery—first, with greatest prevalance at any point in time, and most completely (that is, with the smallest copayments and deductibles). Conversely, consumers have insured those services that are most sensitive to price—such as psychiatric care and dental care—last, with the lowest frequency, and with the largest copayments.

Nearly the same ranking would arise if one assessed the variability of expenses facing uninsured consumers (the other side of the insurance decision coin). Consumers insure most often those categories of expense that pose the greatest financial risk to consumers—large but infrequent and unpredictable expenditures such as hospitalization and surgery—and often leave uninsured those services that pose less financial uncertainty because they are more common and less expensive when occurring—such as dental care or weekly psychiatric visits.

The implication for health insurance markets seems clear. If tax treatment of health insurance led people to reduce their scope of benefits, consumers would first eliminate those services with the greatest price responsiveness in consumption and those posing the least financial uncertainty. Presumably, this would lead to reductions in coverage for

211

such services as dental care, psychiatric care, and other services only recently falling under the insurance umbrella.

Changes in the scope of benefits would produce markedly different consequences for medical markets than changes in deductibles, copayments, or upper limits. Obviously, if the major dimension of adjustment was to remove insurance coverage for some services but leave other coverage unchanged, many of the various health care markets would be unaffected by the change in tax law.

Changing to Prepaid Care. Each of the preceding discussions considers ways consumers might modify a fee-for-service insurance package in the face of a change in tax policy toward health insurance. Deductibles sufficiently large to alter hospitalization rates would impose large financial risk on consumers and would not alter marginal decisions such as length of stay in the hospital. Copayments have some potential for effect, but estimates of how consumers respond to copayment changes in hospitalization do not offer large promise of major effects from copayments plausibly arising from tax policy changes. Changes in upper bounds of coverage could cut off some large expenditures, possibly just shifting those patients into the public sector, but would be unlikely to have substantial effects on most hospitalization decisions. Changes in scope of benefits are not likely to eliminate hospitalization coverage. Thus, none of these alterations will likely provide major changes in patterns of use of hospitals.

Alternatively, consumers could shift to a different way of buying their health care and health insurance—that is, shift into a prepaid group practice, an independent practice association, or other such prepayment plan. In these plans, the incentives to control utilization lie largely with the provider. Evidence accumulates from a variety of sources that such plans produce substantial reductions in expenditure and resource use, particularly in the area of hospital use.[28]

Potentially, one might observe great changes as patients shift from the fee-for-service sector to the prepayment sector, thus increasing the competition between those two sectors of the health care market. If so, the fee-for-service sector would likely respond by finding new cost-containment devices, leading to still better functioning of medical markets and still further reductions in cost increases for hospital and other forms of health care.

Appropriate Policy Response to Lack of Knowledge

Given this rather abysmal state of knowledge about the unfettered consequences of a general change in the tax treatment of health insurance premiums, it seems worth exploring some alternative "fine-tuning" policies the government might consider to achieve more directly the goals of increasing market functioning in health care sectors.

In any discussion of tax treatment of health insurance, the potential issue of "grandfathering" is important. Total elimination of the tax-exempt status would raise large amounts of revenue: most recent estimates suggest that the current tax law costs about $23 billion per year, a sum that would obviously take a large bite out of current federal budget deficits. But this same large bite would be felt by taxpayers, all of whom would see their taxable income rising, their before-tax pay unchanged, and their after-tax income smaller. The most likely political compromise, in order to accommodate those interests that support the current tax treatment, would allow certain base levels of insurance to maintain their tax-exempt status, with taxation on marginal purchases.

A regulatory approach would allow policy makers to tailor the changes in insurance coverage specifically—by establishing detailed specifications for a "standard insurance policy," coverage beyond which would be considered taxable income. Presumably, a sufficient number of people would choose to purchase only the tax-exempt level of coverage so that tax planners could establish the cost of that plan relatively simply, and hence calculate the full value of any additional premiums.

A regulatory mechanism would allow the government to specify more directly the dimensions of change in insurance policies in order best to achieve other desired goals. If tax planners wished to reduce demand in the physician services sector, for example, they could increase the deductibles of many consumers. To do this, the "standard tax-exempt policy" should contain a large deductible. If tax planners wanted to affect hospital length of stay, they would have to manipulate copayments in some way, since deductibles would not affect such decisions.

Alternatively, tax planners could specify "quantity limits" for tax-exempt insurance and then change the relative prices of various types or dimensions of coverage through taxation. Tax planners might, for example, allow tax deductibility of an insurance policy in direct proportion to the size of the deductible in the policy, the magnitude of the copayment chosen, or some other parameter of the policy, rather than keying specifically on the total premium.[29]

Tax-Exempt Premium Rebates. An alternative to taxation of insurance beyond some critical level would be to hold harmless the financial condition of those who currently benefit from the tax-exempt income status of health insurance premiums. To achieve this, tax planners could specify that premium reductions below some specific level could be returned to the employee as tax-free income if he took a lower-cost insurance policy. This technique would eliminate the subsidy to health insurance, while leaving the after-tax income of each person unchanged. By contrast, the taxation scheme would remove the subsidy, but would decrease after-tax incomes of individuals. If done correctly, the tax-rebate idea would not increase federal tax expenditures but would merely redefine the categories in which they were spent.

Operational complexities of a rebate scheme such as this, however, appear considerable. Would firms increase their coverage levels at the last minute in order to make available larger amounts of tax-free income for their employees? As with many ideas, this apparently simple plan contains many "unexploded bombs" that must be defused before the policy becomes safe for promulgation.

Issues of Noncomparability. As simple concepts are set forth to alter the tax treatment of health insurance, complexities and puzzles invariably surface onto the debate. If tax policy incorporates some sort of limits or caps, should they vary by region of the country? By urban/rural distinctions? By family structure? How should they change through time? How should such changes be integrated, if at all, with the deductibility of medical expenses?

Regional variation. The issue of allowing regional variation in the structure of tax-exempt health insurance is fundamentally one of equity. If tax planners have decided, for example, that a deductible of at least $X is sufficient to induce appropriate price consciousness in all consumers, they must only select $X so that it appropriately affects the region of the country with the highest level of medical prices. Any area with lower medical prices will find that deductible larger—compared with medical prices—and hence more of an incentive to shop for lowest prices, curtail demands, etc. (Of course, carried to extremes, this would suggest that no insurance be specified as tax-exempt.)

At the other extreme, one would allow for regional variation in the amount of insurance eligible for tax-exempt status to account for differences in medical costs—for example, using the same percentile of medical expense distributions across all regions.

Family variation. The concept of using percentile-equivalents as a basis for establishing an equitable tax treatment of insurance immediately suggests modifications for family structure. Two issues arise. First, is it fair to large families to allow income exemption for premiums of only a certain amount, when large families face larger total premiums? Second, for income tax treatment based upon per person limits (for example, deductibles), should tax planners account for intrafamily cor-

214

relations of medical expenses when establishing parameters for "allow-able" health insurance plans? Just as one might pick, say, the twenty-fifth percentile across regions, one might pick a deductible structure that allowed tax exemption for any plan that captured at least the twenty-fifth percentile of the size-conditioned distribution of family medical expenditures.

A number of potential complications arise from such tax treatment. For openers, family structure is notoriously difficult to define in general. The tax system's basis of definition, though useful for many tax pur-poses, does not necessarily match well how families spend money on medical care. The option to file tax returns on either an individual or a family basis, for example, would complicate the issue of how to treat premiums for a family policy. How should tax law treat families that reconfigure during the tax year? One simple solution would be to treat the family the same as for other tax law—that is, its constitution on the last day of the tax year. As with other tax issues, incentives posed to individuals and families, in the face of "simple" administrative solutions, may produce unintended results.

Updating through time. Tax planners must also consider how to update the tax treatment of health insurance through time. The issues are far more complex than merely adjusting for changes in a general price level, or for specific medical care costs. All of these issues arise whether the planners want to keep things constant in real terms or to deliberate changes in the level of tax-exempt insurance.

First, should financial levels in the tax treatment of health insur-ance change through time on the basis of a general CPI or a medical price index? The CPI keeps things constant in real terms and seems an automatic candidate for that reason. If tax reformers wish to miti-gate price increases in the medical market, however, indexing the tax treatment of health insurance in some ways to the medical component of the CPI may provide better self-correction in the system. If planners choose initially a deductible of $200 for a tax-exempt plan, for example, then tying that deductible to the medical component increases it faster when the relative price of medical care rises.

A more troublesome issue arises from technical change in medicine. Even though technical change is small in any given year, its cumulative effect can radically disrupt past notions of normal medical practice and its attendant financial consequences. The most obvious arena for this is in the scope of benefits of a standard tax-allowed policy. Is ambula-tory care for illness to be included and, if so, by what sorts of providers? Are treatments by paraprofessionals covered? Should the tax treatment of health insurance encourage use of paraprofessionals? In part, the

215

answer may depend upon one's beliefs about whether paraprofessionals are substitutes or complements for other types of medical care. (The same issue arose in early debates about the desirability of full coverage of ambulatory care versus inpatient care.)

Changing technology can alter the shape of the frequency distribution of medical expenses so that, even if an allowed deductible of $X is updated annually by the medical CPI, it might cut into the frequency distribution of expenses in quite a different location in the future than was contemplated when established. Suppose, for example, that $X were chosen initially to represent the twenty-fifth percentile of the medical expense distribution, and that tax law updated this level annually by the medical CPI. Since the CPI prices out a given bundle of services, technical change could readily move the updated $X deductible to the twentieth, fortieth, or any other percentile rank of future years' medical expense distributions.

Updating the $X by average medical expenses runs other risks. For example, if the frequency distribution becomes more skewed through time so that uncommon, larger expenses weigh more heavily in the average cost, the updated deductible of $X may increase more rapidly than policy makers desired.

An Incidence Issue: Does It Matter Who Faces the Tax Liability?

Past discussions about changes in the tax status of health insurance premiums focused on the individual's tax return, pointing toward declaration of health insurance premiums as taxable income to the employee. The tax incidence clearly falls 100 percent, or nearly so, on the employee.[30] More recent proposals, however, focus on the tax deductibility by firms for health insurance. Under such proposals, firms could not deduct as allowable business expenses the costs of any health insurance exceeding the standard policy defined by law. Such a standard policy could range from nothing at one extreme to the cheapest plan offered by any firm at the other.

Under simple models of labor markets, the incidence of such a tax could be expected to fall, in the long run, on the employee. The firm's willingness to pay for labor would not change with the redefinition of deductible expenses, but the net cost of labor would increase. Firms would reduce demands for labor, and labor would bear the tax burden, at least in the long run. Important differences can emerge, however, at least in the short run.

First, since health insurance policies are a fixed cost per worker, firms would substitute overtime labor for more workers, until new equilibria could be reached. The results would compare with those

216

arising from mandated health insurance for workers, a common part of recent proposals for national health insurance. Recent studies show that mandated national health insurance of "moderate" levels (for example, as proposed by Presidents Nixon and Carter) could temporarily increase unemployment by several percentage points in some industries.[31] The extent to which tax changes could precipitate the same phenomenon would depend largely on the magnitude of increase in after-tax cost of workers, plus any mitigating changes in treatment set forth in the law to phase in the change. Unlike the issue of mandated national health insurance, the proposed tax change would have its largest effect on those firms now with high levels of insurance, whereas small firms with little insurance would be relatively unaffected.

Second, tax increases imposed on firms may be mitigated or eliminated by recent changes in corporate tax law that, in effect, allow them to sell tax losses to those firms with increased tax liability. These provisions of the tax law appear, however, to be under substantial pressure for revision or elimination, so their long-term consequences may be trivial.

Third, tax liability on an employer is of no consequence if the employer faces no positive tax rate. To this extent, employees of not-for-profit corporations and of federal, state, and local governments would comparatively benefit from a change in tax law placing health insurance premium liability on employers. Setting aside issues of horizontal equity, an important number of employees would not face incentives to purchase less health insurance. Since about one-fifth of the U.S. labor force works for government or not-for-profit employers, the choice of placing tax liability for insurance premiums on employers could significantly reduce the overall effect on health insurance coverage and its attendant effects on health markets.[32]

Other Tax Changes: The Tax Deduction for Medical Expenses

The previous discussion focused on proposed changes in tax policy affecting health insurance premiums. Still other proposals have suggested modifying the deductibility of health expenses to increase price sensitivity and price awareness in medical markets. The best evidence suggests that modifying the tax deductibility of medical expenses—to make them less subsidized—would not significantly affect medical markets.

Two steps lead to this conclusion. First, most Americans have considerable health insurance coverage, particularly for large (hospital) expenses. For small expenses, insurance covers only a little of the cost; for larger expenses, however, private health insurance appears to cover approximately three-quarters of all health care costs.[33] This occurs because (1) many policies contain deductibles, effectively eliminating coverage for small expenses, and (2) because coverage for hospital care —invariably a large expense when it occurs—is nearly universal and quite comprehensive.

Second, under current law, consumers may deduct medical expenses exceeding 5 percent of the adjusted gross income (AGI) of the household.[34] After such a deduction, the effective coinsurance rate (the proportion paid by the patient) is $(1 - t)$, where t is the marginal tax rate. Thus, the IRS health insurance plan already has a large deductible and a very large coinsurance, relative to commercially available plans. For those few persons without hospitalization insurance, the IRS plan really does not eliminate patient incentives to shop carefully for care, although it does blur them somewhat. For those who do have health insurance, the IRS plan pays only on the out-of-pocket expenses remaining after the initial plan. As such, because of the 5 percent of income limit, only a few patients are further affected by the IRS plan. For example, a patient with a standard major medical insurance, with a $200 deductible and a 20 percent copayment rate, and with a family income of $20,000, would have to spend $600 out of pocket before the IRS plan paid anything. This would require actual medical expenses of $2,000 above the deductible (to accumulate $400 in addition to the $200 deductible). Even then, with a marginal tax rate of, say, 30 percent, the IRS plan would reduce the effective copayment rate of the individual from 20 percent (the major medical plan rate) to 0.7 x 20 percent = 14 percent. Individuals with higher income would face a higher marginal tax rate, but the out-of-pocket expenses would rise proportionately with income before any deduction could be taken. A person with $40,000 annual income, must spend $1,200 out of pocket before the IRS plan pays anything. A $200 deductible plus $5,000 of direct expenses ($1,000 paid by the individual) would qualify, but even then the effective copayment rate would still not substantially differ from the original major medical plan's 20 percent.

These sorts of calculations illustrate, but do not prove, the stated hypothesis—that is, changing the 5 percent of AGI limit would have little effect on medical markets. The reason, in summary, is that such a change would affect only a few people, and for them the change in effective marginal copayment (in private health insurance plans) would be small.

This conclusion is reinforced by the observation that more and more private health insurance plans contain "stop-loss" or "catastrophic coverage" provisions, limiting the out-of-pocket payments of individuals to some fixed dollar amount—for example, $1,000 to $2,000.[35] For persons with such insurance provisions, raising the 5 percent of AGI floor on deductible medical expenses would be irrelevant. The private plan would have dropped the copayment rate to zero for most individuals before the IRS plan would ever enter, even with a 5 percent limit. Raising that limit to, say, 7 percent of AGI would produce no change in patient incentives, except for a few special areas of treatment such as psychotherapy or major dental work such as orthodontia.

In addition, proposed policy changes might reduce or remove the deductibility of individually paid premiums. Ironically, the better the individual's privately purchased insurance, the less likely he will have out-of-pocket expenses exceeding 5 percent of AGI, and hence the less likely he will benefit from this second type of deduction. Clearly, complex interactions occur between income, medical expenses, and health insurance premium payments, making it difficult to understand fully the consequences for medical market demand from changes in the IRS plan health insurance policy.

Summary and Concluding Remarks

Tax subsidies to health care have accounted for a large part of effective health policy for many decades. Continuing and apparently uncontrollable increases in resource use and prices for health care now lead some health policy makers to question whether to continue these subsidies. In particular, policy makers question the general subsidy of health care and health insurance that arises from treating health insurance as tax-exempt income.

Proponents of a more competitive health care sector foresee two gains from increased taxation of health insurance premiums. Increasing the price of insurance to consumers should reduce insurance coverage and therefore reduce demand for health care, hence reducing pressure on the delivery system and reducing prices, or at least their rate of increase. More price-consciousness among consumers should also lead to better exchange of information among health market participants, thereby enhancing (according to some theories) the competitiveness of health care markets.

Increased taxation of health insurance policies poses grave uncertainties in outcomes, despite the apparent attractiveness of this vehicle for controlling medical costs. Perhaps most important, available knowledge cannot predict the dimensions of adjustment of health insurance policies that might follow a general tax increase. How much consumers might change the scope of benefits, deductibles, copayments, internal limits, or other dimensions of coverage seems unknowable from existing studies. At a larger scale, movement of consumers into alternative health care/insurance systems such as HMOs, IPAs, and other cost-controlling organizational settings could generate still larger changes in the health care market. Yet each of these potential changes could cause substantially different effects on health care markets and costs.

Efforts to tailor consumer responses more carefully—for example, by specifying a standard insurance package, with additions to its coverage being taxable income—add other potential complexities. Should the definition of a standard package vary by region, by family size, or by other characteristics? How should such a package change through time? Tax planners must face these issues before they attempt to grandfather some base level of tax-exempt insurance into a new law. Yet, without some such grandfathering, the political feasibility of achieving a tax law reform to combat health cost increases seems remote: The increase in income taxes arising from a straight removal of the tax-exempt status of health insurance would amount to $23 billion per year in 1982 dollars. This figure seems unlikely to pass muster in the Congress, unless the budget deficit becomes so prominent in politicians' minds that novel revenue sources become viable political alternatives.

Casual choices for complex tax issues likely will introduce important unforeseen complications into both the tax law and the functioning of medical markets. Caution and further analysis will pay large dividends.

Notes

1. The proportion of hospital beds provided through tax-exempt private firms varies considerably through time. Currently, proprietary hospitals account for 11 percent of the nongovernment hospital beds in the United States.

2. Some other fringe benefits maintain tax-exempt or partial tax-exempt status, but they are rare. Life insurance contributions are tax-exempt only up to a maximum coverage. Vacation pay is taxable. Sick leave benefits are generally tax-exempt, as are payments from disability income. But all of these benefits, except vacation, serve to subsidize medical care even further than the straight exemptions discussed above.

3. For example, the donor may derive pleasure from the favorable publicity surrounding his gift. Further, tax law makes such donations deductible, so the individual is paying only a fraction of the cost of his donation, with the Internal Revenue Service paying the remainder. On the other hand, charitable donations may be undersubscribed even if health care is a merit good, because individual B can gain pleasure from knowing that individual X consumes medical care financed by individual A. The tax-deductible status of charitable donations offsets, at least in part, any potential undersubscription to medical charities from this problem.

4. Although repealed by the Twenty-first Amendment, the experiment of

prohibition may have been the most effective public policy ever devised for increasing the health and safety of the population. Perhaps only tobacco consumption has been more broadly implicated in producing deleterious effects on the consumer. Interestingly, until the Sixteenth Amendment, which authorized income taxes, was ratified in 1913, the primary source of federal revenue was excise taxes on alcohol and tobacco.

5. See Charles E. Phelps, *The Demand for Health Insurance: A Theoretical and Empirical Investigation,* R-1054-OEO (Santa Monica, Calif.: The Rand Corporation, 1973); Jan P. Acton, "Demand for Health Care among the Urban Poor, with Special Emphasis on the Role of Time," in Richard N. Rosett, ed., *The Role of Health Insurance in the Health Services Sector* (New York: National Bureau of Economic Research, 1976). An important exception to the unanimity surrounding this belief would be Professor Milton Roemer, who concluded that decreases in health coverage, particularly for ambulatory care, deter people from using medical care until they become substantially more ill, thereby requiring hospitalization, and thus increasing overall medical use. See Roemer et al., "Copayments for Ambulatory Care: Penny Wise and Pound Foolish," *Medical Care,* vol. 13 (June 1975), pp. 457–66.

6. For a fine summary of this literature, see Joseph P. Newhouse, "The Demand for Medical Care Services: A Retrospect and Prospect," in Jacques van der Gaag and Mark Perlman, eds., *Health, Economics, and Health Economics* (Amsterdam: North-Holland, 1981).

7. Joseph P. Newhouse et al., "Some Interim Results from a Randomized Controlled Trial in Health Insurance," *New England Journal of Medicine,* vol. 305 (December 17, 1981), pp. 1501–7.

8. Joseph P. Newhouse, "The Structure of Health Insurance and the Erosion of Competition in the Medical Marketplace," in Warren Greenberg, ed., *Competition in the Health Care Sector: Past, Present, Future* (Germantown, Md.: Aspen Systems Corporation, 1978).

9. For a good discussion of the pertinent issues, see Paul B. Ginsburg, "Altering the Tax Treatment of Employment-Based Health Plans," *Milbank Memorial Fund Quarterly/Health and Society,* vol. 59, no. 2 (1981), pp. 224–55.

10. I do not share this belief. In general, inflation is not caused by increases in the relative prices of some commodities. Inflation is a monetary phenomenon. The only way in which a given commodity's production could contribute to the causes of inflation would be if the resources used to produce that commodity were suddenly used less efficiently. Real output would then fall for the same level of resource use, which would truly add to inflation. This does not seem to be an important aspect of the health care sector.

11. Some persons object to the phrase "tax expenditure" on the grounds that it presumes the government has a right to receipt of the income tax and has decided to "spend" it. I adopt the customary phrase without entering into the political debate over the philosophy of income taxation.

12. Congressional Budget Office, *Containing Medical Care Costs through Market Forces* (Washington, D.C., May 1982).

13. Martin Feldstein and Elizabeth Allison, "Tax Subsidies of Private Health Insurance: Distribution, Revenue Loss and Effects," in *The Economics of Federal Subsidy Programs*, pt. 8, A Compendium of Papers Submitted to the Subcommittee on Priorities and Economy in Government of the Joint Economic Committee, 93rd Congress, 2nd session, July 1974, pp. 977–94.

14. Bridger M. Mitchell and Charles E. Phelps, "National Health Insurance: Some Costs and Effects of Mandated Employee Coverage," *Journal of Political Economy*, vol. 84, no. 3 (1976), pp. 553–71.

15. See Alain Enthoven, *Health Plan* (Reading, Mass.: Addison-Wesley, 1980); Newhouse, "The Demand for Medical Care Services"; and Martin Feldstein, "The Welfare Loss of Excess Health Insurance," *Journal of Political Economy*, vol. 81, no. 2, pt. 1 (March/April 1973), pp. 251–80.

16. See, for example, Feldstein, "The Welfare Loss of Excess Health Insurance."

17. See Charles E. Phelps, "Demand for Reimbursement Insurance," in Rosett, ed., *The Role of Health Insurance in the Health Services Sector;* and Phelps, *The Demand for Health Insurance.*

18. Still further, eliminating the subsidies may raise the apparent price of some medical services by eliminating the masking effects of the subsidy that hid the true resource costs of the services. Exposing true price is a "good"; nevertheless, there might be the appearance of increased prices, just the opposite of at least one major intended effect of the policy change.

19. See Phelps, *The Demand for Health Insurance*; Phelps, "Demand for Reimbursement Insurance"; H. E. Frech III, "Market Power in Health Insurance, Effects on Insurance and Medical Markets," *Journal of Industrial Economics*, vol. 27 (September 1979); Gerald S. Goldstein and Mark V. Pauly, "Group Health Insurance as a Local Public Good," in Rosett, ed., *The Role of Health Insurance in the Health Service Sector"*; and Martin Feldstein and Bernard Friedman, "Tax Subsidies, the Rational Demand for Insurance and the Health Care Crisis," *Journal of Public Economics*, vol. 7 (1977), pp. 155–78. A dissenting estimate can be inferred from Victor R. Fuchs and Marcia J. Kramer, *Determinants of Expenditures for Physicians' Services in the United States, 1948–68* (New York: National Bureau of Economic Research, 1972).

20. As noted above in footnote 5, an important exception to this belief is found in Roemer et al., "Copayments for Ambulatory Care." But substantial evidence to the contrary exists. See Jay Helms, Joseph P. Newhouse, and Charles E. Phelps, "Copayments and Demand for Medical Care: The California Medicaid Experience," *The Bell Journal of Economics*, vol. 9, no. 1 (Spring 1978), for a summary of pertinent literature. For strong evidence that the "Roemer effect" does not work as he initially hypothesized, see Newhouse et al., "Some Interim Results from a Randomized Controlled Trial in Health Insurance." The consequences for health status of the insured population are still under investigation.

21. Suppose that there are two types of buyers—insured and uninsured—and that the insured buyers are much less sensitive to price than the unin-

sured buyers. Then a seller, desiring to raise his price, faces the trade-off of losing price-sensitive customers. It would seem, from this way of framing the question, that not only would the relative numbers of insured and uninsured buyers in the market be important, but also their comparative elasticities of demand, the effects of any spatial monopolies on pricing, and the role of advertising.

22. Alan Schwartz and Louis Wilde, "Competitive Equilibria in Markets for Heterogeneous Goods under Imperfect Information: A Theoretical Analysis with Policy Implications," *The Bell Journal of Economics*, vol. 13, no. 1 (Spring 1982), pp. 181–93; Schwartz and Wilde, "Intervening in Markets on the Basis of Imperfect Information: A Legal and Economic Analysis," *Pennsylvania Law Review*, vol. 127 (1979), pp. 630–82.

23. Kenneth J. Arrow, "Optimal Insurance and Generalized Deductibles," *Scandanavian Journal*, 1974, pp. 1–42.

24. James Lubitz, Marian Gornick, and Ron Prihoda, "Use and Costs of Medicare Services in the Last Year of Life" (U.S. Department of Health and Human Services, Health Care Finance Administration, Office of Research and Statistics, September 21, 1981; mimeographed).

25. Ibid.

26. See Richard Zeckhauser, "Medical Insurance: A Case Study of the Tradeoff between Risk Spreading and Appropriate Incentives," *Journal of Economic Theory*, vol. 2, no. 1 (1970), pp. 10–26; Kenneth J. Arrow, "Welfare Analysis of Changes in Health Coinsurance Rates," in Rosett, ed., *The Role of Health Insurance in the Health Services Sector*.

27. The welfare loss from health insurance increases with the elasticity of demand for the insured medical service.

28. See Harold Luft, "Assessing the Evidence on HMO Performance," *Milbank Memorial Fund Quarterly/Health and Society*, vol. 58 (Fall 1981), pp. 501–36. But all of the studies Luft reviewed face potential contamination by self-selection of unusually healthy (or unusually sick) people into prepaid plans. If so, the differences he observes would not carry over to a general population. Data from Rand's Health Insurance Study will provide estimates from a randomized trial, available by 1983, that should avoid this problem.

29. In effect, an insurance policy is a bundle of many characteristics. Pricing the policy becomes an exercise in "hedonic prices," much like pricing automobiles of various characteristics. If the hedonic prices are known, tax policy could also establish changes in the relative prices of the various dimensions of the insurance policy directly. This whole approach to altering tax treatment of insurance would seem quite complicated, particularly given the lack of specific knowledge about the benefits of a particular tax policy.

30. See discussions and references in Mitchell and Phelps, "National Health Insurance."

31. Ibid., and Charles E. Phelps, "National Health Insurance by Regulation: Mandated Employee Benefits," in Mark V. Pauly, ed., *National Health Insurance: What Now, What Later, What Never?* (Washington, D.C.: American Enterprise Institute, 1980).

32. Alain Enthoven is the source of this insight.

33. Charles E. Phelps, "Statement of Charles E. Phelps, Ph.D.," in *National Health Insurance—Implications,* Hearings before U.S. Congress, House of Representatives, Committee on Interstate and Foreign Commerce, Subcommittee on Public Health and Environment, 93rd Congress, 2nd session, 1974.

34. Recent congressional action raising the cutoff from 3 percent to 5 percent should provide a small experiment to test the accuracy of this discussion.

35. But even these policies often contain upper bounds of insurer liability —for example, $250,000.

12

Administrative Problems with Proposals for Health Care Reform

Sean Sullivan with Patricia W. Samors

This chapter considers administrative issues arising from the possible enactment of a competitive health care proposal. For illustrative purposes, and because it is the most comprehensive proposal, H.R. 850, introduced by Congressman Richard A. Gephardt (Democrat, Missouri), is discussed here because it embodies the procompetition approach to reform of the health care financing and delivery systems. Other proposals are also discussed, however, especially S. 433, introduced by Senator David Durenberger (Republican, Minnesota).

The first part of the chapter summarizes the significant sections of H.R. 850. Then the issues are discussed under eight topical headings: qualification of plans; limits on tax-free employer contributions; employee refunds; tax credits; Medicare reform; Medicaid reform; deregulation; and impact on small business. A summary and conclusions make up the final part of the chapter.

Synopsis of H.R. 850—Gephardt Bill

The Gephardt bill would make sweeping changes in the health care delivery and financing system, using a combination of regulation and incentives to promote a more competitive market for health care services and thereby to restrain increases in health care costs. The most important features of the bill are summarized as follows:

1. Employer contributions for health care can be excluded from employee income only if the employee joins a qualified plan, and then only up to a specified dollar ceiling (exclusion limitation amount). (*a*) The exclusion limitation amount is determined by average federal Medicare expenditures for a transitional period, and then by average premiums paid to qualified plans in the same health care area and for

the same actuarial category. (*b*) Current or guaranteed levels of benefit contributions above the exclusion limitation amount are "grandfathered."

2. Employees who select qualified plans with premiums that are less than the employer's maximum contribution amount for all plans receive the difference in tax-free cash refunds (up to a limit). (*a*) The refund is available only to employees who choose qualified plans. (*b*) Employers' maximum contribution amounts must be equal for all plans.

3. Plans are qualified by the Secretary of Health and Human Services. (*a*) Qualified plans must provide specified basic health care services, allow open enrollment (subject to limits on the number of high-risk people), establish a single annual premium for each actuarial category in each health care area, and limit out-of-pocket expenditures for a member to a fixed amount determined by the secretary. (*b*) Qualified plans must also be certified as financially able to meet their obligations to their members by a Health Benefits Assurance Corporation (HBAC) established within the Treasury Department. The HBAC also administers a fund to ensure delivery of benefits to enrollees of bankrupt plans.

4. Self-employed people and people whose employers do not contribute to health plans for them are given a tax credit equal to the premiums they pay for membership in a qualified plan, up to the exclusion limitation amount. (*a*) The credit is approximately equal to the government's tax subsidy to workers whose employers contribute to their health plans. (*b*) The credit is refundable to the extent it exceeds the individual's tax liability.

5. Medicare recipients who elect to do so receive direct health care contributions in the form of vouchers from the Secretary of Health and Human Services, to be applied to the premium of the qualified plan of their choice. (*a*) During a transitional period the amount of the voucher is determined by average per capita Medicare expenditures; thereafter, it is determined by average premiums paid to qualified plans in the same health care area by those in the same actuarial category. (*b*) Individuals making the election are assured of the basic services and catastrophic coverage required of qualified plans. They are also eligible for tax-free refunds if they choose plans that cost less than the amounts of their vouchers. (*c*) Once more than 50 percent of Medicare recipients have elected to receive direct contributions, the existing Medicare program under Title XVIII of the Social Security Act is discontinued.

6. After the competitive system envisaged by the bill has had a few years to become established, states can choose to opt out of the Medicaid system. (*a*) The Secretary of Health and Human Services issues vouchers to low-income people (determined according to appli-

cable poverty guidelines and adjusted for regional cost-of-living differences if the secretary so decides) in the states that so choose. The vouchers equal the sum of average premiums paid by members of qualified plans in the same actuarial category in the same health care area plus average out-of-pocket expenditures incurred by those members. They may be applied to any qualified plan in the area. (*b*) States that opt out of Medicaid must contribute to the cost of health care for low-income people an amount equal to their 1981 expenditures under their Medicaid plans, indexed for inflation. These states are not eligible to receive any payments under Title XIX of the Social Security Act.

7. All federal and state laws that require review of providers' expenditures, of their services, or of the prices they charge are repealed and/or preempted. (*a*) The bill eliminates the Professional Standards Review Organization (PSRO), uniform reporting, capital expenditure limitation, and hospital utilization and bylaw provisions of the Social Security Act, and amends the customary charge limitation and reasonable cost provisions. (*b*) The bill also substantially abolishes the health maintenance organization (HMO), health planning, and health resources development provisions of the Public Health Services Act, and modifies the Hill-Burton Services provision. (*c*) The bill seeks to replace economic regulation of health care delivery with the restraints imposed by competitive forces. Reasonable cost reimbursement—a prime element of federal regulation—would be replaced gradually with the private market system of prospective premiums as Medicare and Medicaid recipients opted for inclusion.

Administrative Issues Raised by H.R. 850

The rest of this chapter describes the administrative burdens and dilemmas that would follow passage of the Gephardt bill and suggests possible ways to handle some of them. The existing system, however, already contains a complex regulatory apparatus (HSAs, PSROs, etc.), much of which would be dismantled if the Gephardt bill were passed. And without a market reform bill of some kind, the likely alternative response to the continual cost spiral is more "command and control" regulation of the sort represented by the ill-fated Carter hospital cost-containment bill. The Gephardt bill is a blueprint for comprehensive change, and criticizing particular features of such a sweeping proposal is easier than putting one together in the first place. Gephart's bill is only slightly less comprehensive than Alain Enthoven's Consumer Choice Health Plan and would be a meaningful reform proposal even in a whittled-down version.[1] So it is necessary to weigh his scheme for restructuring incentives in the health care marketplace against the likely alternatives to such "structured" competition even while indicating problems with it.

Qualification of Plans. The Gephardt bill and several other so-called procompetition bills require health care plans to be "qualified" in order for employer contributions to them to retain their tax-free status for employees. The qualification procedure under Gephardt imposes new burdens on both the government and private insurers.

The Secretary of Health and Human Services (HHS) is assigned the principal role in determining whether a plan is qualified. He must act on plan applications within thirty days of receipt and provide written explanation and opportunity for a hearing to applicants whose plans he does not approve. Before the secretary can approve a plan, however, a newly created Health Benefits Assurance Corporation (HBAC) must certify that the plan is financially sound enough to meet its obligations during its initial year. In order to do this, the HBAC—which would be located in the Treasury Department—must tell HHS what information it needs to make its determination, get the information from HHS, and notify HHS and the applicant within twenty days of receipt of the application by HHS. This arrangement seems unnecessarily cumbersome, and could be made less so either by locating the HBAC at HHS or by having the secretary make the judgment of financial soundness himself. This would reduce intragovernmental paper work and place full responsibility for qualifying plans in the department that has been assigned most of it anyway.

That responsibility grows heavier with the charge to issue regulations defining "medically high-risk individuals" and specifying the factors to be used in determining whether a plan would have a disproportionate number of these people compared with other plans in the same health care area. Health care areas are also to be defined by the secretary, based on Office of Management and Budget (OMB) designations for urban areas within Standard Metropolitan Statistical Areas (SMSAs) and his own judgment, given a list of criteria for nonurban areas. The secretary must then approve any limitation on the number of such high-risk people that a plan must accept if he deems it necessary to prevent the plan from suffering unfairly from such risk selection vis-á-vis its competitors.[2]

Under the Gephardt bill, the secretary is also given the onerous task of reviewing brochures of all qualified plans for conformance with the bill's information requirements. He must then prepare pamphlets stating the terms of all qualified plans in each health care area and distribute them annually to all eligible people. Given the importance assigned by Enthoven and others to information disclosure, this burden may be unavoidable; given the numbers of people, health care areas, and plans, it is also enormous.

In addition to qualifying plans, the secretary is responsible for disqualifying them. Any disqualification would have to be made within twenty-one days of receiving notice of a change in the plan's basic services or out-of-pocket expenditure limits that puts it out of conformity with the bill's standards. He must also disqualify a plan that violates the antitrust provision of the bill, which prohibits any plan sponsor from sponsoring more than one qualified plan in any health care area. Because a violation of these provisions is also made a violation of the Sherman Antitrust Act, the Justice Department or the Federal Trade Commission (FTC) presumably becomes involved as well. As with the earlier over-lapping roles of HHS and Treasury, it makes better sense to locate all authority for carrying out a particular responsibility in one place. In this instance, either the Justice Department or the FTC seems better qualified than HHS to deal with antitrust questions.[3]

The list of chores to be performed by health plans seeking qualification is formidable. In their applications, plans must show that they meet the bill's requirements to provide specified basic health care services, allow open enrollment of all eligibles in their health care areas (subject to limits on the number of defined medical high-risk people), set annual premiums at the start of the plan year that are the same for all people in each actuarial category in each health care area, and limit members' maximum out-of-pocket expense to the "maximum permissible financial participation amount" determined by the secretary. Plans must hold general enrollment periods and, under certain conditions, accept members at other times as well. The open enrollment requirement guards against risk selection by plans that do not want to insure high-risk people; conversely, plans can get the secretary to limit the number of high-risk people they must accept, to protect them against excessive adverse risk selection. These provisions aim to assure that the higher-risk population in each health care area will be able to get health insurance, and that risks are spread fairly among the qualified plans in the area. The tax incentive provisions of the bill may, however, generate more adverse selection than the secretary can handle under the qualification provisions, necessitating a further scheme of risk pooling.

Plans must report annually to the secretary their number of members and the premiums they are charging each actuarial category in each health care area. This places a heavier burden on insurers offering plans in many areas. They must also report any proposed reductions in covered health care services or in out-of-pocket expenditure limits, so that the secretary can determine if they still meet the requirements for qualified plans.

The most detailed, and perhaps most vexatious, reporting requirements concern the brochures that plans must file each year with the

229

secretary. These brochures must contain a long list of items, including services to be provided, methods of provision, rules for out-of-pocket expenditures, premiums to be charged, etc. As noted earlier, the secretary must approve these brochures by determining that they contain all necessary information and do not contain any misleading statements. Burdensome as these requirements may be, reformers stress the importance of consumers having good information in order to make rational choices.

The Gephardt bill also requires the plans to report to the new HBAC. They must provide whatever financial information it requires to conduct its reviews of their financial status. Beyond this merely procedural requirement, though, is an obligation to contribute a per capita payment to the HBAC, to go into a protective fund. The fund is to be used to meet a plan's obligations to its members for the rest of a plan year if it should fail. This provision puts insurers and the government in the guarantor business—hardly a new one for either, but potentially entailing large administrative costs if plan failures exceed expectations. Even if they do not, the fund is an added cost of doing business for qualified health plans. Given the risks involved in establishing a new plan and making it viable, consumers may need such assurance to choose these plans over "safer" established insurance plans.

The bill imposes another new administrative burden on health plans. They must provide the right to arbitration for individuals with unresolved grievances—either over denial of membership in a plan or over terms or conditions of the membership agreement. The bill does not mention costs, but it is likely that plans would bear them—adding further to the cost of doing business.

The qualification requirements of the Gephardt bill are detailed enough to impose definite burdens on regulator and regulated alike. Some burden is probably unavoidable, because any scheme to develop a more competitive marketplace for health care will involve at least a modicum of regulation—of "product" quality, if nothing else.

Many believe that this bill involves more than a modicum of regulation. The minimum required benefits package eliminates any market for lesser coverage. Enthoven, explaining his Consumer Choice Health Plan, which the Gephardt bill comes closest to representing, thinks that a minimum benefit provision is necessary to limit plans' opportunities for preferred risk selection and consumers' opportunities for free riding—buying minimal insurance when well and switching to more comprehensive coverage when sick. The Gephardt bill tries to handle the former problem by requiring qualified plans to offer annual open enrollment periods, but this aggravates the latter problem—which would be better met either by allowing individuals to switch plans less frequently or by "penalizing" them in some manner for switching too frequently. This would lighten the administrative load on both HHS and the plans as well as reduce the opportunities for free riding without vitiating the open enrollment principle. In this regard, under the Federal Employees Health Benefits Plan—probably the closest existing system to the kind contemplated by the bill—only about 6 percent of federal employees switch plans during the annual open season.

The language of the bill is not clear about how employer self-insurance arrangements are to be treated under the qualified-plan concept. Health Insurance Institute statistics suggest that nearly 20 percent of all health insurance coverage is in this form—up from only 5 percent as recently as 1975. The Health Insurance Association of America, the trade association of large commercial insurers, estimates that more than 25 percent of all group health benefits are self-insured. And a survey of more than 500 companies by Hay Associates shows that nearly 40 percent are either self-insured or combine self-insurance with some degree of commercial coverage. (Hay surveys mostly large firms, which are more likely to self-insure.) If self-insurers are required to become qualified plans under the bill, they may lose most of the advantages they currently enjoy. The Employee Retirement Income Security Act (ERISA) exempts them from all state regulation of insurance plans, enabling them to avoid premium taxes and reserve requirements; this exemption would presumably continue. But if the Gephardt bill means that self-insurers must offer the minimum benefits package and catastrophic coverage on an open enrollment basis to nonemployees in their health care area while their own employees are free to enroll in other plans, then self-insurance becomes impractical.

The Durenberger bill specifically allows for self-insurance as one of its three required options, but the Gephardt bill leaves the question unanswered. Given the extent of self-insurance, it is likely that big companies will not meekly accept its elimination. It could probably survive the minimum benefits requirement, but would have to be exempt from open enrollment and, consequently, from risk pooling outside the experience group. This raises another knotty issue concerning risk selection. Self-insurers exempt from open enrollment could have a significant cost advantage over health plans in their health care areas if their employee groups were relatively healthy, and much of the intent of the bill could be defeated by a further rush of employers into self-insurance to escape its reach. This could leave qualified plans holding a large bag of high-risk people. If employees were free to join other plans, however, and if there were more attractive plans in the area—because of either better benefits or lower premiums that would allow employees to receive refunds—the cost advantage might disappear.

And if an employee group were relatively unhealthy, the healthier members would probably find more attractive plans—and leave their employer with its own problem of adverse selection.

Employers, whether they would continue to self-insure or not, would all have to bear some burden of administering the general open enrollment periods for their employees. Although their responsibilities would not be so great as those of the government in administering open season for federal employees (because HHS would bear part of it), they would have to keep track of all the plan switching in order to direct their contribution to the plan of each employee's choice. Of course, companies have to do this now, but in most cases they are dealing with one insurer and, perhaps, a federally qualified HMO. In the new environment, they could be dealing with many more plans, which would complicate their job.

Unlike the Durenberger and Hatch bills, the Gephardt bill does not require employers to offer a multiple choice of plans. Instead, it takes them out of the decision-making process entirely by allowing their employees to choose any qualified plan available in the area. They are required to make their contributions to whatever plans their employees choose, creating the potentially large administrative burden just discussed. Some analysts would not go directly to a wholly consumer-centered health care system, as the Gephardt bill does, but would leave the employer some choice about how many and which plans to offer its employees. Employers would still be moved to offer multiple choice by their employees' desire for options that would allow them to receive tax-free cash refunds, but they would retain some control over the size of their administrative load by not having to offer every qualified plan in every area where they have employees. One analyst would put a maximum as well as a minimum limit on the number of plans an employer could offer. The burden of informing employees about all the plans offered could then properly be switched back from the Secretary of Health and Human Services to the employers, because only they would know just which plans they were offering to employees in each area.

A final administrative creature of the Gephardt bill is a U.S. Health Court and Health Court of Appeals. The Health Court is to have jurisdiction over all civil claims and disputes arising under the bill, as well as the power to appoint a receiver to administer any plan that it has determined to be unable to meet its obligations for the rest of the year. The Appeals Court, of course, is to hear all appeals from the Health Court. Constructing a special judicial system for a program that is supposed to be an alternative to command-and-control regulation seems contrary to the spirit of the promarket reforms. It is difficult to imagine that the very existence of such a legal apparatus would not encourage its use. This would add to the costs of health insurance with very little likelihood of producing any substantial offsetting benefits other than to the legal rather than the medical profession.

Limits on Tax-Free Employer Contributions. The Gephardt bill, like the Durenberger bill, the Hatch bill, and most other procompetition approaches, imposes a ceiling on the amount of an employer's contribution to a qualified plan that will not be taxed as income to an employee (if the plan is not qualified, the entire contribution becomes taxable income to the employee). The Gephardt bill's method for determining this exclusion limitation amount, however, is more complex than the method employed by either the Durenberger bill or the Hatch bill.

Under the Gephardt proposal, responsibility for making the determination belongs, again, to the Secretary of Health and Human Services. During the first three years after the bill takes effect, the exclusion limitation amount is the average per capita expenditure for an aged individual under Medicare during 1981, adjusted for inflation. Under this bill a separate calculation is made for each health care area, so that regional differences in medical costs are accounted for, whereas they would not be under a single national limit. After the first three years, the limit is the weighted average premium for qualified plans selected during the previous general enrollment period by people in the same actuarial category and health care area, again adjusted for inflation. Making the Medicare calculation for the first three years is burdensome enough, although it can at least be done by manipulating data that already exist somewhere. But HHS would have to develop a whole new data base before it could make the calculations of weighted average premiums of all qualified plans by actuarial category and health care area. This would be a major task in itself.

Simplicity and equity often collide in the design of new regulatory schemes. A single national tax cap, as proposed in the Durenberger bill, would be much simpler to administer. That bill would establish a first-year limit of $125 per month for family coverage, effective in 1984 and indexed for inflation in succeeding years. Such a cap would eliminate the need for HHS to build a data base and make calculations for all the health care areas every plan year. It would also simplify matters for employers with multiple locations, who under the Gephardt scheme would have to keep track of separate contribution limits for each health care area in which they operate and identify any taxable amounts on employee W-2 forms. In sum, the administrative simplicity of a national cap makes it appealing to employers and HHS alike.

The problem with a national ceiling is that it would discriminate against employees in high medical cost areas and those in higher-risk actuarial categories by allowing employees in lower-risk categories and those in low medical cost areas to purchase more generous tax-free benefits. This equity problem can be dealt with only by sacrificing simplicity and varying the cap by region and actuarial group, as the Gephardt bill does.[4]

Regional and actuarial differences in tax caps would also create administrative complications for the Internal Revenue Service (IRS). A single national cap would be easy for the IRS to check against tax returns. Many different caps, however, would require the IRS to check returns by health care areas.

Another problem with the contribution limit arises from the variety of mechanisms now used by employers to price and finance employee health benefits. In some instances, employers would find it difficult to determine an accurate monthly cost per employee. Employers who self-insure either fully or partly may not know what their true insurance costs are; they know only that they are saving money by avoiding state insurance taxes and regulations. In such cases, it would be difficult to calculate the amount of the employer's contribution for health benefits and, therefore, to determine employees' tax liability, if any. It may prove necessary for someone—probably the IRS—to develop rules for calculating the value of employer contributions in such situations.

Refunds. Employees who choose health care plans with premiums that are less than the maximum amount their employer contributes toward the premium of any health plan are entitled to cash refunds that are tax-free up to an amount that is the lesser of $500 (indexed for inflation between 1981 and the applicable year) or the difference between the employer's maximum contribution and the exclusion limitation amount.

The Durenberger bill also offers refunds, but taxes them as income. The refunds are to be paid by the employer, who is assigned the administrative chores of developing a data base for tracking employees' choices of plans and calculating both the amount of any refund to which they are entitled and the amount of the refund, if any, that is taxable. The IRS's role with respect to employer contributions was discussed earlier. It will also have to develop a data base and programs for checking the tax status of employee refunds, a task that is complicated, again, by having separate tax caps for each actuarial group in each health care area.

Tax Credits. The Gephardt bill seeks to end the unfair tax treatment of people who purchase their own health insurance. It establishes a tax credit in the amount of the premium paid to a qualified plan up to the applicable exclusion limitation amount set by HHS for the person's health care area and actuarial category. If a person's tax credit exceeds his tax liability, he is eligible for a refund. This accords such people the same tax treatment given employees whose employers make contributions for them. The IRS will presumably have to administer the credit itself, using the same data base as for the employer contribution limitation and the employee refund provisions.

Medicare. Reform of the Medicare system is part of the Gephardt scheme. Each person eligible for Medicare may elect to take, in lieu of any benefits under Title XVIII of the Social Security Act, a health care contribution in the form of a voucher from the Secretary of Health and Human Services. The secretary is to set the amount of the contribution for the first three years equal to the average per capita Medicare expenditure for the aged and disabled categories in 1982, adjusted for inflation. In succeeding years the amount is to equal the weighted average of the premiums of qualified plans selected by members within each actuarial category in a health care area during the prior year, adjusted for inflation. These calculations are the same as those made to determine employers' exclusion limitation amounts, and they do not impose any additional burden on HHS.

The bill's ultimate aim is to phase out entirely the existing Title XVIII Medicare program. This would happen when HHS determines that more than 50 percent of Medicare eligibles have elected to receive the direct contributions in lieu of their normal Medicare benefits. Eliminating the Medicare program with its voluminous regulations would confer an administrative blessing on HHS which administers them and on hospitals and physicians that must comply with them. William Hsiao studied the comparative cost of administering the Medicare program and the Federal Employees Health Benefit Program, which has some features similar to the system that the Gephardt proposals would try to establish; he found Medicare administrative costs to be about 25 percent higher.[5]

People who elect to receive the voucher may present it to qualified plans in their health care areas as full or partial payment of the plan's premium for individuals in that actuarial category. If the face value of the voucher exceeds the applicable plan premium, the individual is entitled to a refund of the difference. Plans are required to accept the vouchers as payment from individuals they enroll, and they are entitled to present them to HHS with information on the individuals' actuarial categories and health care areas and to receive payment of the amounts specified on them.

Medicare beneficiaries are given two kinds of incentives to opt for the vouchers in place of their present benefits: (1) they will be assured of limits on out-of-pocket expenses—catastrophic coverage that qualified plans must provide but that is lacking under Medicare; (2) they can receive tax-free refunds if they choose plans with premiums that are less than the amounts of their vouchers. It is not certain, of course, that 50 percent of Medicare eligibles will respond to these incentives, and HHS could end up running the Medicare system indefinitely. Also, another form of adverse selection could operate to take the healthier Medicare eligibles out of the system and leave it with the costlier ones. This could defeat the objective of getting Medicare costs under control, an important concern for the federal government.

But the burden of running a voucher system alongside the current Medicare system is small, and an effort must be made to bring Medicare within the new system if health care reform is not merely going to redistribute costs between the private and the public sectors. This could happen if the Gephardt incentives selected out many younger, healthier employee groups into prepaid health plans, but left the aged, disabled, and needy to drive up costs even faster in the fee-for-service and cost-reimbursement sector. Walter McClure believes that the chances for getting Medicare recipients to switch are enhanced if initial attempts are concentrated in areas where the competitive market is developing successfully.[6] A gradualist approach could be implemented by starting with demonstration projects in selected areas. The political process, however, is more likely to attempt Medicare reform before anything else. Unless a broader private market is established first, however, there would probably not be enough health plans around to choose from, and those that did exist would not be seeking high-cost enrollees from Medicare.

Medicaid. Medicaid reform is delayed under the Gephardt bill until four years after the rest of the bill goes into effect. States can opt out of the existing Medicaid system, in which case they receive no federal payments under Title XIX of the Social Security Act and they agree to maintain the same level of contribution to health care for Medicaid eligibles as they did in 1981, adjusted for inflation. Thus, a state could choose to freeze its real Medicaid expenditures at the 1981 level.

Eligible individuals in states that make this election are entitled to direct health care contributions in voucher form if their incomes do not exceed the income poverty guideline applicable to their states under Title II of the Community Services Act of 1974. The Secretary of Health and Human Services may make adjustments in these income poverty guidelines if he determines that differences in the cost of living among the states necessitate them.

The secretary must also determine the amount of the health care contribution, which is to equal the sum of the weighted average of premiums paid to qualified plans in the same health care area by members in the same actuarial category during the previous year's enrollment period and the average out-of-pocket expenditures incurred in the second previous plan year by those members, this sum to be adjusted for inflation. Qualified plans must accept health care vouchers toward payment of their "adjusted" premium for the individual's actuarial category and health care area. This adjusted premium equals the plan's premium for other members plus the average out-of-pocket expenditures those members are projected to incur during the year. The purpose of this provision is to provide these low-income people with full dollar coverage. Plans then submit the vouchers to HHS for payment, but they are entitled only to the amount of the adjusted premium if it is less than the voucher amount. If a plan so elects, it can share any savings from lower than projected out-of-pocket expenditures with the government in exchange for the government's sharing of higher than projected out-of-pocket expenditures.

The Medicaid proposals would bring the poor into the new health care marketplace with fully subsidized purchasing power, if the states so choose, whereas the choice for the aged and disabled rests with Medicare recipients themselves. Some states might decline to participate because they would be given increased responsibility for the cost of nursing home care, but many would probably regard this as a reasonable trade for freezing other Medicaid costs (in real terms) and freeing themselves from their present administrative burdens at the same time. These burdens would be shifted to HHS, which would have to run the voucher program, but there could be a net reduction in the overall government administrative burden.

Deregulation. The Gephardt bill wipes out a sizable chunk of the existing regulatory setup, in keeping with its promarket slant. It takes the federal government out of the business of promoting and regulating HMOs, and also preempts any state regulations that would interfere with the establishment of alternative delivery systems—such as prohibitions against the corporate practice of medicine and requirements of state qualification of health plans. It also scraps the local health planning apparatus and leaves providers free to respond to the market forces that it hopes to stimulate. This prospect is unsettling to payers, insurers, and providers alike because it would replace familiar mechanisms for cost containment with unfamiliar mechanisms of a competitive marketplace. It also raises issues of possible conflict with the authority of the states to regulate the activities of insurers and providers.

The administrative burdens of complying with the requirements of

237

earlier federal laws would, of course, be eliminated as well, to be replaced by the various burdens imposed by the Gephardt bill itself. Some detractors of the bill object that in the name of the free market it imposes more regulation on the health care industry than exists now. The bill does not establish a compulsory scheme of national health insurance with the associated regulatory apparatus of the command-and-control model proposed by Senator Edward Kennedy (Democrat, Massachusetts), but it does embody a comprehensive national approach to establishing the private market as the model. To do this, it sets the rules for all the market participants, which entails a new set of regulations with a new set of burdens—chiefly for employers, plan sponsors, and the government. Hospitals, however, come away with a lighter administrative load than they bore under the old rules.

The Gephardt bill does one other thing to promote fair competition by setting the same ground rules for every one; the bill eliminates the advantage that Blue Cross/Blue Shield plans enjoy in half of the states —their exemption from premium taxes imposed on commercial health insurance plans. This step would not lower anyone's costs directly— indeed, it would raise costs for the Blues—but it could lower costs indirectly by enabling commercial plans to compete more effectively in areas that the Blues now dominate.

Small Business. Special mention must be made of the problems that enactment of the Gephardt bill would cause for small business. Neither the Gephardt bill nor the Durenberger bill requires any employer not contributing to employee health insurance before to do so now (the Hatch bill does have such a requirement and is thereby a compulsory health insurance bill for employers). Any employer who is contributing to employee insurance would, however, have to meet the requirements of the bills. Although the Gephardt bill does not require an employer to set his maximum contribution amount at any particular level, it does require him to administer the open enrollment provision for his employees. The cost of doing this would be more difficult for a small business to absorb, and for some it might even mean the difference between staying in business or not being able to offer any health benefits at all. The experience with pension benefits under ERISA may be instructive here.

Small businesses also experience a high rate of employee turnover, in part because they employ many seasonal and part-time workers and secondary wage earners. The bill's provision for continuity of coverage —requiring continued employer contributions up to ninety days after termination of employment—could impose heavy costs on many marginal businesses and even threaten their survival.

The bill's requirements may have to be eased for businesses below a certain size, or of a certain nature—for example, businesses that are seasonal in their operations. Employees of such businesses could be partially covered by the tax credit provision.

Summary and Conclusions

The Gephardt bill would try to reform the entire health care system, reestablishing it on a single basis of individual consumer choice instead of its present dual basis of group purchase for those who are employed and Medicare/Medicaid for the elderly, disabled, and poor. It would change the dominant financing mechanism from retrospective cost reimbursement to prospective fixed premiums for a defined set of basic benefits, thereby putting providers at risk and giving them incentives to deliver health care services more efficiently. Consumers would be given double incentives to choose the most economical providers: first, by taxing employer contributions to health care plans above a certain dollar limit as income to employees; second, by rewarding the choice of plans costing less than the limit with tax-free cash refunds. Government and employers would share the burden of administering this scheme for employees. The bill would also place those who purchase their own health insurance on an equal footing by providing them tax credits equivalent in value to the income exclusion for employer contributions. Finally, it would use vouchers and the same tax incentives to lure Medicare recipients out of the old cost-reimbursement system, and it would offer to states other incentives to pull out of Medicaid and let the poor be brought into the voucher scheme as well. If everyone responded, there would be a single market for health care, with consumers offered choices of qualified plans. Whereas other bills such as Durenberger and Hatch would mandate a choice of at least three separate plans in each area, the Gephardt bill would rely on the demand-side incentives to elicit the supply-side response needed to make competition viable. McClure is not so sanguine about the prospects for such a self-generating response. He suggests that federal financial help in the form of temporary tax incentives or limited grants and loans for targeted development of alternative delivery systems may be needed to get the competitive reaction going.[7] Gephardt eschews any such financial involvement.

These changes would be sweeping, although the participants are given time to prepare themselves (the bill would become effective January 1, 1984). Many analysts would prefer to make the changes in increments rather than all at once. Either way, they raise two overriding administrative concerns—the procedural issue of complexity and the structural issue of adverse selection.

Any of the procompetition proposals would create administrative burdens, but the Gephardt bill introduces the most complexity. Much of it arises from the decision to set a different employer contribution limit for each actuarial category in each health care area, meaning that there would be hundreds of different limits for HHS, for employers with multiple locations, and for the IRS to keep track of in administering the tax-related provisions of the bill. The opposite model of simplicity—sacrificing some equity—would be the Durenberger provision for a single national limit. Other possibilities were discussed, but the issue remains critical to the administrative feasibility of the Gephardt bill.

The other principal concern is the degree of regulation introduced by the elaborate apparatus of the Health Benefits Assurance Corporation and the Health Court; this could be administrative overkill in the name of consumer protection.

Notes

1. Alain Enthoven, *Health Plan* (Reading, Mass.: Addison-Wesley, 1980).

2. This adverse selection problem is discussed in chapter 10 of this volume: Sean Sullivan and Rosemary Gibson, "Tax-Related Issues in Health Care Market Reform."

3. The issue of antitrust action against collusive provider efforts to block competition is considered in chapters 15 and 16 of this volume: Clark Havighurst, "The Contributions of Antitrust Law to a Procompetitive Health Policy," and William Kopit, "Health and Antitrust: The Case for Legislative Relief."

4. This issue is discussed further in chapter 10 of this volume: Sean Sullivan and Rosemary Gibson, "Tax-Related Issues in Health Care Market Reform."

5. William Hsiao, "Public versus Private Administration of Health Insurance: A Study in Relative Economic Efficiency," *Inquiry*, vol. 15 (December 1978).

6. Walter McClure, *Comprehensive Market and Regulatory Strategies for Medical Care* (Excelsior, Minnesota: Interstudy 1979), p. 198.

7. Ibid., p. 197.

Part Four

Federal Policy Reform:
Regulatory and Legal Issues

13
Health Care Delivery and Financing: Competition, Regulation, and Incentives

Rosemary Gibson and John B. Reiss

State and federal regulations have affected significantly the development of competition in the health care delivery and financing system. In this chapter, we explore the extent to which both existing and proposed regulations could inhibit the realization of the basic goals embodied in the proposed procompetitive legislation. We also examine the extent to which the proposed bills may inadvertently stifle the competitive incentives they are trying to stimulate because they impose an alternative regulatory framework. We analyze the proposed health care reforms to see whether they complement, supplement, or are inconsistent with existing regulations. The state and federal regulations highlighted for discussion are illustrative rather than exhaustive.

The thrust of this chapter is to analyze a broad variety of state health care regulations, evaluating modifications that may need to be made in order to breathe life into a market-oriented health care cost containment strategy. The current organization of the health care market —and the body of government regulations governing the actions of market participants—often encourages insurers, providers, and consumers to ignore cost considerations. The system's stimuli have encouraged competition on the basis of quality and quantity of health services. The procompetition proposals, however, envision service price competition among providers and premium competition among insurers (both called price competition hereafter). The thrust of the proposals is to alter existing incentives and encourage providers to reduce costs for a given quality or enhance quality for a given cost and make consumers cost sensitive. Specifically, the proposals intend to:

• Encourage *consumers* to be cost conscious in their purchase of insurance. Changes in the current open-ended tax subsidy are expected to affect insurance coverage, deductibles, and copayments.

• Encourage *insurers* to offer differentiated products by requiring employers to offer a choice of plans with various premium and benefit levels.

• Encourage insurers to bear down on *providers* to offer services that are competitive on the basis of price as well as quality. Fixed-dollar employer contributions and vouchers for public program beneficiaries (with employee and beneficiary supplementation for any additional cost) are designed to force insurers to exercise cost control over providers.

One of the current health care reform proposals, H.R. 850, offered by Congressman Richard A. Gephardt (Democrat, Missouri), also attempts to alter the existing incentives in the health care delivery and financing system by changing current state and federal regulations. Section 302, for example, would preempt "any provision of law, regulation or administrative action of State or unit of local government which prevents or impedes the reforms of the health care delivery system implemented by the program created." Thus, through preemption, H.R. 850 implicitly recognizes that various state statutes and regulations are barriers to competition. The potential scope of preemption implied, and the difficulty of deciding how far it should extend, have not been addressed.

To develop a competitive health care market, the necessary ingredients include a sufficient number of buyers and sellers so that each buyer or seller is a "price taker." For market participants to be price takers, three general requirements exist:

• free entry and exit of capital, labor, and other resources to and from the relevant market

• knowledgeable buyers who can assess the benefits of the product they are purchasing

• sensitivity of consumer purchases to the price of the good or the service

To assess the effects of federal and state statutes and regulations (both being law) on the establishment of price, product, and quality competition in health care markets, it is useful to see how such laws affect these and related aspects of a truly competitive market. For discussion purposes, state and federal laws are organized according to their effect on consumers' demand for, and suppliers' provision of, health care services.

244

State and Federal Laws Affecting the Demand for Health Care Services

The demand for care is affected in a number of ways by the procompetition legislation. H.R. 850, for example, would establish minimum benefit requirements, which might be raised (or lowered) over time thereby increasing (or decreasing) coverage and hence the use of health services. At the same time, the bill would truncate tax subsidies related to the purchase of health insurance, which is expected to reduce the use of medical services.

Under existing public programs—Medicare, Medicaid, CHAMPUS, Veterans Administration, and others—the demand for health care services is determined by eligibility requirements, the scope of benefits offered, and the extent of cost sharing. Under H.R. 850, the elderly could elect either to choose benefits of plans offered by the competitive system or to continue under the existing Medicare program. With vouchers or a less regulatory approach than is currently in use, demand would be determined by eligibility for, and the value of, the vouchers—including any limits established for this use. The poor would be included "after the competitive system has become well-established, and if a State so elects, [under] a direct contribution equal to the average health care expenditure in the area."[1] Since the latter amount may be greater than the government is paying for its beneficiaries, some elderly and most of the poor probably would continue under systems comparable to the present. A crucial issue is whether uncovered care would be provided to those with inadequate coverage and, if so, who would pay for it.

Some of the existing laws relating to the demand for health services that would be affected by the procompetition proposals include those concerning access to services by low-income persons, consumer information, and health insurance regulation.

Access. A competitive model may create problems with respect to equal access to medical care. In the past, regulations have been developed to ensure that health care facilities are accessible to people who might otherwise have problems obtaining care. In part, the health planning regulations (particularly certificate of need) were developed to ensure more equal distribution of health care facilities by locating services in areas where economic demand might be too low to induce providers to undertake the necessary activities.

Other regulations used to ensure access are those associated with the use of federal funds—for example, the Hill-Burton free care and community service rules. The free care rules, rewritten to higher standards in 1979, require that a hospital or other facility that has received federal funds provide a certain value of free care to indigent persons in their service areas each year. Any institution that accepts federal funds also has been required to provide "community service," which means they cannot discriminate on any basis. Other federal rules affecting access include the provisions of the federal Civil Rights Act as well as certain provisions with respect to age. Among the most potentially costly requirements are the "access to the handicapped" regulations. Many states have adopted similar rules.

If competition alone is to govern access to health care, many of these rules that force providers to give "free" care will have to be eliminated. Consequently, some beneficiaries of these rules may be denied access. If the various rules requiring access regardless of ability to pay are maintained, facilities located near higher concentrations of needy populations will be placed at a competitive disadvantage compared with those not so located.

Information Flow. For competition to work effectively, potential consumers of health care services need to be informed fully about available medical treatments and their associated risks and benefits, other services available from different providers for treating the same health care problems, and the relative merits as well as all the costs involved. Federal and state rules governing the confidentiality and privacy of information and restrictions on advertising are all potential inhibitors of effective competition.

The rules forbidding access to information from Professional Standards Review Organizations (PSROs), reinforced by restricted interpretations of the Freedom of Information Act and similar statutes and regulations, severely inhibit the public's access to information about the quality of care provided by hospitals and physicians. The codes of ethics of various professions, which generally prohibit providing public information about the quality of care provided by those practitioners, normally have been sustained as legitimate private acts by the courts and have not been challenged by the government. All of this makes it difficult for consumers to exercise rational choice.

In competitive markets, the incentives on health care providers to restrict the availability of information concerning personal health status indicators—particularly differences in mortality and morbidity rates among institutional and individual providers—will be greater than the incentives to reveal that information, because of potential malpractice claims and for reasons of competitive advantage. Since the health care product, unlike other products, is unknown to consumers, the likelihood that service competition will work without such information is negligible. Even premium competition will be inhibited without such information.

Therefore, an important issue underlying the development of a competitive approach is the extent to which confidentiality and privacy laws will be repealed and the role government will play in enhancing the flow of medical and health information. Section 205(b) of H.R. 850 requires insurers to make reports on reductions of coverage and increases in cost sharing to the Health Benefits Assurance Corporation (HBAC). Whether HBAC could define the term "coverage" broadly and thereby force insurers to provide helpful medical information is doubtful. It is, however, the only statutory provision in H.R. 850 that offers any basis for making such information available.

Health Insurance Regulation

Several legislative proposals would cap the amount of an employer's contribution to a health plan that employees could exclude from income for federal tax purposes. Some of these proposals also would require employers to offer a choice of plans and allow employees who select low-cost health insurance to reap the savings. These proposals are attempts to encourage competition among insurers on the basis of premiums and benefit packages. Yet tax incentives and multiple-choice, while necessary to encourage competition, may not establish sufficient conditions for a more competitive insurance industry. Existing regulations may stop health insurers from competing on an equal footing.

The health insurance industry consists of two types of firms. Commercial insurers, which number about 300, constitute about half the industry. They include profit-seeking firms and mutual insurers. Blue Cross and Blue Shield (the Blues), often referred to as hospital and medical service corporations, make up the balance of the industry. The role of the Blues in the insurance industry has been discussed at length in the economics and legal literature.[2] H. E. Frech contends that, though the commercials are competitive, the Blues' organizational structure inhibits competition. "Assisted by the national associations, the firms collude on geographic market areas. Further, Blue Shield and Blue Cross plans for the same area rarely compete."[3] In some states the Blues have a relatively small market share, whereas in other states they hold 80 percent of the market.

Health insurance regulation was assigned to the states by the McCarran-Ferguson Act of 1945. Insurance regulations vary among the states and for categories of insurers: commercials, Blues, and self-insurers. Commercial insurers are subject to laws under the state insurance code, whereas the Blues generally are governed by special enabling legislation. The commercials and Blues are subject to financial and benefit requirements, whereas self-insurers, because of the Employee Retirement Income Security Act (ERISA) exemption, are not subject to state health insurance regulations.[4] Financial requirements include initial solvency requirements for the start-up of business, reserve requirements, limitations on the instruments in which insurers can invest, premium regulations, and premium taxes. Benefit requirements stipulate the extent of coverage and the providers who must be reimbursed for various categories of services.

Premium Taxes. A major difference in state treatment of the commercials, Blues, and self-insurers is the level of the premium tax. States impose varying premium taxes on commercial insurers, which are generally higher for foreign (out-of-state) companies than for domestic ones. Some states impose premium taxes on the Blues, whereas others require payments such as a flat fee per contract. In general, half of the states impose no tax on the Blues, whereas almost all of the states impose a tax of approximately 2 percent on domestic commercial insurers and a higher tax on foreign ones.

The anticompetitive impact of the premium tax differential has been documented in the economics literature. A 2 percent premium tax differential has been found to give the Blues cost advantages over the commercials—an advantage of more than 30 percent for Blue Cross plans and more than 20 percent for Blue Shield plans.[5] Moreover, the self-insurers, which are exempt from the premium tax, have a clear cost advantage. According to one estimate, premium taxes in California for one major employer amounted to $2 to $4 a month per covered employee, depending on the comprehensiveness of the plan.[6] These expenditures could otherwise be used to add a vision or drug plan or to reduce the employer contribution. Thus, a competitive system requires that all categories of insurers be taxed equally.

Reserve Requirements. Commercial insurers and the Blues must abide by reserve requirements designed to ensure that the companies possess sufficient assets to meet future insurance obligations. Premium reserves reflect liabilities for losses that have not occurred but for which premiums have been paid.

The states show little consistency in their treatment of reserves. Michigan, for instance, has not delineated premium reserve requirements for commercials, but has set a guideline of 12 percent of premiums as a reserve. Other states, such as Wisconsin, have an explicit requirement for computing premium reserves. In Illinois, the reserve requirements are the same for the commercials and the Blues.

Reserve requirements constitute a cost to the employer. "This cost results from the time lag between the date the premiums are collected from the employer and the date the claims are honored by the insurer."[7] Both the insurer and the employer earn interest on the reserve amounts. Since the reserves can total between 20 and 30 percent of annual premiums, the cost of reserves can be significant and can contribute to a competitive advantage for self-insurers.

Thus, a competitive system requires consistent treatment of the reserve requirement for all insurers.

Investment Regulation. State insurance codes often identify the type and volume of investments the commercials and Blues can make. Regulations regarding investment portfolios are generally the same for both. In Oregon, companies may not invest more than 10 percent of assets in common stocks. Other states prohibit companies from investing more than 20 percent of assets in corporate bonds or debentures.

Self-insurers, again because of the ERISA preemption, are not subject to investment regulation. As is true with reserve requirements, employers who self-insure may be able to accumulate better earnings from funds without restrictions on investment instruments. Consequently, these rules also need to be made consistent for all insurers.

Initial Solvency Requirements. State health insurance codes require insurers to deposit with the insurance commissioner all or part of the amount required in the solvency standard. These requirements vary widely among the states and by type of commercial company (stock or mutual). Massachusetts requires $100,000 capital for the start of stock companies only. In Michigan, stock and mutual companies must have $1 million of capital and a surplus of $500,000. In New York, mutual companies must have 500 applications with collected premiums amounting to $20,000 and an initial surplus of $150,000 to start business.

The Blues were established under special enabling legislation exempting them from the initial capital requirements applicable to commercials. States have set separate, less stringent requirements for the Blues. Illinois has initial capital requirements for Blue Cross of $1.5 million compared with $2 million for commercials. In Maryland, the Blues must have at least $100,000 of initial capital, whereas the commercials need $250,000. Michigan required $10,000 in initial capital for the Blues; that has recently been raised to $500,000, though it is being contested in the courts. The commercials are required to have $1 million in initial capital.

Although the requirements for the commercial insurers are clearly more stringent, the extent to which the initial solvency requirements inhibit commercial insurers from entering the market is unclear. As is true with reserve requirements and investment regulation, however, costs are incurred for funds that could otherwise be invested at higher earnings. Consequently, the advantage accorded self-insurers again is evident.

Premium Regulation. The commercials and the Blues are subject to different approval processes for the setting of premiums. States generally do not approve rates for commercials, although the filing of rate information is, or can be, required. In some states, insurance commissioners can reject an insurance policy premium if the plan's benefits are unreasonable relative to the premium charged.

The National Association of Insurance Commissioners (NAIC) has established benchmarks that most states apply to determine the reasonableness of the benefits and the premiums charged. Most states scrutinize rates for individual policies rather than group policies, because buyers of group insurance are believed to possess greater expertise in evaluating the premiums charged for given benefit packages. Some states, such as New York and West Virginia, have established specific standards for individual and group policies. In New York:

> These are generally in the form of loss ratios which measure the amount of premium returned to claimants in the form of benefits. In general, the standards require a minimum of 50 percent loss ratio for individual policies sold to persons under age 60 and 60 percent for persons age 60 or over.[8]

Unlike the commercials, the Blues normally are subject to a formal premium review process, although the criteria for rate approval are often only general. In Connecticut:

> No such corporation shall enter into any contract with subscribers unless and until it has filed with the insurance commissioner a full schedule of the rates to be paid by the subscribers and has obtained said commissioner's approval thereof. The commissioner may refuse such approval if he finds such rates to be excessive, inadequate or discriminatory.[9]

In Colorado, the premium review process has been used as leverage to alter the Blues' operations. When the Blues requested a rate increase, the state approved the increase in exchange for the Blues' scaling back the number of policy choices offered.

The extent to which premium regulation of the Blues affects the level and competitiveness of premiums in the health insurance industry is uncertain. Yet, the issue of creating incentives for competitive premiums becomes more pressing under the proposed legislation that establishes a federal premium-setting process.

Mandated Benefits. Many states impose mandated benefits on the commercials and the Blues, whereas self-insurers are exempt from such requirements. Generally, the trend in the states has been to expand the benefits that carriers must either offer or make available to consumers. An example of one of the fastest growing benefit areas is mental health, alcoholism, and drug abuse. During 1979, thirty-four new state laws were enacted requiring mandatory or optional coverage for such services.

Exemption from mandated benefit laws affords a competitive advantage for self-insurers and has created a further incentive for employers to self-insure.

> ERISA contains language specifically stating that ERISA preempts any State law or regulation covering employee benefit plans. To date, various court decisions would appear to indicate that such preemption applies to non-insured, but not insured benefits. That explains in large part the rush to non-insured plans which can take advantage of the ERISA preemption umbrella and write uniform multistate benefits.[10]

In addition to imposing mandated benefits, several states have enacted comprehensive or catastrophic health insurance coverage for individuals who otherwise would be unable to purchase private health insurance because of financial considerations or records of high utilization. In Connecticut, every carrier offering individual health insurance in the state must make available an individual comprehensive insurance plan to all residents who are not eligible for Medicare. Group insurers must also make available comprehensive group plans to all employers with three or more employees. In some states, the legislation specifies deductibles, copayments, and annual out-of-pocket limitations that must be observed for a plan to qualify as comprehensive or catastrophic.

In the case of Connecticut, the original legislation called for self-insurers whose plans cover three or more employees to allow those who terminate employment to convert to a traditional plan offering individual comprehensive health care. Because of court cases in Minnesota and Hawaii, however, which invalidated state laws that attempted to regulate self-insurance, Connecticut voluntarily withdrew the provision. In another instance, Connecticut tried to impose a premium tax on self-insurers that was determined subsequently to be contrary to ERISA. In the Hawaii case, the Hawaii Prepaid Health Care Act, which sets minimum benefit standards for employer health insurance plans, was found not to be applicable to the Standard Oil Company's self-insurance plan.

In other states, the law is vague. In Michigan, firms offering administrative services only (ASO) are not prohibited by law, yet there is no clear statutory authority for companies to engage in ASO contracts.

Consequently, legislation has been introduced in the state legislature specifically to authorize the use of ASOs.

As in other cases discussed, the ERISA exemption creates a competitive edge for self-insurance.

Proposed Legislation. A key issue in the procompetition debate is the potential impact of the proposed legislation on the growing self-insurance markets. H.R. 850 would preempt the McCarran-Ferguson Act to make health insurance regulation an activity of the federal government, in particular by using the Health Benefits Assurance Corporation. The regulatory framework to be established is especially important for what is not said about self-insurance. One issue is whether and to what extent self-insured employers should be required to participate as underwriters of pool coverage and to bear adverse pool experience. Without such a requirement, insurers argue that the incentive is for employers to self-insure to avoid bearing the costs of high-risk groups or individuals who elect pool coverage, thereby requiring insured employers to finance high-risk persons. Self-insurers argue that their reduced expenses arise from positive steps they have taken to reduce health benefit costs, not from selection factors. Self-insurers urge that aid to high-risk persons should be subsidized from broader revenue sources, not from a "surtax" on employee benefits through creation of pool coverage.

Another issue concerning self-insurance and two of the procompetitive proposals—S. 433, introduced by Senator David Durenberger, and S. 139, introduced by Senator Orrin B. Hatch—is whether self-insurers, who usually offer a single plan from one source, would be required to offer employees a multiple choice of plans. Such mandated provisions, it is argued, would legislate what self-insurers attempt to avoid—namely, higher administrative costs. Even with multiple-choice provisions, self-insurers would have a competitive advantage over traditional insurers if they continue to be exempt from regulation.

Under H.R. 850, the HBAC would "establish for each plan year for each health care area in which it is located, an annual premium for each of the actuarial categories without regard to health status or utilization of services." At the same time, the bill would preempt state laws that would "regulate or limit the premium or price charged." The extent to which federal premium setting would differ from existing state procedures is uncertain, though H.R. 850 requires HBAC to "establish . . . an annual premium" that is more stringent than current state laws providing for the approval of premiums. The degree to which the HBAC regulations would apply to self-insurers and allow for competitive pricing among insurers remains to be seen. Discriminatory taxes would be preempted by H.R. 850—that is, "any tax on the premiums charged by a qualified plan to the extent that it is greater than the tax imposed on other health insurance plans" would be eliminated. According to this provision, the Blues' premium tax advantage would be eliminated, though it is unclear whether self-insurers would be subject to premium taxes.

The HBAC would also "review once every three years the financial ability of each plan to fulfill its obligations to its members." It would "determine the amount of funds that may reasonably be predicted to be needed in each plan to fulfill the obligation." Issues arise about the kinds of reserve requirements and initial capital requirements that would be mandated in federal legislation to ensure financial soundness as well as to encourage new entrants into the insurance industry. Moreover, the degree to which self-insurance would be included in the proposed regulatory framework and the effect of proposed regulations on the growth of self-insurance is unclear.

A key issue in the procompetitive legislation is the effect of setting minimum benefit requirements for qualified plans. Although the initial benefit packages may include basic coverage that should be available to all, it is argued that "including a mandatory basic benefits provision in a legislative package designed primarily to stimulate more competition among insurers could, ironically, turn out to be an inadvertant, backdoor approach to a 'regulatory-style' comprehensive national health insurance program."[11] H.R. 850 illustrates this potential situation. The legislation defines basic health care services that could be expanded as a result of special interest lobbying. Indeed, the trend in the states to require more benefits and to reimburse new categories of providers could be replicated on the federal level. Encouraging competition may require legislation mandating clear descriptive language for benefits if it is likely to be harmed by mandated benefits.

In general, the ERISA exemption for self-insurers may have to be repealed if competitive markets are to be achieved. The existence of the exemption may, however, give corporations more leverage in the marketplace, which could assist "business coalitions" in developing effective market strategies for reducing health care costs.

State and Federal Laws Affecting the Supply of Health Services

Free Choice of Provider. A major thrust of the procompetition bills addresses the present system of payment for health services, which provides few incentives for consumers to choose the most efficient providers. According to Mancur Olson, there is "freedom to choose the most expensive of the available alternatives without having to pay extra."[12] In response to the absence of a payment mechanism that rewards the cost-conscious provider, the Hatch and Durenberger bills would require that consumers be offered a multiple choice of plans. With caps on the tax subsidy and multiple-choice offerings, insurers would be encouraged to contract with the most efficient providers in efforts to lower premiums to compete with other insurers. It has been speculated that attempts to limit coverage to services provided by only the more efficient providers would be prohibited by state provisions granting free choice of providers.

These free-choice provisions require third-party payers to pay licensed providers for services rendered in accordance with their lawful scope of practice and covered by an insurance agreement. In Utah, state law mandates "that the right of any person to exercise full freedom of choice in the selection of a duly licensed [provider] shall not be restricted."[13] Other states, such as Tennessee, have enacted less encompassing laws that prevent insurers from discriminating against specified categories of providers—for example:

> Whenever any policy of insurance issued in this state provides for reimbursement for any service which is within the lawful scope of practice of a duly licensed chiropractor, the insured or other person entitled to benefits under such policy shall be entitled to reimbursement for such services, whether such services are performed by a duly licensed medical physician or by a duly licensed chiropractor, notwithstanding any provision contained in such policy.[14]

There is a trend for states to require that insurers reimburse providers previously excluded. In 1977 and 1978, three states—New York, Maryland, and Louisiana—enacted statutes requiring payment of social workers. In 1979, nineteen states enacted free-choice provisions requiring payment for occupations such as nurse midwives and podiatrists. At least thirty states have enacted statutes allowing psychologists to bill patients or insurers directly. In New Jersey, employers are prohibited from excluding psychologists' care from insurance coverage if psychiatric care is covered. The expanded coverage requirements may partially explain why the number of psychologists involved in private health care practice increased 50 percent over the past five years.[15]

In some states, free-choice provisions are applicable to the commercials but not to the Blues. In Illinois and Colorado, where the Blues have been established to deal with providers directly, the state does not mandate that the Blues pay various types of providers as it does for the commercials. The absence of a free-choice statute does not preclude a patient from receiving benefits from a provider who has not contracted with the Blues, though payment by the Blues may be at a lower rate. The Blues point out that they have been ahead of state mandates in terms of expanding benefits and paying for new categories of providers.

254

Although free-choice provisions have prevented insurers from discriminating between physicians and other classes of providers, such as podiatrists, chiropractors, and osteopaths, it is questionable whether these state laws would permit insurers to contract with only the more efficient members of a providers' group. The ability of insurers to discriminate within a class is a linchpin of the procompetitive proposals.

The extent to which free-choice provisions would have a chilling effect on insurer-initiated cost containment is speculative at this point. The provisions could be read to guarantee the insured unrestrained free choice of a provider, thereby precluding the organization of closed-panel plans except under special provisions of state or federal law, such as for HMOs. In most states, however, the statutes provide that "the policy may not require that the service be rendered by a particular hospital or person."[16] These provisions have been interpreted to allow insurers to exclude physicians who do not abide by cost-containment efforts so long as some choice is left to the insureds. Whether the range of choice needed for state statutes is consistent with procompetition requirements has to be determined. Clarifying language could be added to state statutes to remove potential problems.

Occupational Licensing. Section 302(b)(2) of H.R. 850 provides an automatic preemption of state and local laws, regulations, or administrative actions which require that "various types of health care services be delivered only by specific categories of health care professionals." This provision recognizes the need for easier entry to, and mobility in, the health care occupations for a competitive system to take root.

Licensing of occupations is a state responsibility. State laws require that only licensed persons may practice the relevant professions. Applicants for licensure must fulfill criteria of education, experience, and competence.

Since the late 1960s, new health care occupations, including physician assistants, psychiatric social workers, and nurse practitioners, have entered the labor market. As these new health personnel have been trained (with the federal government having contributed more than $50 million toward their training by the mid-1970s), numerous state laws have been enforced that delineate their legal scope of practice and specify their market entry requirements.

Most states rely on independent licensing boards for each health care occupation. California, for example, has eleven different boards for the allied health professionals, resulting in a fragmented regulatory apparatus with little policy coordination. Several states, such as Minnesota and Michigan, have established agencies to coordinate the various boards. The trend toward coordination of licensing activities is illus-

255

trated by New York, which relegates licensing boards to an advisory capacity with state agencies performing the licensing functions.

A major function of the boards is to regulate market entry through licensure and to impose market exit through disciplinary procedures for unprofessional, incompetent, or irresponsible practice. In some states, the licensing boards lack sufficient resources to undertake vigorous disciplinary policy. Moreover, there is growing concern that the licensing boards are acting as defenders of the licensed occupation, not as supporters of quality health care.

A second function of the boards is to interpret and enforce the statutory scope-of-practice provisions for the health occupations. Some observers contend that the scope-of-practice issue is one of the most important facing state licensing boards and other public agencies concerned with regulating health care professionals. There is evidence of growing tension among the licensed occupations as each seeks to broaden its scope of practice at the expense of others and simultaneously to block the substitution of one profession for another. Consequently, some tasks that can be performed competitively by professionals with less training and skill are precluded from being performed by members of those professions.

Regulations defining the scope of practice for physician assistants illustrate the tension between the goal of preserving quality care and that of increasing access and lowering costs. Forty states have enacted statutes governing physician assistants, which define the scope of physician supervision, diagnostic competence, and prescribing power. Although specific services are designated as within the authorized scope of practice (and these vary from state to state), supervisory requirements often are not delineated clearly and differ widely from "over the shoulder" to "reasonable proximity." On an ad hoc case-by-case basis, state agencies and boards are responsible for interpreting the law.

The extent to which the restrictions and uncertainties explain physicians' reluctance to use physician assistants and other auxiliary health personnel is unclear. In eight states, the scope-of-practice statutes provide that physician assistants may perform only those tasks delegated to them by the physician with whom they work. Accordingly, the physician, rather than the state or licensing board, defines the scope of the assistant's activity. These statutes add to the liability of physicians who employ new health professionals. Nurse practitioners contend that some insurers refuse to sell malpractice insurance to physicians who hire them. When insurance coverage is available, the risks associated with hiring new health personnel are reflected in the cost. The actual effects of malpractice liability on inhibiting the use of new health professionals, highlighted by the delegatory statutes, remains to be seen.

256

States' definitions of the scope of practice have ramifications for federal reimbursement policy under Medicare and Medicaid. Medicare is reluctant to reimburse new health professionals, in part because state laws regarding the authorized scope of practice are so inconsistent. States set the tone for federal Medicaid policy, as illustrated by the Medicaid regulations permitting reimbursement of new health professionals licensed by a state.

Vague statutes, which may have chilling effects on the regulated, often are interpreted by protective licensing boards to inhibit health professionals from performing particular tasks. Specific regulations directly inhibit the substitution of one kind of health care provider for another. Both activities block competition among occupations. Indeed, a broader issue in occupational licensing is the extent to which restrictions on the use of ancillary health professionals may frustrate the development of innovative delivery systems staffed by such providers.

Quality Controls. In attempting to promote adequate care for patients, various jurisdictions have established controls purporting to ensure the delivery of high-quality care to patients. At the federal level, the major relevant rules are the Medicare "conditions of participation." States' licensing statutes often include similar requirements. According to H.R. 850, "nothing contained . . . in this Act shall be construed to preempt a State or local subdivision therein from taking an action, whether by law, regulation or administrative determination, which is intended to and does in fact promote the quality of health care services, personnel, equipment or facilities." Do the preemption requirements of H.R. 850 apply to these rules? How is the promotion of quality care "in fact" to be measured?

The Medicare regulations have many sections that set standards for the governing body of institutions, require various committees, establish academic and other qualifications for personnel, and specify detailed requirements ostensibly designed to ensure quality care for patients. These rules have never been tested to see whether the criteria established actually result in better patient care. The rules are developed by consensus seldom related to factual bases. These rules, by establishing qualifications for personnel, limit entry into those markets and protect the status of those already engaged in the relevant technical areas because they include grandfathering provisions. The rules are based on process standards because "outcomes cannot be measured." There is rarely a demonstrated relation between the process standards and the outcomes for patients. The benefits are seldom known, though frequently believed.[17]

Examples of the requirements include that the "circulating nurse" in an operating room must be a registered nurse (RN). Recently, the Department of Health and Human Services (HHS) attempted to change the rule so that a person with appropriate technical training could fulfill those activities. The opposition from the nursing profession and others persuaded the department to withdraw the proposed change. Clearly, requiring an RN to circulate is far more expensive than using some lesser-skilled individual. Although the opposition to the change was couched in terms of the care for the patient, some people with expertise in the area claimed that the change would not alter the quality of care. In fact, there is no evidence on either side of the issue. Restricting the activity to RNs raises the cost and creates for them a monopoly market position.

A similar result occurred for the "nursing home conditions of participation" requirement that, if a nursing home did not have a registered dietician as an employee, it had to have a dietary consultant. This led to the creation of an entirely new industry of dietary consultants. When HHS attempted to rescind the requirements in the proposed 1980 amendments, the dietary consultant industry opposed the proposed changes so vigorously that the department withdrew them. There is no evidence that the requirement for dietary consultants results in better care for patients. It has, however, created a new class of "health" professionals with an interest to protect.

The states have developed rules for the Medicaid program and for other patients in hospitals and nursing homes that are similar to the conditions of participation. New Jersey, for example, has highly detailed rules about the number of hours of care to be given nursing home patients. Although these may be valuable in eliminating or reducing abuse, there is little current evidence that the benefits outweigh the costs. Certainly, that issue has not been studied objectively, and the necessity for such rules has not been established without question.

Building Codes and Fire and Life Safety Codes. Building and fire and life safety codes have been established by federal, state, and local governments to ensure the safety of physical environments. The existence of these standards limits market entry and inhibits the potentially desirable consequences of encouraging competition. The costs of these standards must be weighed against the benefits associated with improved safety. Do the preemption requirements of H.R. 850 apply to these rules?

When the Hill-Burton construction program was developed by the federal government, comprehensive building requirements were established for facilities funded by that program; these requirements have become more detailed over the years. The Hill-Burton code has been adopted by many states, with and without modifications, and has been applied to the construction of all health facilities. Other building codes

258

exist at the state and local levels, which have inconsistent standards. Building codes frequently have criteria inconsistent with those of the fire and life safety codes.

The underlying principle has been that, because many patients in hospitals are relatively immobile, they have to be given considerable protection. This is a sound principle, but in practice the protection may have been carried well beyond the point where added costs are justified by commensurate benefits. Frequently, parties with a self-interest in construction have developed these standards. Building standards committees generally have included architects, building component manufacturers, fire safety officials, and others with a vested interest in the construction of the buildings and in improving safety, no matter what the cost. Cost-effectiveness studies of the code standards developed have never been undertaken. Without doubt, these standards have been effective in eliminating multiple death fires in hospitals. The question is whether such fires could have been reduced or eliminated at significantly less cost. Meanwhile, the cost for new construction of a hospital bed now exceeds $120,000. The magnitude of the costs has to deter new entries into the marketplace.[18]

Many standards for which there is little evidence of justification are found in the "minimum requirements of construction and equipment for hospital and medical facilities." Standards include the rate of transfer of air in operating rooms, currently required to be twenty times per hour, whereas it may be that twice per hour would be sufficient to keep infection rates at current levels.[19] A gratuitous rule specifies the height of windows above the floors and below the ceilings. More important are the costly requirements of massive fire-resistant walls, floors, and ceilings.

Hospitals tell innumerable stories of conflicts between building and fire inspectors regarding the location of fire extinguishers in elevator shafts. Such levels of detail in rules governing fire safety and construction are likely to add little to patient safety; they certainly raise costs and thereby reduce opportunities to compete.

Limits on Product Availability. Various drugs and devices are prohibited by either the Food and Drug Administration (FDA) or state rules on grounds that they lack medical safety and efficacy. Few advocates of competition have proposed that restrictions on the availability of products as they relate to medical safety and efficacy should be abandoned, even though the ultimate logic of a competitive model is that consumers, having been given full information on the subject, should be able to choose to purchase any goods and services.

One limit on product availability already discussed is the refusal of insurers to pay for certain services on behalf of program beneficiaries or

259

insurance policy holders. Other limits relate to the licensing statutes for health personnel. If certain products or services are provided by people with particular skills, and such persons are not allowed to provide them under the health practice acts of various jurisdictions, the product or service will not become available.

H.R. 850 proposes that minimum insurance benefits be established by the HBAC. If HBAC makes determinations concerning products for which insurers must (or must not) make payment, it will establish product availability. This may be accomplished either by financial limits or by direct exclusions. The effect of benefit policy on the development of new medical technologies could be significant.

Certificate of Need. Certificate-of-need (CON) statutes have been enacted by all states except Louisiana. H.R. 850 proposes to repeal the Health Planning and Resources Development Act of 1974, which required the states to enact CON statutes. Such repeal would eliminate the federal requirements (already much modified by the Omnibus Budget Reconciliation Act of 1981) but not the state statutes. Because the latter do restrict market entry, hospitals and other existing providers in many states will fight to keep the state statutes in place. As states have to accept more of the financing burden for Medicaid, and other health and welfare programs, they will be looking for any method to reduce those burdens and may decide CON is a valuable tool.

CON was developed initially to control capital expenditures by health care facilities. Because many people believed that health care facility purchases of new plant and equipment were not constrained by the payment system, direct controls on such expenditures were deemed necessary. Although several states (New York, New Jersey, and Massachusetts among them) had developed statutes well before the federal government became involved, most CON statutes have been adopted as a result of the Health Planning and Resources Development Act.

The CON statutes vary in detail from state to state, but all have to meet minimum federal requirements promulgated by the Secretary of Health and Human Services under the Public Health Service Act (Title XV, section 1532). These include review of all new institutional health services and of any capital expenditures for equipment or plant exceeding $150,000 (raised to $500,000 by the 1981 Reconciliation Act). The sanction for noncompliance is withdrawal of various federal health funds from the state.

Only state governments, however, have the authority to invoke the regulatory powers needed to implement CON programs.[20] State sanctions for noncompliance with CON laws range from injunctive relief to withholding of licenses or payment for services.

CON removes capital investment decisions from the immediate power of the potential investor and allows other groups, acting through the power of the state, to limit the extent of capital investment taking place. Since the system relies on agencies having broad interest group representation, the investment decisions cease to be market decisions and become subject to the many different motivating forces that affect the interests of those participating in the decision-making process. It is inherent in the decision-making process and in the nature of the planning agencies that the interests of existing facilities are protected. The agency's task is to limit expansion, hence entry. Because of the different interests in the various states, entry controls are likely to differ. Indeed, the distribution of proprietary hospitals, with their heavy concentration in the South and West and almost complete absence in highly regulated states, indicates that different entry patterns do exist. Product differentiation and diversification of production methods possibly also are caused by attempts to avoid the effects of CON rules.

CON may have limited the effect of the present perverse financing incentives that seem to foster more and more spending. If price-competitive payment systems are established, however, CON will inhibit their success in allocating resources to reflect market forces.

Planning Rules. A number of states have developed, in addition to CON, a series of "planning rules" that set standards for developing particular services. These rules may be implemented through the CON or state rate-setting processes.

New Jersey, for example, established a series of planning rules to promote the regionalization of various health care services to reduce their cost and improve their quality. These include neonatal intensive care, cardiac catheterization, cardiac surgery, burn centers, and other specific services. One aspect of the rules required that certain levels of activity for a covered service had to be met before a CON would be considered for any change in that service. In many instances, the rules require that existing services be reviewed to determine whether they should be allowed to continue. These rules tend to inhibit competition in the sense that they restrict the entry of providers doing "small" numbers of procedures. However, they may enhance competition between "large" producers and thus be consistent with procompetition proposals. Such rules raise the issue of how procompetitive proposals will ensure that price and premium competition will not produce unacceptable reductions in quality of care not necessarily subject to malpractice complaints.

The principles underlying the planning rules relate to both the quality of care and its cost. Thus, the cardiac surgery rules were developed with the assistance of many cardiologists and cardiac surgeons

261

in the state. That, in itself, raises questions about the market-limiting activity involved. The standards eventually agreed upon included the requirement that at least 150 procedures a year must be undertaken in a facility before it could continue to perform heart surgery. Various standards were required relating to staffing patterns, equipment requirements, and other aspects of the provision of the service. Because the state was responsible for setting reimbursement rates for Blue Cross and Medicaid (at the time the rules were developed, now for all payers), these rules were enforced by the ability to withhold payment for the service involved.

The rules were developed in an environment in which most any service delivered to a patient was paid for by the relevant third-party payer. The theory underlying the rules was that patients were in no position to judge either the adequacy or the cost of the service being made available. Acting on behalf of the consumer, the state in cooperation with interested parties developed standards to overcome the consequences of both the lack of consumer information about quality and the failure of the market to respond to differences in the cost of delivering the care.

The existence of such rules in a price-competitive system might inhibit institutions from responding to relevant market forces. If the competitive system provides consumers with adequate information about quality and cost, and if they are faced by economic incentives that make them weigh the cost of the service against other uses of their income, the existence of planning rules might inhibit the desired competitive results. For price competition to lead to the desired results, however, change in the information available to consumers is a prerequisite. Amended versions of planning rules may be necessary to provide the appropriate information to consumers.

Payment. A crucial issue in payment for health services is the extent of cost shifting between public (government) and private payers and its effects on competition among insurers and providers.

Under public programs, regulations concerning Medicare and Medicaid reimbursement have contributed to substantial cost shifting from payers that reimburse costs to payers that pay charges. Because of controlled payments for Medicare and Medicaid, hospital payment differentials of 20 to 50 percent have developed in some states between patients covered by Medicare and Medicaid and those insured by the Blues and commercial companies. Any insurer paying charges may absorb a still larger proportion of health care expenditures as budget cuts reduce Medicare and Medicaid payments.

Cost shifting also results from Blue Cross "discounts." The discount arises when Blue Cross reimburses hospitals on the basis of "reasonable" costs rather than charges. As in the Medicare and Medicaid programs, Blue Cross excludes some expenses such as bad debts from the allowable cost base and finds other expenses "unreasonable." These uncompensated costs are passed on to non-Blue Cross subscribers who pay charges.

The discount ranges from 2 to 30 percent in Newark, New York City, and Pittsburgh, although the average discount is approximately 8 to 15 percent.[21] This discount creates a significant competitive advantage over commercial insurance companies. The extent to which the discount represents a return to the Blues for services they offer—such as assured revenue to hospitals, open enrollment, etc.—is subject to debate. In a procompetitive world in which insurers would be vying for arrangements with providers, discounts would be accorded to insurers offering attractive packages to providers. The issue for the procompetition discussion is the degree to which the discounts reflect anticompetitive regulatory advantages as opposed to an advantage accorded by the exchange of services for payment.

Government tends to use retrospective cost-based reimbursement which, within certain constraints, means that providers are repaid for any expenditures they incur. This approach is antithetical to competition. Many private payers pay charges billed by a provider—increasingly, up to a limit based on the "usual and customary rate." Copayments and deductibles do force patients to share in some costs now, but these requirements are not consistent for any payer across all settings and providers, so they have adverse effects on price/premium competition. For instance, many third-party payers pay the full cost of acute inpatient care, but a lower and lower proportion of costs as the setting changes from inpatient to outpatient to the home. Thus, the financial incentives encourage use of the highest cost setting.

Currently, various payers use different payment schemes. Prospective payment schemes usually involve setting a price or budget for a future period so that providers have to work against a target. Even though such prospective financial targets are not set by market forces in many instances, they do have economic incentives similar to those of a market.

Payment systems are the key to the development of any price-competitive model. Indeed, the concept of reimbursement is incompatible with competition. Of course, a prospective or any other payment system may have the characteristics of reimbursement if there is no effective limit to the prospective price paid for providing care. A prospective payment system usually is designed so that charges are set for an array of services to be offered patients, with patients able to choose among services, weighing the prices involved. In order to make choices, patients must have considerable information about the quality and necessity of the services.

Alternative payment methods will have different sets of incentives, but each will have direct effects on the delivery of care:

• Payment of billed charges will have incentives dependent upon the circumstances under which the charges are set. If the fees result from competition, the incentives are those of such markets. If providers can collude or otherwise set fees, payment of billed charges ratifies those decisions.

• Payment on a per diem basis encourages the use of more days, especially because later days of care are less costly to provide. Depending on how the charges for the day are developed, such a system could encourage or discourage the use of ancillary services.

• Payment by the case should reduce the number of days provided and the use of ancillary services. Subject to malpractice constraints, this approach could reduce the quality of care.

• Payment of fixed budgets to institutions (also to individual providers if it became politically possible) places the burden of rationing care squarely on the provider. Fixed resources have to be distributed over the patients presenting themselves for care.

Prospective or retroactive adjustments applied to any of these approaches will modify the incentives. A "fixed prospective budget" with retroactive adjustments, for example, ceases to be fixed.

An example of a case-based payment scheme is the New Jersey Diagnostic Related Groups (DRG) system, under which payment by public and private payers is determined by the patient diagnosis. A DRG-type system of payment is also under consideration by the HHS for the Medicare program. The primary economic incentive is the possibility of earning a profit if the costs of providing the services are below the agreed-upon payment for the case. This particular aspect of the DRG system is similar to a market model in which the supplier makes a profit if the price at which the market will "clear" is greater than the cost of producing the commodity or service. Direct controls could exist in such a system and might include controls on whether particular cases are paid for, whether certain cases would be treated in an outpatient rather than an inpatient setting, and so on.

Any payment system can incorporate direct controls as well as economic incentives to encourage desired behavior. Indeed, setting parameters may be necessary to maintain price competition.[22] Indeed, if consumers cannot be informed adequately, then establishing a market-like payment system may create results as if there were a competitive market. Payment for incurred costs, however, is always incompatible

264

with competition, so the Medicare and many states' Medicaid rules need to be changed.

The decision to pay for services of individuals with particular skills is another way of affecting resource allocation through market decisions. Licensing statutes, by affecting the decision to pay for paraprofessional as well as physician services, affects the nature and type of services delivered. It is not possible to buy less expensive services if their provision is illegal. Serious consideration must be given to eliminating or severely restricting the relevant state rules.

Exemption from Taxation. Many health care providers have established corporate purposes that grant them tax exemption under the relevant federal and state statutes. This tax exemption usually extends to income taxes, property taxes (though there is some potential for change in this area), and excise, sales, and other use taxes. In addition, many state and federal statutes and regulations give health care providers access to the tax-exempt bond market.

To the extent that all health care providers have the option to incorporate under tax-exempt principles, the choice to be exempt or nonexempt clearly hinges on matters other than the competitive position of the provider. The availability of a tax-exempt status changes the power of health care providers in general to gain access to resources, vis-à-vis other manufacturers or providers of services in the economy as a whole. This may lead to excessive use of the national resources for health care. Since much of the concern about developing price competition in the health care industry is to create an environment more like that alleged to be true for the rest of the economy, the maintenance of tax exemption for either capital or operating purposes places the industry on a different footing from all others. If the purpose of inducing competition in health care is to reduce total expenditures and total resources allocated to that activity, then serious consideration must be given to the elimination of tax exemption.

Within the industry, tax exemption has no effect on the competitive position of similarly situated ventures. Between exempt and nonexempt facilities, *ceteris paribus,* the exempt can charge lower prices than the nonexempt, putting it in a more favorable competitive position. But *ceteris paribus* does not hold true. Proprietary hospitals perceive advantages from that status which may counter, to some extent, their lack of a tax-exempt status. The requirements that must be met to reach tax-exempt status inhibit activities proprietaries deem desirable. Thus, on balance, it is not clear that tax exemption is per se anticompetitive. In fact, depreciation allowances, investment credits, and other tax expenditures available to proprietary hospitals may moot the whole issue in real terms.

265

Conclusion

Statutory proposals intended to increase competition over price, premium, and product in the health care delivery system must change the behavior of both consumers and providers of health care to be effective in practice. The issue raised in this chapter is whether existing and proposed regulations will allow incentives for providers, consumers, and insurers to take root.

Past experience shows that consumers demand more health care as eligibility for, and coverage of, government programs expands and as the benefits of private health insurance increase. Examples include the increased use of acute inpatient care by the elderly after the passage of Medicare and the increased use of alcoholism and mental health treatment programs as states required insurers to include these benefits. Regulation requiring that people who cannot afford care be given access eliminates the constraints of market forces. Statutory and regulatory controls on the flow of information to patients, in the name of privacy and confidentiality, inhibit the development of the necessary knowledge base for consumers to make choices about either the price they should pay for health care services or the premiums for particular kinds of policies. Health insurance regulations inhibit the development of product and premium competition. Thus, an agenda for reform requires that most of these rules need to be eliminated or changed for competition to thrive.

The supply of health services has a history of response to the market environment. For example, the almost nonexistent payment for home health services along with full coverage of inpatient care has led to the development of highly sophisticated acute care inpatient facilities and little provision of home health services. Altering these incentives should improve the balance between care in institutional and noninstitutional settings. Various laws, however, restrict the necessary changes in the supply of health services. Free-choice-of-provider provisions, which may be construed to prohibit payment plans designed to encourage efficient provision of care, can keep prices higher than they would be otherwise. Occupational and facility licensing may inhibit the development of competing skills or facilities with lower prices. Quality controls and building and life safety codes also limit entry into the industry, even if they improve the quality of care. Other controls on supply reduce the potential for competition to occur over service price, products, or premiums.

The laws discussed in this chapter should be modified or in some cases eliminated unless there is a factual basis establishing that such controls achieve their desired results in the face of their clear anticompetitive attributes. A fundamental question in the procompetition debate is the extent to which the existing and proposed regulatory framework will allow for more efficient allocation of health care resources reflecting the choices of consumers. Moreover, the extent to which procompetition proposals can contain health care costs is a function not only of the response of consumer demand to procompetition incentives but also of the willingness to alter the regulatory framework to allow more flexibility, pluralism, and balance between the benefits and costs of regulation.

Notes

1. H.R. 850, section 4 (2)(D).

2. H. E. Frech III and Paul B. Ginsburg, "Competition among Health Insurers," in Warren Greenberg, ed., *Competition in the Health Care Sector: Past, Present, and Future* (Washington, D.C.: Federal Trade Commission, March 1978), pp. 168–72; H. E. Frech III, "The Regulation of Health Insurance" (Ph.D. dissertation, University of California, Los Angeles, September 1974); Nancy (Greenspan) Thorndyke, "The Effects of Regulation in the Private Health Insurance Market" (M.A. thesis, University of North Carolina, 1976); and Ronald J. Vogel and Roger D. Blair, *Health Insurance Administrative Costs,* U.S. Department of Health, Education, and Welfare, Social Security Administration, Office of Research and Statistics, Staff Paper No. 21 (Washington, D.C., 1976), pp. 250–84.

3. H. E. Frech III, "Blue Cross, Blue Shield, and Health Care Costs: A Review of the Economic Evidence," in Mark V. Pauley, ed., *National Health Insurance: What Now, What Later, What Never?* (Washington, D.C.: American Enterprise Institute, 1980), p. 251.

4. The Employee Retirement Income Security Act of 1974 governs employee welfare benefit plans, which include any plan or program sponsored by an employer or employee organization that provides health insurance benefits. ERISA preempts state laws that have a regulatory impact on employee benefit plans yet leaves untouched state laws that regulate the business of insurance. The courts have prohibited states from requiring self-insurers to abide by regulations applicable to traditional insurance, such as reserve requirements and minimum benefits.

5. Frech, "Blue Cross, Blue Shield, and Health Care Costs," p. 252.

6. Glen Slaughter, "Why Non-Insure? Pro and Con on Going It Alone," *Employee Benefits Journal,* vol. 4 (Spring 1979), pp. 20–21, 29–30.

7. Glenn R. Markus, *Self-Insured Health Benefits—Trends and Issues* (Washington, D.C.: Congressional Research Service, April 15, 1981), p. 6.

8. Glenn R. Markus and Valerie Hauch, *State Regulation of Private Health Insurance* (Washington, D.C.: Congressional Research Service, May 1, 1972), p. 71.

9. Ibid., p. 99.

10. Warner B. Clarke, "Can Self-Insurance Save You Dollars?" *Pension World,* vol. 15 (February 1979), pp. 58, 60.

11. Jack A. Meyer, "Health Care Competition: Are Tax Incentives Enough?" in Mancur Olson, ed., *A New Approach to the Economics of Health Care* (Washington, D.C.: American Enterprise Institute, 1982), p. 429.

12. Mancur Olson, "Introduction," in Olson, ed., *A New Approach to the Economics of Health Care*, p. 6.

13. Utah Regular Session, House Bill No. 66, 1977.

14. Tennessee Regular Session, Senate Bill No. 64, 1981.

15. Mark N. Dodosh, "Psychiatrists Fight against Further Inroads by Psychologists in Mental Health Markets," *The Wall Street Journal,* August 20, 1981.

16. See Clark Havighurst, "Role of Competition in Cost Containment," in Warren Greenberg, ed., *Competition in the Health Care Sector* (Washington, D.C.: Federal Trade Commission, March 1978), pp. 372–75.

17. See John B. Reiss et al., *The Reform of Regulations in the Department of Health and Human Services: Proposals for Change,* Final Report of the Office of Health Regulation to the Secretary, Department of Health and Human Services, January 1981.

18. Ibid., "Analysis of Certain Construction Standards."

19. Ibid.

20. See, for example, National Gerimedical Hospital and Gerontology Center v. Blue Cross, No. 80-802 (S.Ct. June 15, 1981).

21. Roger Feldman and Warren Greenberg, "The Relation between the Blue Cross Market Share and the Blue Cross 'Discount' on Hospital Charges," *Journal of Risk and Insurance* (June 1981).

22. Note the activities of the Bureau of Competition, Federal Trade Commission.

14

Legal Issues Arising under the Consumer Choice Proposals

Lynn E. Shapiro

During the first term of the 97th Congress, three bills designed to increase competition in the health care industry were introduced. These bills—Gephardt,[1] Durenberger,[2] and Hatch,[3] and other proposals, such as one now being developed by the Reagan administration—are collectively referred to as the "consumer choice proposals." They are intended to be "competitive" alternatives to previously advanced "regulatory" solutions for containing inflation in the health care sector of the economy.

The theory underlying the consumer choice proposals is that a more competitive health insurance market will result in a more efficient health delivery system. Insurers are subject to greater competition and, as a result, put pressure on health care providers to be more cost conscious in rendering health care services.

Although each bill has its own particular approach for injecting competition into the health care industry, these proposals have some common denominators, most notably their use of the federal tax laws to create a more competitive climate. All three proposals, for example, would limit the extent to which an employer's contribution for health insurance is treated as nontaxable income to the employee. Many agree that existing tax law encourages the purchase of inefficient and unnecessary health insurance coverage. Thus, providing a limit on this tax-free benefit is designed to make the purchaser of health insurance more cost conscious.

The consumer choice proposals are also designed to encourage the

NOTE: I wish to thank the members of the AEI Legal Issues Task Force and the staff of AEI for their constructive comments and guidance in writing this chapter. I also want to thank William Kopit and Robert Moses of the firm Epstein, Becker, Borsody, and Green, P.C., for their assistance and encouragement in preparing this chapter.

269

purchase of health insurance plans that provide for cost sharing—copayments and deductibles—by the insured. It is anticipated that greater cost sharing by the insured will make the patient more cost conscious in seeking health services under the insurance plan chosen.

Finally, the consumer choice proposals would require the employer to make equal contributions to all plans offered in order to provide the employee with an incentive to purchase only as much insurance as he or she needs, as well as to create greater competition among health insurance companies and alternative health care financing systems. If an employee chooses a plan with a premium that is less than the employer's contribution, that employee would be entitled to a corresponding rebate or equivalent benefits. If the premium is greater, the employee would have to make up the difference.

The structure of the consumer choice proposals clearly creates a range of legal issues. The purpose of this chapter is to raise and examine some of these issues as they arise under the various proposals. In particular, the chapter examines the effect such proposals would have on areas of existing law that are not specifically addressed in the proposals and, as a result, have not received much attention in the procompetition debate to date. The discussion of each area is preceded by a summary of existing law in that area. It is hoped that, by raising these relatively technical issues at this early stage in policy development, costly litigation that may impede the success of any new proposal ultimately enacted into law may be avoided.

The chapter is directed primarily at the three consumer choice proposals currently before Congress, but many of the problems raised are found in other consumer choice proposals as well.

The chapter is divided into the following four sections:

- federal-state conflict
- interactions with federal-state antitrust laws
- nonhealth statutes and issues
- health-related statutes and issues

Questions regarding federal-state relations under the consumer choice proposals are raised in the first section. Questions regarding the interaction of consumer choice proposals with federal and state antitrust laws are raised in the second section. Questions arising out of statutes that do not exclusively concern health programs but that may nonetheless interact with the consumer choice proposals are raised in the third section. Finally, questions regarding the interaction of existing health programs with the consumer choice proposals are raised in the fourth section.

Federal-State Conflict

The Extent to Which State Insurance Laws May Conflict with the Consumer Choice Proposals and the Legal Consequences of Such Conflicts. Historically, states have been the predominant arena for legislating insurance laws. State insurance laws may dictate the types of benefits a health insurance plan must offer, as well as the terms and conditions of such offerings. The consumer choice proposals, however, also seek to shape the benefits and offerings of health insurance plans. Therefore, the issue that needs to be addressed is the extent to which the consumer choice proposals' requirements will override state law, as well as the extent to which existing state insurance laws and other state laws of similar import must still be heeded.

According to the Supreme Court, state law must give way to federal legislation where a valid "act of Congress fairly interpreted is in actual conflict with the law of the State" under the doctrine of supersession.[4] Such actual conflict is most clearly manifest when the federal and state enactments are directly contradictory on their face. Under such circumstances, federal law will supersede state law where compliance with both is a literal impossibility.

State and federal laws need not, however, be directly contradictory on their face for the federal law to supersede. The actual conflict may be more subtle. Thus, state law must be invalidated if its effect is to discourage the conduct that federal action seeks to encourage. In the case of *Nash* v. *Florida Industrial Commission,* for example, the Supreme Court invalidated a state unemployment compensation law insofar as it denied benefits to otherwise eligible applicants solely because they had filed an unfair labor practice charge with the National Labor Relations Board.[5]

The legal principle of preemption is different from supersession. Under the principle of preemption, if Congress has validly decided to "occupy the field" for the federal government, then state laws will be invalidated even if they are consistent with federal law. Unless the federal law specifically addresses the issue of preemption, the question whether the federal law preempts state action is one of statutory construction by a court of law. Even when it is clear that preemption applies, the limits of that preemption are also an issue.

Historically, the power to regulate insurance has been among the police powers of the state. Indeed, as will be discussed more fully subsequently, 15 U.S.C. sections 1011 and 1012(a) of the McCarran-Ferguson Act specifically state that the business of insurance shall be subject to the laws of the states, and that silence on the part of the Congress shall not be construed to impose any barrier on the regulation or taxation of such business by the states.

The Supreme Court, however, has also held that, when Congress exercises a granted power in a field that states have traditionally occupied, and unmistakably evinces its intent to exclude the states from exerting their police power in that field, the federal legislation may displace state law under the Supremacy Clause.

The state insurance law often stipulates certain benefits that must be offered, and it may also specify eligibility requirements. Moreover, states have been particularly active in the area of regulating insurance premiums. States also regulate the creation and operation of health maintenance organizations (HMOs). Therefore, if increased competition among health insurance plans is the desired objective for any consumer choice proposal, legislators will need to address the extent to which state activity in regulating insurance may stifle that objective. Hence, any attempt by Congress to develop a consumer choice proposal should address the extent to which Congress intends to preempt the state's rights to legislate in these areas.

Much can be learned regarding the issue of preemption of state insurance law from *Hewlett-Packard Co.* v. *Barnes,* a case brought by the state of California challenging the constitutionality of the Employee Retirement Income Security Act of 1974 (ERISA).[6] In this case, a number of employers and employee benefit organizations brought suit to enjoin the California Commissioner of Corporations from requiring them to comply with California's Knox-Keene Health Care Service Plan Act of 1975. The plaintiffs argued that this state law, which regulates health maintenance organizations, was preempted by the federal ERISA law.

ERISA has two relevant paragraphs that attempt to define the scope of its preemption of state law. The first paragraph provides that ERISA "shall supersede any and all state laws insofar as they may now or hereafter relate to any employee benefit plan."[7] A second paragraph provides that "nothing in this subchapter shall be construed to exempt or relieve any person from any law of any State which regulates insurance, banking or securities."[8] While the state of California argued that the Knox-Keene Act was an insurance law exempt from the ERISA preemption paragraph, the plaintiffs argued that such an interpretation would frustrate the purposes of ERISA. The court of appeals held that, despite the fact that the Knox-Keene Act dealt with insurance, ERISA preempted this state law. Hence, even when Congress provides legislation addressing the issue of preemption, its scope is still subject to litigation and interpretations by a court of law.

All three consumer choice proposals mandate, to some extent, that in order to obtain the favorable tax treatment, the health insurance plan must include a minimum amount of benefits. Such federal requirements might conflict with existing state law requirements regarding minimum benefits. None of the proposals is mandatory, however, and thus one would need to argue that the federal law is inconsistent with state law in this area. Therefore, unless the consumer choice proposal explicitly preempts certain aspects of state regulation of the insurance industry, it is possible that a health insurance plan would need to satisfy both federal and state requirements in order to be qualified and in order to do business in the relevant state.

Only one of the present consumer choice proposals specifically addresses this issue of supersession or preemption of state law. In particular, section 302(a) of the Gephardt proposal provides as follows:

> Any provision of law, regulation or administrative action of any State or unit of local government which prevents or impedes the reforms of the health care delivery system implemented, or the program created, under this Act is preempted as of the date of the enactment of this Act.

Section 302(b) then lists specific categories of law preempted, including corporate practice, premium setting, plan arrangements, capitalization, and marketing. Section 302(c), however, qualifies and limits the scope of the preemption clause with the following:

> Nothing contained in this section or elsewhere in this Act shall be construed to preempt a State or local subdivision therein from taking an action, whether by law, regulation, or administrative determination, which is intended to and does in fact promote the quality of health care services, personnel, equipment, or facilities.

Although these provisions attempt to address this complex issue, unless Congress is more specific, much room is still left open for interpretation through litigation, similar to what happened with the ERISA statute. For instance, does a state's health planning law "prevent or impede the reforms of the health care delivery system" created by this bill, or does it constitute a law designed "to promote the quality of health care services, personnel, equipment or facilities," and as such is not preempted? Similar issues can be raised regarding state licensing of hospitals, nursing homes, health professionals, and various other state health laws not specifically mentioned in the bill.

The states and private parties will likely litigate this issue, since they have a strong interest in maintaining their right to regulate the insurance industry. Therefore, unless the legislators provide greater specificity in this area of preemption, it will be left to the courts to interpret the scope of federal preemption. Such interpretations may or may not be consistent with legislators' policy objectives.

One factor that the courts would certainly consider is the McCarran-Ferguson Act and the federal legislative preference it creates in favor of state regulation of insurance. This issue is not typically addressed in the consumer choice proposals. Indeed, even the Gephardt proposal, which does amend the McCarran-Ferguson Act, does so only with respect to its applicability to antitrust laws. Another frequently overlooked section of McCarran-Ferguson should, however, be addressed by legislators who are developing consumer choice proposals. The relevant section provides as follows:

> No Act of Congress shall be construed to invalidate, impair, or supersede any law enacted by any State for the purpose of regulating the business of insurance; or which imposes a fee or tax upon such business, *unless such Act specifically relates to the business of insurance.*[9]

The legal climate surrounding the act's passage was summarized by Justice Thurgood Marshall in *Securities & Exchange Commission* v. *National Securities, Inc.*:

> [The Act] was passed in reaction to this Court's decision in *United States* v. *South-Eastern Underwriters Assn.,* 322 U.S. 533, 64 S.Ct. 1162, 88 L.Ed. 1440 (1944). Prior to that decision, it had been assumed, in the language of the leading case, that "[i]ssuing a policy of insurance is not a transaction of commerce." *Paul* v. *Virginia,* 8 Wall. 168, 183, 19 L.Ed. 357 (1869). Consequently, regulation of insurance transactions was thought to rest exclusively with the States. In *South-Eastern Underwriters,* this Court held that insurance transactions were subject to federal regulation under the Commerce Clause, and that the antitrust laws in particular, were applicable to them. Congress reacted quickly. . . . The McCarran-Ferguson Act was the product of this concern.[10]

Although the act was passed primarily in response to *South-Eastern Underwriters,* an antitrust case, its scope appears to be much broader than the antitrust area. Congress was also concerned with the overall regulatory picture, including "collection of premiums, general regulations, the issuing of licenses, and many other aspects of the business.[11] Thus, state tax laws relating to the business of insurance are expressly covered by 15 U.S.C. sections 1011 and 1012. Indeed, these two sections speak of "regulation" of the insurance business, and that term is certainly not limited to antitrust regulation. Moreover, cases have held that the scope is broader than the antitrust area.[12] Clearly then, Congress wanted to ensure that no future federal legislation enacted under the Commerce Clause and not specifically related to insurance would be construed as an implied repeal of the McCarran-Ferguson Act.

Thus, the McCarran-Ferguson Act returned to the states the power to regulate the business of insurance. If Congress intends to invoke its Commerce Clause powers to occupy part of the field of insurance regulation, the existence of the McCarran-Ferguson Act is yet another reason to say so expressly.

While it may appear obvious that any of the consumer choice proposals would constitute an act that "specifically relates to the business of insurance," it is at least arguable that, as long as the proposals do not specifically address this issue, they would be restricted by McCarran-Ferguson. As previously mentioned, for example, in *Hewlett-Packard Co.* v. *Barnes* the state of California argued that, under this section of McCarran-Ferguson, the Employee Retirement Income Security Act should not be construed in a way that violates the policy of reserving to the states the power to regulate insurance unless ERISA "specifically relates" to insurance. ERISA itself was silent on this point. Consequently, it required extensive litigation on this and other issues before the courts held that ERISA did specifically relate to insurance.

The Extent to Which the Consumer Choice Proposals Will Affect State Governments, Both as Employers and as Sponsors of Qualified Plans. Although all three proposals concern the employer's responsibilities in the offering of health insurance plans, none of them addresses the issue of whether "employer" includes state and local governments. As a result, state and local governments may be subject to the same obligations imposed upon other employers. This may not be the intended result. The Federal Health Maintenance Organization Act of 1973, for example, contains requirements for state and local government employers that are different from those for private employers.

In addition, many of the proposals are vague in addressing who may be a "sponsor" and whether any special considerations should be made if the state is the sponsor. The Gephardt proposal, however, does define sponsor as follows:

> The term "sponsor" means, with respect to a qualified plan, the person, partnership, association, agency of government, or other entity which is legally responsible for fulfilling the obligations of the plan. An entity may be a sponsor of more than one qualified plan in one or more health care areas.

Consequently, a state may be a sponsor of a qualified health plan under the Gephardt proposal. Therefore, the major issue that needs to be

275

addressed is whether and by what authority the federal government can dictate to a state what it can and cannot do as an employer or sponsor under a consumer choice proposal. The leading case in this area is *National League of Cities* v. *Usery*.[13]

In *National League of Cities,* the Supreme Court held that extension of the minimum wage and overtime provisions of the Fair Labor Standards Act (FLSA) to state and local government employees was not a permissible exercise of Congress's power under the Commerce Clause. The Supreme Court reasoned that the Tenth Amendment and principles of federalism inherent in the Constitution place an affirmative limitation on use of the commerce power to regulate the conduct of the states as states. In particular, the Court stated:

> One undoubted attribute of state sovereignty is the States' power to determine the wages which shall be paid to those whom they employ in order to carry out their governmental functions, what hours those persons will work, and what compensation will be provided where these employees may be called upon to work overtime.[14]

Hence, the specific holding of the case was that "insofar as the challenged [FLSA] amendments operate to directly displace the States' freedom to structure integral operations in areas of traditional governmental functions, they are not within the authority granted Congress by Art. I, § 8, cl. 3 [the Commerce Clause]."[15] In so holding, however, the Court expressed

> no view as to whether different results might obtain if Congress seeks to affect integral operations of state governments by exercising authority granted it under other sections of the Constitution such as the spending power, Art. 1, § 8, cl. 1, or § 5 of the Fourteenth Amendment.[16]

In fact, in a case immediately following *National League of Cities,* referred to as *Usery* v. *Charleston County School District of Charleston County, South Carolina,* the court of appeals held that the decision in *National League of Cities* did not preclude applying the provisions of the Equal Pay Act to state and local governments.[17] The court reasoned that this statute is viewed as an exercise of Congress's power to adopt legislation enforcing the Fourteenth Amendment's guarantee of equal protection of the law, and under this view "there is no doubt that application of its provisions to state and local governments is a valid exercise of Congress' constitutional authority."[18]

In light of this case law, it would appear that extending the definition of employer or sponsor to include state governments as well may violate the federalism principles espoused in *National League of Cities.* However, does the fact that consumer choice proposals are legislated via Congress's taxing authority, as opposed to the Commerce Clause in *National League of Cities,* defeat the relevance of this case law? Does the fact that these proposals are not as compulsory as the FLSA also defeat the relevance of this case law? These questions are not easily answered. They may need to be resolved by litigation only.

Interactions with Federal-State Antitrust Laws

Whether the Consumer Choice Proposals Are in Conflict with or Complement the Federal and State Antitrust Laws. Essentially, federal and state antitrust laws are designed to promote competition by prohibiting unreasonable restraints of trade and unfair trade practices. Primary among the many practices that have been found to be unreasonable restraints of trade are those that have been considered to be "per se violations" of the antitrust laws—price fixing, market allocation, group boycotts, and tie-ins. These forms of restraints ordinarily are treated as per se violations of the antitrust laws because their mere existence constitutes a threat to free competition. In the health care field, however, many courts have applied "rule of reason" analysis to concerted activities that might have been treated as per se violations in other industries.[19]

An agreement between competitors that affects the price of their goods or services is ordinarily per se illegal as price fixing. Although actually setting the price of goods is the most obvious type of price fixing, other arrangements such as agreements to limit production, prohibit credit sales, and regulate price advertising also have been classified as price fixing.

Similarly, agreements that specifically divide territories and/or allocate customers are not the only arrangements that are condemned as per se illegal market allocations. For example, an assignment of areas of primary responsibility and certain trademark licensing systems have been found to be per se violations.

Concerted refusals to deal, or group boycotts, also generally constitute per se violations, particularly when it is demonstrated that the actors wield power in the marketplace. Thus, a joint refusal by physicians to deal with a hospital or health maintenance organization would be illegal. Some courts, however, have permitted inquiry into the reasons behind a boycott where no anticompetitive intent is shown.

Tie-ins occur when a seller ties the sale of one product or service to the sale of another. A manufacturer or dealer, for example, might require the purchaser of medical equipment to purchase a service contract as a precondition to purchasing the equipment. This type of arrangement is usually found to be per se illegal because it forces a purchaser to buy an additional, perhaps unwanted, service in order to obtain the desired product.

Other practices might also constitute unreasonable restraints of trade. For example, courts have examined the drafts and organizational membership restrictions in professional sports to determine their legality. In order to determine whether these practices constitute an antitrust violation, courts undertake a detailed inquiry into the reasonableness of the challenged practice under the circumstances.

Monopolies and mergers (and other acquisitions) are special classes of restraints that have acquired their own set of analytical rules. Even in these areas, however, the antitrust laws serve the same purpose: preventing the exercise of market power by one or more firms in a concentrated market.

Price discrimination has also been given special statutory treatment. Under the Robinson-Patman Act, it is unlawful "to discriminate in price between different purchasers of commodities of like grade and quality" when such discrimination has a substantial adverse effect on commerce. Price differentials that solely reflect "allowances for differences in the cost of manufacture, sale or delivery resulting from the differing methods or quantities in which such commodities are . . . sold or delivered" are permitted. The Robinson-Patman Act applies only to goods, however, and not to services.

There are several statutory and judicially created exceptions and defenses to the application of the antitrust laws. These exceptions recognize the conflict between the antitrust laws and federal and state policy in certain areas, and might be applicable in certain circumstances in the health care industry.

Activities that would otherwise violate the antitrust laws, but that are necessary to carry out a federal statutory scheme, may be upheld under the doctrine of implied repeal. This doctrine is premised on the theory that Congress must have intended a limited repeal of the antitrust law to the extent that a subsequently enacted regulatory statute and the antitrust laws are "clearly repugnant." Similarly, under the federal supersession doctrine, a federal regulatory statute may override the application of a state antitrust act, insofar as they are in actual conflict.

As a general rule, preemption of the antitrust laws under either the implied repeal doctrine or the supersession doctrine is not easily accomplished. Recently, in *National Gerimedical Hospital & Gerontology Center* v. *Blue Cross*, the Supreme Court held that the national Health Planning and Resource Development Act was not so inconsistent with the federal antitrust laws as to repeal them. The Court noted, however, that the Health Planning and Resources Development Act may immunize certain specific activities from scrutiny under the antitrust laws.

Congress created an important exception to the antitrust laws for the business of insurance by enacting the McCarran-Ferguson Act. This exception was primarily to permit cooperative rate making and other activities required to be undertaken in connection with the underwriting of risks. It is important to recognize, therefore, that all activities of insurers are not exempt under McCarran-Ferguson; only those activities that constitute the "business of insurance" are protected. Furthermore, under McCarran-Ferguson, group boycotts by insurers are subject to the antitrust laws even if they constitute the business of insurance. There is also the possibility that otherwise exempt activities may be illegal under state antitrust laws.

The courts have also created a defense to the antitrust laws for certain actions taken in response to the commands of the state. This defense, known as the state-action or *Parker* v. *Brown* defense, recognizes that the Sherman Act was intended to regulate private rather than government practices. A two-pronged standard has evolved to determine whether a particular practice falls within this defense. In order to be a defense from the antitrust laws, a restraint must be clearly articulated by state policy and actively supervised by the state.

The constitutional right to petition the government has also resulted in an exception to the application of the antitrust laws. Under the so-called Noerr-Pennington doctrine, concerted action to persuade a government body or official to act in a specific manner does not violate the antitrust laws, even if the underlying motive is anticompetitive. This immunity is not unlimited, however; mere sham invocations of the right to petition are not protected. For example, collective efforts to lie to executive officials and collective efforts to exercise undue and improper influence on administrative officials have not been protected.

Assuming that the consumer choice proposals are designed to promote a competitive marketplace, it is desirable for these proposals to complement, rather than conflict with, existing federal and state antitrust laws. In this regard, the Gephardt proposal makes it unlawful for a nongovernmental sponsor of a qualified plan to control, be controlled by, or be affiliated with any other sponsor of a qualified plan located in the same area. This is an example of a consumer choice proposal complementing the policy of the antitrust laws.

The Gephardt proposal also includes specific provisions that declare certain sponsor activity subject to antitrust scrutiny. Thus, the Gephardt proposal states that policies of insurance or reinsurance offered to qualified plans and to persons providing such policies will be subject to federal antitrust law scrutiny "regardless of whether such business or persons are regulated by State law." Consequently, consumer choice insurance policies would not be able to hide behind the McCarran-Ferguson business-of-insurance exception to avoid antitrust law application.

It is unclear, however, to what extent this provision may render all such activities illegal with regard to insurance or reinsurance offered to both qualified and nonqualified plans. Moreover, this provision arguably is intended to repeal the state-action doctrine, since it apparently provides for preemption of state law. Furthermore, the legislators may want to revise this language, since at present it may be broadly interpreted to repeal McCarran-Ferguson for all activities of qualified plans, and this may not be the intent.

The Hatch proposal, on the other hand, contemplates certain joint activities that may violate the antitrust laws. Section 1924(a) requires all carriers to enter into arrangements either with the state "or with other carriers" to provide catastrophic illness insurance to individuals who are not eligible for group coverage or government programs. This provision clearly contemplates invocation of either the state-action or the implied-repeal defense, but it does not specify the scope of the activities that would be covered by the defense.

Except for the above, no direct legal conflict appears to exist between the consumer choice proposals and the antitrust laws; nonetheless, there may be an indirect conflict, to the extent that the current antitrust laws are inadequate in promoting free enterprise in the health care industry. This may frustrate the goal of the consumer choice proposals. Therefore, the issue that needs to be addressed is whether the existing application of antitrust laws to the health care industry will enhance or stymie the competitive environment designed by the consumer choice proposals.

In addressing this issue, conflicting viewpoints were expressed by the members of the AEI Legal Issues Task Force. This debate is reflected in chapters 15 and 16 of this volume, written by two members of the task force—Clark C. Havighurst and William G. Kopit.

In summary, Kopit takes the position that the peculiar situations in the health care market and the lack of judicial guidance about what may violate antitrust law create a chilling effect on the numerous competitive activities that most would classify as laudatory or at worst benign. Although the problems in applying antitrust law to the health care industry are not created by the consumer choice proposals, Kopit asserts that these problems, if not solved legislatively at the outset, create a potential incompatibility between the consumer choice proposals and antitrust law that could serve to reduce substantially any beneficial competitive impacts that such proposals could have if enacted.

On the other hand, Havighurst takes the position that the health care industry, even under the proposals, "fits easily" within the mainstream of traditional antitrust analysis and that any doctrinal uncertainties that exist are ultimately attributable "not to policy doubts or to notions that health care is a unique undertaking, but to the complexities of applying antitrust principles in unusual factual circumstances." Instead of legislative solutions to clarify these unknowns, as espoused by Kopit, Havighurst would rely on the court system to clarify these issues.

Nonhealth Statutes and Issues

The Extent to Which the Consumer Choice Proposals Would Affect the Collective Bargaining Obligations of Employers and Union Representatives under the National Labor Relations Act. In brief, the National Labor Relations Act (NLRA) grants employees the right to organize and to bargain collectively with their employers through representatives of their own choosing.[20] Collective bargaining under the NLRA includes the requirement that an employer and the majority representative of his employees meet at reasonable times, confer in good faith about certain matters, and put into writing any agreement reached if requested by either party. These obligations are imposed equally on the employer and on the employees' collective bargaining representative. It is an unfair labor practice for either party to refuse to bargain collectively with the other. That obligation does not, however, compel either party to agree to a proposal by the other, nor to make a concession to the other.

The duty to bargain covers all matters concerning wages, hours of employment, or other conditions of employment. These are called "mandatory" subjects of bargaining about which the employer, as well as the employees' representative, must bargain in good faith. These mandatory subjects have been held to include, but are not limited to, such matters as pensions, bonuses, and group insurance. "Nonmandatory" subjects are matters other than the wages, hours, and other conditions of employment; the parties are free to bargain and to agree about these matters. Neither party, however, may insist on bargaining on such subjects over the objection of the other party.

The NLRA is administered and enforced principally by the National Labor Relations Board. The presidentially appointed five-member board is an independent agency that decides cases involving charges of unfair labor practices and determines employee representation questions that are submitted to it.

Several issues arise under the NLRA when examining the consumer choice proposals in light of the collective bargaining obligations imposed upon employers and the employees' representatives. For instance, what are the respective roles of the employer, union representative, and employee if an employer offers multiple health plans? In other words, would the individual employee or the union possess the right to choose from among competing health insurance plans?

These issues previously arose after the passage of the Federal Health Maintenance Organization Act of 1973. Under that law, an employer, under certain circumstances, is required to offer a federally qualified HMO as an alternative to his traditional health insurance policy. This is commonly referred to as an employer's "dual choice" obligation. The HMO law, as originally passed, however, did not address the issue of whether the unionized employer satisfies his dual-choice obligation by merely offering it to the union representative. After years of debate and confusion, the federal law was amended to provide that the union representative has the authority to accept or to reject the offering of an HMO on behalf of all represented employees.

A literal reading of some of the consumer choice proposals suggests that the employer would not be obligated to offer a plan first to a collective bargaining representative, although the proposals are not completely clear on this point. Legislators need to address whether the union representative should be given the sole power to decide these matters, whether he should merely have the right of first refusal, or whether the employee alone should be presented with the option. The Hatch proposal, for example, does provide the collective bargaining representative with the right of first refusal. Related to this question is the issue of whether the union's right of first refusal might reduce substantially the amount of competition that otherwise would be created if unionized employees had the right to choose health insurance plans on an individual basis.

In light of the employer's obligation under some of the consumer choice proposals to provide equal contributions to the different plans offered, several further issues arise. First, can the employer's contribution amount differ between union and nonunion employees? Second, what impact will different bargaining units have? Third, how does this new obligation affect existing collective bargaining agreements that are not currently subject to renegotiations? Would the passage of a consumer choice proposal unilaterally amend these outstanding agreements? Legislators should provide for an express resolution of this problem as, for example, the grandfathering of these new employer obligations, in light of existing collective bargaining agreements.

Finally, although group insurance has been held to be a mandatory subject for collective bargaining, it is not absolutely clear whether the qualified plans would necessarily fall within the mandatory category. Furthermore, if there is a dispute regarding the offering of a qualified plan, it is unclear whether that should be deemed a labor dispute subject to the NLRB's jurisdiction or subject to the jurisdiction of the health courts described in the Gephardt proposal, or possibly subject to the jurisdiction of both.

Whether the Employer's Contribution for the Employee's Health Insurance to a Nonqualified Plan May Be Deemed "Wages" for Purposes of the Employer's Obligations under the Federal Wage and Hours Laws. The consumer choice proposals would make the employer's contributions for the employee's health insurance taxable income unless the plan meets the statutory requirements. The Gephardt proposal, for example, provides that the employer's contributions are nontaxable only if the premium payment for each employee is made to a qualified plan and does not exceed the average premium paid for basic services in the health care area. Therefore, if the employer fails to offer a qualified plan, or if the employer's contribution exceeds permissible limits, each employee must include such amounts in his taxable income. The conversion of premium payments from a tax-exempt benefit to taxable income, however, may have implications beyond merely subjecting the employee to federal income tax liability.

If the fringe benefit does become subject to federal income tax, an issue arises whether the employer's contribution constitutes a wage for purposes of the employer's obligations under a variety of federal wage and hour laws. In other words, the employer's health insurance contribution that is beyond the tax-free limit may also be included as part of the wage rate for computing minimum wage and overtime payments under any of these statutes. A further issue is whether such consequences are desirable.

The Fair Labor Standards Act of 1938, for example, requires certain employers to pay their employees a specified minimum hourly wage and to pay them at one and one-half times their regular wage rate of pay for hours worked in excess of forty per week.[21] A series of federal laws address the wage rate for employees working on government contracts. The McNamara-O'Hara Service Contract Act of 1965, for example, establishes that the employer must pay certain minimum wage rates and fringe benefits to employees working on service contracts and subcontracts with the federal government.[22] The Davis-Bacon Act has similar requirements for federal government contracts for the construction or repair of public works.[23]

If it is determined that taxable health insurance contributions are to be included in wage rates, then policy makers must also consider that the definitions of critical terms such as "employer" and "wage" vary among these statutes. Hence, the economic consequences of having the contribution included as a wage for any one of these statutes may be different from those under another statute.

Finally, a similar analysis could be made for the application of the employer's contribution to the Federal Unemployment Tax Act (FUTA) and the Federal Insurance Contributions Act (FICA).

Whether the Consumer Choice Proposals Are Inconsistent with the Employer's Obligations under ERISA. Title I of ERISA defines employee benefit plans in broad terms to include "employee pension benefits plans" as well as "employee welfare benefit plans."[24] Section 3(1) of the act defines a welfare plan as any plan or program established or maintained by a sponsoring employer or employee organization that provides employees with medical, surgical, or hospital care benefits and disability, accident, sickness, death, or unemployment benefits, among other items. Therefore, the employer's offering of a qualified plan under the consumer choice proposals would fall within the meaning of a welfare plan under ERISA.

For purposes of this chapter, the most relevant section of ERISA concerns the employer's obligations with respect to the offering of health insurance plans. In particular, ERISA imposes upon employers extensive reporting and disclosure requirements in offering health insurance plans. In outline form, some of the principal requirements include the following:

1. Reports to the Department of Labor (DOL) and the Internal Revenue Service (IRS).
    a. Annual report must be filed by the employer with IRS on or before the last day of the seventh month following the end of the plan year.
    b. The summary plan description (SPD) must be filed with DOL within 120 days after a law is adopted.
    c. Material modifications in the SPD must be filed with DOL within 210 days after the last day of the plan year in which a material modification in the terms of the plan or in other matters is made.

2. Disclosure to plan participants and beneficiaries.
    a. The summary plan description must be distributed to each participant within 90 days after becoming a participant or within 120 days after a plan is adopted.
    b. The summary of material modifications in the SPD must be distributed to each participant within 210 days after the end of the plan year in which the material change is adopted or occurs.
    c. The summary annual report (SAR) must be distributed to

each participant and beneficiary within nine months after the end of the plan year to which it relates.

d. Copies of the SPD, the latest annual report, and plan documents must be made available for examination by plan participants and beneficiaries.

e. Upon the written request of a plan participant or beneficiary, he or she must be furnished with a copy of the most recent or updated SPD, annual report, and plan documents.

In light of these requirements under ERISA, three main issues arise. First, under the Gephardt proposal, although employers have no reporting requirements, qualified plans have to submit information to the Secretary of Health and Human Services—information that is very similar to what the employer currently submits to the Department of Labor under ERISA. Therefore, to the extent that such information is now being reported to the federal government, it may not be necessary to require such additional regulation of qualified plans.

Second, it is debatable whether such reporting and disclosure requirements stifle or enhance a competitive environment. If legislators decide that the requirements stifle competition, they may wish to delete some of those that would apply under existing law.

Finally, it is possible that the Secretary of Labor's administration of ERISA will interfere with the effective administration of competition proposals by the Secretaries of Treasury and Health and Human Services. In the event of a conflict, it should be clarified which statute should prevail.

The Extent to Which the Consumer Choice Proposals Interact with the Freedom of Information Act. Neither the Durenberger proposal nor the Hatch proposal requires health insurance plans to submit information to the federal government, nor do they include vouchers or other forms of government payment that might support the contention that the plan or even the employer is acting as a federal agency for purposes of the Freedom of Information Act (FOIA). Consequently, very few FOIA implications are inherent in these proposals.

The Gephardt proposal, however, raises FOIA issues by creating a new entity—the Health Benefits Assurance Corporation. It requires qualified plans to submit financial information to the corporation, and it involves giving vouchers to private entities.

In summary, FOIA is designed to give the public maximum access to information in the files of federal agencies.[25] It requires federal agencies to make available to the public all information held by them, unless the information falls within one of the nine statutory exemptions.

285

With respect to the consumer choice proposals, the relevant exemptions include:

- matters related solely to the internal personnel rules and practices of an agency
- matters specifically exempted from disclosure by statute
- trade secrets and commercial or financial information obtained from a person and considered privileged or confidential

Upon receipt of a request by any person, the agency must determine whether the requested material falls within one of the exemptions. If an agency refuses an FOIA request, the requester may sue to enjoin the withholding of information. The burden is on the agency to prove that the material falls within one of these exemptions.

Lack of thorough consideration of the implications of FOIA for new programs or agencies can result in significant legal difficulties in administering the program. The Professional Standards Review Organization (PSRO) program provides examples of such difficulties. Established as private organizations under federal grants to carry out utilization review of Medicare and Medicaid services rendered, PSROs collect a substantial amount of data on patients, practitioners, and providers. From the beginning, PSROs believed that most of their data should be kept confidential and, in fact, that the program's success was dependent on such confidentiality. Moreover, the PSRO law required all data to be held in confidence except as allowed or required by the Secretary of Health and Human Services by regulations.

Nevertheless, in 1979, a consumer group in Washington, D.C., successfully brought suit in federal district court under FOIA for the release of a substantial amount of PSRO data. In reaching its decision, the district court found both that PSROs should be considered federal agencies for purposes of FOIA and that none of the FOIA exemptions applied to the requested PSRO data. The PSROs had claimed that they were not federal agencies, but instead simply contractors receiving federal grants. Furthermore, they had claimed exemptions for the data requested on the basis of section 552(b)(3), material specifically exempted by statute; section 552(b)(5), intra-agency letters or memoranda not normally discoverable in civil court proceedings; and section 552(b)(6), personnel and medical files, the disclosure of which would constitute a clearly unwarranted invasion of personal property. In rejecting all of the PSRO's claims, the district court judge stated that he sympathized with their dilemma, but that the statutory language of the PSRO law was not strong enough to protect the data against the FOIA claim and any changes would have to come from Congress.

Although the PSROs finally won this case in the court of appeals, this does not discount the extensive time and expense that has been incurred to resolve this issue for the PSROs in the courts. This costly litigation could possibly have been avoided if the PSRO law had addressed this issue.

With respect to the Gephardt proposal the Health Benefits Assurance Corporation is specifically designated as a federal agency. Therefore, this new entity would probably constitute a federal agency for purposes of FOIA. As a result, the information it compiles may be available to the public.

With respect to the information this corporation collects, the Gephardt proposal requires each qualified plan to submit to the corporation such financial information as is necessary for the corporation to review the plan.

In light of the type of information that will be collected by the corporation, the major FOIA issue concerns the type of confidential information to be gathered under these proposals and how it will be protected. For example, to what extent is it desirable to allow competitors access to financial information, and what effect will such access have on the competitive environment? If confidentiality is desired, is it sufficient to rely merely on an agency's determination of whether the information falls within the meaning of one of the FOIA exemptions or should such matters be specifically anticipated in the competition legislation? If complete confidentiality is desired, the consumer choice proposal should be explicit in specifying what information to be submitted by a health plan is not subject to FOIA.

Furthermore, if an insurance company accepts a voucher, one could possibly argue that the company is thereby acting as a federal agency for purposes of FOIA. This was essentially the argument directed against the PSROs. While the Gephardt proposal does state that the mere receipt of a voucher does not make the qualified plan a federal agency, other proposals do not address this issue. Therefore, the consumer choice proposal may need to specify that receipt of a voucher does not make the entity a federal agency "for purposes of FOIA or any other federal statute."

Finally, many such issues under FOIA may also arise under the freedom of information acts adopted by the states. Therefore, even if the legislators limit access to a plan's financial information in order to promote competition, its competitors may have access to the same information under the state's FOIA. To avoid this result, state FOIAs would need to be preempted by federal law.

The Manner in Which the Health Court System as Proposed in the Gephardt Bill Would Fit into the Existing Federal and State Judicial Systems. Article III of the U.S. Constitution provides for the establishment of the federal judicial system, which is implemented and governed by Title 28 of the United States Code. The states have parallel constitutional and statutory underpinnings for their respective judicial systems.

With respect to the consumer choice proposals, the Gephardt proposal would establish a U.S. Health Court and Health Court of Appeals (trial court and court of appeals). These additions to the federal judicial system would have exclusive jurisdiction over all disputes and claims of a civil nature that would arise under the proposed legislation. The proposal includes provisions for the appointment, tenure, and salaries of the judges; the manner for handling trials; and the jurisdiction of the two courts.

The main legal issue arising out of this provision is how these courts would fit into existing federal and state judiciary systems. One issue is the possible overlap of jurisdiction between the health courts and the NLRB. Another issue is whether the health court could accept jurisdiction in a case if it included matters under the act as well as matters arising under another statute but generated by the same episode. Would the court have to parcel out those claims not arising directly under the act?

Legal Issues regarding the Health Benefits Assurance Corporation Created by the Gephardt Proposal. Section 222 of the Gephardt proposal establishes a Health Benefits Assurance Corporation within the Department of the Treasury. The HBAC is responsible for determining which health care plans are qualified to participate in the competitive system created by the legislation and for monitoring plans already qualified. The HBAC would also have the power to make financial investigations of plans both before and after qualification, and it would have the authority to establish a protective fund to cover subscribers in the event a plan defaults on its obligations. If the HBAC finds that a plan is unable to fulfill its financial obligations, it is also authorized to apply to the U.S. Health Court for the appointment of a receiver for the plan. The Gephardt proposal further provides that the HBAC would be tax-exempt, would have the power to sue or be sued, and would constitute an "agency" under the Administrative Procedures Act.

The first issue to be addressed is whether HBAC's location in the Department of Treasury will cause jurisdictional problems within the federal government, particularly with the Department of Health and Human Services (HHS). This might be avoided if the Gephardt proposal provided greater specificity in its section on the HBAC's duties and functions.

Second, what are the criteria for approving a "qualified plan"? The Gephardt proposal requires HBAC to determine whether the plan has "sufficient financial ability to fulfill its obligations to its projected membership as a qualified plan during its initial plan year." The proposal, however, provides little guidance about the meaning of these terms. The legislation, or at least the legislative history, should address this issue.

Third, the Gephardt proposal provides that, during the period a receiver has been appointed, no bankruptcy proceeding may be commenced under federal or state law and any proceeding commenced before appointment of the receiver shall be suspended. Is this provision intended to supersede state bankruptcy laws?

Health-Related Statutes and Issues

The Extent to Which the Consumer Choice Proposals Will Affect the Medicare Program. Before examining the extent to which the consumer choice proposals will affect the Medicare program and any legal issues arising therefrom, a brief summary of the Medicare program is in order.

The Medicare Amendments to the Social Security Act, passed in 1965, established a health insurance system for eligible elderly and disabled individuals (end-stage renal disease patients were added later) in which the federal government functions as an insurer.[26] Medicare is an exclusively federal program providing two different types of health insurance.

Part A, which is financed through the social security payroll tax paid by employees and employers, provides hospital insurance in the form of reimbursement for inpatient hospital, skilled nursing, home health, and other related forms of care. Under Part A, providers must meet certain criteria established by regulation to be eligible for reimbursement, and then are reimbursed to the extent of the lesser of their customary charges or their reasonable costs in providing covered services.

Part B, supplementary medical insurance, is an optional program that pays for physicians' fees and other outpatient services. To qualify for Part B coverage, individuals must pay a monthly premium, although additional financing from general revenues is needed to cover the costs of this program.

Physicians and suppliers who accept assignment under Part B are reimbursed 80 percent of their customary fee, subject to the limitations that it be no more than the prevailing fee in the area and that it be

289

reasonable. Once a provider or physician has agreed to participate, except for any deductible or coinsurance for which the beneficiary is responsible, the Medicare payment constitutes payment in full. If the physician or supplier does not accept assignment, then the beneficiary is reimbursed for 80 percent of the "reasonable charge" of the covered service.

Medicare is administered at the federal level by the Health Care Financing Administration (HCFA) of HHS. Administration is accomplished through fiscal intermediaries and carriers (generally private health insurance companies) who are under contract with the federal government and, as such, act as its agents. The intermediaries and carriers perform day-to-day administrative tasks, verify expenditures and services, determine reimbursable costs and charges, and make payments to providers and practitioners. In addition, both the Medicare law and implementing regulations contain provisions for monitoring the program for fraud and abuse on the part of participating providers and practitioners.

The Durenberger proposal has no direct effect on the Medicare program, although the proposal does define the minimum benefits a qualified plan must provide as those provided under Medicare. The Hatch proposal adds catastrophic protection to existing Medicare coverage but does not otherwise alter the current program. Thus, neither the Durenberger nor the Hatch proposal would substantially change the Medicare program as it now operates.

On the other hand, the Gephardt proposal provides Medicare recipients an option of remaining with the present Medicare program or choosing to receive the benefits of qualified plans offered by a competitive system. Medicare beneficiaries who choose the new system would be provided a health care voucher in an amount equal to the average cost of plans purchased by Medicare beneficiaries. Moreover, qualified plans under this proposal would be required to provide benefits greater than those currently covered by Medicare, such as coverage for outpatient drugs and for an unlimited number of hospital days. If an aged or disabled beneficiary chooses a plan costing less than the value of the voucher, the beneficiary is rebated the difference. Hence, the Gephardt proposal would change the Medicare program substantially.

In examining any Medicare voucher proposal, a number of legal issues arise. First, although the Gephardt voucher proposal specifically applies only to aged and disabled persons, other proposals do not specify whether they are intended for the chronic end-stage renal disease (ESRD) beneficiaries as well as for the aged and disabled persons. This issue is important because ESRD persons have different Medicare eligibility requirements and different reimbursement systems from the aged or disabled beneficiaries.

290

Second, a voucher system should specify the employer's obligations with respect to the Medicare employed population. Will beneficiaries be required to opt only for Medicare or the Medicare voucher, or will the employer be required to cover them until they are no longer employed?

Third, under the present Medicare program, the federal government is the primary payer in almost all situations when a beneficiary has double coverage by Medicare and private insurance. Private insurance companies are able to recoup funds from the Medicare program for covered Medicare services. (This is referred to as "coordinating benefits.") Under the Gephardt proposal, a Medicare beneficiary has the option, "in lieu of receiving benefits pursuant to the provisions" of the Medicare program, to receive a voucher for the purchase of private insurance from a qualified plan. However, unless the quoted language is deemed to amend the section of the Medicare law that makes the federal government the primary payer, then the private plan purchased by vouchers might, nonetheless, be able to coordinate benefits with the Medicare program. In order to avoid this consequence, the voucher proposals should include an amendment that denies the federal government primary-payer status for a plan purchased with vouchers.

Finally, in light of recent budgetary constraints as well as concern for the financial soundness of the Medicare trust funds, the voucher proposal should address its source of funds. Although the Gephardt proposal relies on appropriations, there is still the need to address how the appropriations will relate to the expenditure of the Medicare trust funds under the current Medicare program.

The Extent to Which the Consumer Choice Proposals Will Affect the Medicaid Program. The Medicaid program provides reimbursements from the federal government to the states so that they share the costs of providing medical care to low-income people.[27] Although the program is noncompulsory, currently all states participate except Arizona, which has a demonstration project only. In order to qualify for federal reimbursement, a state's program must, at a minimum, cover the state's welfare population. States may choose to extend coverage to those individuals who do not qualify for public assistance but who cannot afford health care. Similarly, states are required to offer certain specified services, but may choose to offer additional services. In an effort to reduce interstate differences in income and level of welfare payments, the program was designed so that the federal share of state Medicaid expenditures would vary from about 50 to 80 percent, depending on the state's per capita income.

In a manner similar to the Medicare program, states may contract with the fiscal intermediaries of their choice. Medical care providers are reimbursed directly for services rendered to Medicaid patients. Subject

291

to limitations imposed by participating states (for example, length-of-stay limitations), Medicaid generally follows Medicare with respect to reimbursement for inpatient hospital services, unless an exception is specifically approved. With respect to long-term care facility services, Medicaid pays on a modified reasonable cost basis. The recent amendments to the Medicaid program, however, provide the states with greater flexibility in determining reimbursement methodologies. With regard to physician services, reimbursement is generally less than for Medicare and varies from state to state. Unlike Medicare, Medicaid assignment rules are mandatory for all who choose to participate. As with Medicare, Medicaid programs are monitored for fraud and abuse.

Neither the Durenberger proposal nor the Hatch proposal refers to the Medicaid program. The Gephardt proposal, however, does establish a Medicaid voucher system, similar to the one for Medicare beneficiaries, so that the poor can also participate in selecting a competitive health care plan from the private sector. Four years after enactment of the Gephardt proposal, states may elect the voucher system instead of Medicaid. This election is revocable. Under the voucher system, individuals below the poverty line would receive a voucher for an amount based on average costs of plans for other purchasers in the same geographic area and actuarial category. For the near poor, the voucher is reduced in value one-half the amount that income exceeds the poverty line.

The legal issues raised by a Medicaid voucher system are similar to those mentioned for the Medicare voucher system. For instance, what is the source of funding? Will there be federal/state matching payments? In addition, if the definitions of poor and near poor for the voucher system are inconsistent with present Medicaid eligibility requirements, the legislative drafters may need to consider the administrative problems of having two Medicaid plans.

Whether the Consumer Choice Proposals Will Affect the Operations of the PSRO Program. The congressional purpose for establishing PSROs was to assure that health care services for which payment is made through the Medicare, Medicaid, and Maternal and Child Health programs conform to appropriate professional standards and are delivered in the most effective, efficient, and economical manner.[28] PSROs must be nonprofit professional associations whose membership is composed solely of licensed doctors of medicine or osteopathy engaged in the practice of medicine or surgery in the designated PSRO service area. PSROs are required to review federally funded services that are provided in hospitals and other inpatient settings to assure that they are medically necessary, meet professionally recognized standards of care, and are appropriately provided in the most economical setting. To make these determinations, each PSRO must develop standards and criteria for the diagnosis and treatment of the cases it reviews. Failure of the practitioner or provider to satisfy these criteria may result in denial of Medicare or Medicaid reimbursement, as well as further sanctions.

Neither the Durenberger proposal nor the Hatch proposal refers to, or would appear to affect, the PSRO program. Consequently, under those proposals the PSRO program is expected to continue to operate as it does now.

Under the Gephardt proposal, however, both the PSRO program and the requirement that hospitals conduct utilization review under the Medicare program would be repealed. Nevertheless, under this proposal, in order for a plan to be qualified, it must provide basic health care services, which are further defined to include clinical, institutional, and other health services. The proposal specifies, however, that basic health care services do not include a service that is not "medically necessary." Therefore, if a consumer choice proposal wishes to limit coverage to medically necessary services but repeals the PSRO law and hospital utilization review, it is unclear what organization or entity other than the attending physician would have the responsibility for making these decisions. Furthermore, it is questionable whether qualified plans can be evaluated by this criterion without the use of some peer-review mechanism.

Conclusion

In this chapter, we have examined some of the legal issues that may arise under a consumer choice proposal. In particular, we have examined in some detail those current statutes and case law that would interact with a consumer choice proposal. These existing laws included both health and nonhealth statutes and issues. It is hoped that, by raising these technical legal issues at this early stage in policy development, the questions can be resolved through explicit statutory language or legislative history and that, as a result, costly litigation that may impede the success of any new proposal ultimately enacted into law may be avoided.

Notes

1. H.R. 850, National Health Care Reform Act of 1981, introduced by Congressman Richard A. Gephardt (Democrat, Missouri) on January 16, 1981.

2. S. 433, Health Incentives Reform Act of 1981, introduced by Senator David Durenberger (Republican, Minnesota) on February 5, 1981.

3. S. 139, Comprehensive Health Care Reform Act, introduced by Senator Orrin B. Hatch (Republican, Utah) on January 15, 1981.

4. Savage v. Jones, 225 U.S. 501, 533 (1912) (dictum).

5. Nash v. Florida Industrial Commission, 389 U.S. 235 (1967).

6. Hewlett-Packard Co. v. Barnes, 571 F.2d 502, cert. denied 439 U.S. 831 (1978).

7. 29 U.S.C. § 1144(a).

8. 29 U.S.C. § 1144(b) (2) (A).

9. 15 U.S.C. § 1012(b). Emphasis added.

10. Securities and Exchange Commission v. National Securities, Inc., 393 U.S. 453, 458 (1969).

11. 91 Cong. Rec. 481–82 (1945), remarks of Senator Radcliffe.

12. For example, Cochran v. Paco, 606 F.2d 460 (5th Cir. 1979).

13. National League of Cities v. Usery, 426 U.S. 833 (1976).

14. Ibid., 426 U.S. at 845.

15. Ibid., 426 U.S. at 852.

16. Ibid., at note 17.

17. Usery v. Charleston County School District of Charleston County, South Carolina, 558 F.2d 1169 (4th Cir. 1977).

18. Ibid., 558 F.2d at 1170.

19. The Supreme Court's decision in the pending case, *Arizona* v. *Maricopa County Medical Society,* No. 80-419, may resolve the issue of whether rule of reason is applicable to all allegedly anticompetitive activities undertaken in the health care field or whether per se analysis is appropriate in some cases.

20. 29 U.S.C. § 151 et seq.

21. 29 U.S.C. § 201 et seq.

22. 41 U.S.C. §§ 351–357.

23. 40 U.S.C. § 276(a) et seq.

24. 29 U.S.C. § 1001 et seq.

25. 5 U.S.C. § 552.

26. 42 U.S.C. § 1395 et seq.

27. 42 U.S.C. § 1396 et seq.

28. 42 U.S.C. § 1320(c) et seq.

15

The Contributions of Antitrust Law to a Procompetitive Health Policy

Clark C. Havighurst

The strategy of reforming the health care industry through competition depends crucially upon private initiatives that could easily fail to materialize if the antitrust laws do not effectively inhibit private restraints of trade. During the long era, ending in the mid-1970s, when the antitrust laws did not much influence the behavior of health care providers, anticompetitive practices and attitudes became entrenched in the industry and allowed provider interests to shape the system to their liking and economic advantage. In the early 1970s, the uncontrolled costs of the noncompetitive, provider-dominated system prompted public dissatisfaction and demands for extensive regulation, which was generally perceived to be the only way to improve the industry's performance. Only when the antitrust laws began to be applied to govern provider conduct did it become at all realistic to contemplate competition as another policy option. Because of changes that antitrust law has helped to bring about in the competitive environment, one can now reasonably believe that changes in consumers' incentives and market opportunities, such as those projected by today's market-reform strategists, could improve the efficiency with which the health care industry uses society's resources.

This chapter reviews the doctrines of antitrust law on which a national procompetition strategy in the health services industry must depend to ensure the integrity of markets. It seeks to show that the antitrust effort in this sector fits easily within the mainstream of the antitrust tradition and that such doctrinal uncertainties as have existed were ultimately attributable, not to policy doubts or to notions that health care is a unique undertaking, but to the complexities of applying antitrust principles in unusual circumstances. It is argued that legal uncertain-

NOTE: Work on this chapter was supported by Grant No. HS04089 from the National Center for Health Services Research, U.S. Department of Health and Human Services.

ties arose primarily from the courts' limited experience in appreciating competition's role in markets characterized by extensive insurance coverage and by serious consumer information problems. Although courts and enforcement agencies have sometimes deferred to the medical profession and been hesitant to impugn the health care industry's self-regulatory paraphernalia, little likelihood remains that such deference will be given a legitimate place in the analysis of antitrust issues in this industry. Now that basic issues have been clarified, the courts can be expected to enforce the law against physicians and other health care providers as they do against other business enterprises. Thus, it seems safe, in making health policy for the 1980s, to depend upon antitrust law to facilitate private responses to new consumer demands for cost containment.

A Heritage of Trade Restraints

The first eighty-five years after enactment of the Sherman Act in 1890 saw little application of antitrust principles to the medical profession. Some lawyers, seeking to explain this inactivity, deduced that an implied antitrust exemption must exist for the "learned professions" (whoever they might be) and rationalized this elitist conclusion by arguing that the professions were not engaged in trade or commerce, to which the federal antitrust laws exclusively applied. Although this putative exemption was embodied more in inactivity than in precedent, occasional judicial dicta did support the notion that the rules of free enterprise should be applied either not at all or with diminished force to the organized professions. Thus, medicine's own special position was apparently recognized by the Supreme Court in a 1952 antitrust case.[1] Though finding that the government had failed to prove professional sponsorship of a boycott of a type that would ordinarily constitute a clear Sherman Act violation, the Court went out of its way to indicate a tolerant disposition toward such restraints if undertaken by professional bodies:

> We might observe in passing, however, that there are ethical considerations where the historic direct relationship between patient and physician is involved which are quite different than the usual considerations prevailing in ordinary commercial matters. This Court has recognized that forms of competition usual in the business world may be demoralizing to the ethical standards of a profession.[2]

Such apparent deference to professionalism probably reflected attitudes then prevalent in the society as a whole.

As a practical matter, the medical profession's de facto antitrust immunity probably owed much less to judicial belief in professional altruism than to the inability of federal law to reach localized conduct not affecting interstate commerce. Thus, in the famous 1943 case of *American Medical Association* v. *United States,* where jurisdiction was fortuitously not a problem, the Sherman Act was enforced against organized physicians with surprising rigor, yielding criminal convictions of the American Medical Association (AMA) and a local medical society.[3] In that case, the claim was made that a physician boycott against a health maintenance organization (HMO) was intended to protect patients' interests and to eliminate unethical professional practices. In vigorously rejecting this claim of professional immunity, the court of appeals stated: "[A]ppellants are not law enforcement agencies . . . and although persons who reason superficially concerning such matters may find justification for extra-legal action to secure what seems to them desirable ends[,] this is not the American way of life."[4] This language, as well as the result reached, suggests that deference to the medical profession was far from universal and that any immunity enjoyed by the profession was incomplete. Careful analysis of the case law confirms that jurisdictional factors were legally more important than professional status in insulating physicians from antitrust attacks.

Despite the assessment by the court of appeals in the *AMA* case that "the American way of life" does not countenance private regulation, the American public has frequently tolerated the assumption of public responsibilities by professional groups, ignoring the conflict of interests that such groups bring to self-regulatory endeavors. Thus, during the period when the professions were not subject to systematic antitrust oversight, professional groups in medicine developed ethical rules curbing advertising and other commercial practices. Many of the practices thus proscribed might have benefited consumers by breaking down some of the market power that an individual physician naturally possesses by virtue of patients' ignorance, their difficulty in shopping for alternative providers or treatments, and their reluctance to economize on health expenditures, especially when insurance covers all or most of the expense. Although professional codes of ethics have often been defended as a check on physicians' exploitation of their individual market power, they have also been instrumental in maintaining and strengthening such power and in legitimizing its perpetuation by seeming to curb its use. Thus, the profession's collective inhibitions on professional advertising and on express or implied disparagement of other professionals fostered the very consumer ignorance on which the claim of self-regulatory power depends. Such ethical principles embodied intraprofessional recognition of each doctor's sphere of influence over a particular clientele and implied social and other penalties for competitive behavior. Finally, ethical disapproval

297

of "contract practice"—that is, the provision of services under an arrangement with a lay-controlled middleman—inhibited physician cooperation in the organization of alternative financing and delivery systems.

The precise extent of the medical profession's success in curbing providers' competitive behavior cannot be known, but the techniques employed by the profession were well chosen. Even though the profession's ethical principles were not universally enforced or enforceable, their existence conditioned the behavior of those physicians who valued their professional relationships and organizations. The Supreme Court has observed, in another context, that, among a cartel's sanctions, "experience has shown [business honor and social penalties] to be the more potent and dependable restraints."[5] In another case involving a price-fixing plan by real estate brokers that lacked visible enforcement mechanisms, the Court observed that "[s]ubtle influences may be just as effective as the threat or use of formal sanctions to hold people in line."[6] Because the profession's ethical rules were most likely to affect the conscientious physician, they had the additional advantage, from the professional point of view, of ensuring the fulfillment of the prophecy used to justify their adoption—namely, that commercialized practice would primarily attract the profession's less respectable members.

In addition to maintaining an ethos systematically discouraging to commercially motivated conduct, the medical profession has also dominated the strategic points where innovation might enter the system. By dominating accreditation programs, organized medical interests kept the educational system for both physicians and nonphysicians largely in conventional channels, thus perpetuating a professionally approved ideology of medical care and an orthodox hierarchical conception of the delivery system. Systems providing personnel credentials—including state licensing boards and occupational and specialty certification programs in both medicine and allied fields—were also presided over in ways that discouraged threats to the profession's vital interests. Finally, hospital medical staffs have been organized—in compliance with profession-inspired accreditation standards—so that physicians can exercise a strong collective influence over their respective institutions. Although the medical profession's self-regulatory controls have undoubtedly averted some commercial abuses and enhanced the overall quality of care, their most significant effect has probably been to prevent precisely the types of experimentation, input substitution, and economizing reforms that theorists now expect competition to inspire.

Nonenforcement of the antitrust laws was, until recently, also the rule with respect to hospitals and other institutional providers of health services. As in the case of professional services, the localized character of institutional providers and their apparent lack of a substantial impact on interstate commerce long contributed to inactivity on the antitrust front. In addition, uncritical attitudes toward nonprofit firms and diffidence in the face of providers' quality-of-care claims probably diverted enforcement agencies into other areas and, by promising to influence judges, must have discouraged private litigants with potentially meritorious cases. As also occurred with respect to professional services, the absence of an antitrust threat allowed institutional competitors to become accustomed to resolving their differences through discussion and consensus rather than through competition in the marketplace. Thus, hospital planning councils, which had many of the earmarks of hospital cartels, undertook at an early date to reduce competition for philanthropic support and to allocate service responsibilities in local markets in ways minimizing competition. Where necessary, nonprofit institutional providers could use their presumed dedication to the public's interest in quality health care to justify acting collectively to suppress unwanted entrepreneurship. Thus, in a case that the Federal Trade Commission (FTC) eventually failed to win because of its limited statutory jurisdiction over nonprofit firms, hospitals in Kansas City boycotted commercial blood banks that threatened to disrupt the hospitals' own monopoly over blood supplies.[7]

Perhaps the most important development in the health care industry from the 1930s onward was the growth of private health insurance in response to consumers' demand for financial protection against the need for increasingly beneficial but also increasingly costly health services. Recognizing both this demand and the potential demand-increasing effects of extended insurance coverage, providers moved collectively to ensure that such financial protection would be provided in ways that did not threaten their interests. Thus, in what seemed to be forward-looking reforms, providers developed local Blue Cross (hospital) and Blue Shield (physician) service plans as devices for relieving consumers' cost concerns without creating large competitive buyers that might force providers into intensified economic competition. Hospitals used their close relationship with Blue Cross plans to foster a payment system based on retrospective cost reimbursement, thereby ensuring that each hospital could recover its costs without triggering price competition between low-cost and high-cost institutions. In similar fashion, the medical profession at first induced Blue Shield plans to confine their paid-in-full coverage to low-income persons, thus allowing professionals to continue the monopolistic practice of price discrimination by charging more affluent patients in accordance with their ability to pay. Ultimately, a system of "usual, customary, and reasonable" fees was adopted, giving fuller protection

299

to the middle-class consumer while avoiding both price uniformity and price competition.

In addition to sponsoring their own financing plans, provider groups collectively defined and enforced principles for identifying insurance schemes with which providers could ethically cooperate.[8] Physicians were thus able to ensure that commercial insurers, whom they could not directly control, would face serious risks if they sought to force physicians into accepting cost controls and competitive pricing. Perhaps the best-documented instance of physicians' dictating to independent financing plans appeared in the unsuccessful 1952 antitrust case quoted above as the high-water mark of judicial deference to physicians' motives.[9] In that case, Oregon physicians, by establishing and promoting a Blue Shield plan and discouraging cooperation with independent health plans, forced the latter to cease their efforts to police professional fees and utilization.[10]

Not only did the era of nonenforcement of the antitrust laws in the health care industry give rise to private attitudes and practices unfavorable to competition, but it also allowed anticompetitive traditions and attitudes to permeate public policy toward the industry. Many industry preferences for restraining commercial practices and for structuring insurance protection found expression in state laws. Moreover, the federal Medicare program's Parts A and B were modeled, respectively, after Blue Cross and Blue Shield plans and embodied the industry-approved concepts of cost reimbursement and customary fees. Such legal, regulatory, and programmatic barriers to innovation and competition currently prevent a full realization of a national procompetition strategy. Although the federal antitrust laws offer a limited basis for challenging some state laws inconsistent with the maintenance of competition,[11] their major potential value lies in terminating private-sector practices that, however time-honored and well intended they may be, are incompatible with competition. As the foregoing discussion shows, a substantial agenda awaited antitrust enforcers and other potential antitrust litigants when their attention was finally directed to the health care industry.

The Antitrust Explosion

The Supreme Court's 1975 decision in *Goldfarb* v. *Virginia State Bar*[12] decisively rejected the idea that the "learned professions" are exempt from antitrust scrutiny. Together with subsequent cases involving both hospital and professional services,[13] *Goldfarb* also made jurisdictional requirements substantially easier to satisfy in cases involving health care. With the courthouse threshold cleared of these doctrinal obstacles, private antitrust plaintiffs and the FTC touched off a minor explosion of antitrust litigation and considerable apprehension in the health care

300

industry. The FTC, in addition to recognizing the doctrinal significance of the *Goldfarb* case, was moved to act by intense public concern about health care costs and by the unsettled state of public policy toward the industry. Its early investigations would not have led very far, however, if real antitrust problems had not been uncovered. The closer the commission staff looked, the more it appeared that many professional and other concerted activities that had long been accepted as both desirable and inevitable had a darker side and served the industry as bulwarks against unwanted change.

Although the *Goldfarb* case opened all professions to new scrutiny, the health care industry spawned more than its fair share of the new litigation. In part, this reflected the extent to which industry participants had become accustomed to dominating their economic environment and were unwilling to relinquish control. Because local groups of competitors have either not appreciated their new legal responsibilities or have feared legal liability less than the consequences of changing their traditional ways, voluntary compliance has not been sufficient to obviate a great deal of litigation. Moreover, the complexity of the health care market, with its wide variety of public and private financing and regulatory mechanisms, has frequently made the implications of antitrust law less than clear, necessitating lawsuits to convince providers that the law is against them. Some providers have even invoked the antitrust laws to attenuate what they regard as undue competitive pressure, suing insurers over their hard bargaining or their refusals to cover high-cost services. Because these cases, of which there have been a great number, reflect the commonly held but increasingly discredited belief that antitrust law is intended to protect small businessmen against hard competition (rather than to foster such competition), extensive litigation has been necessary to establish the legitimacy of insurer bargaining and selectivity in covering providers' services. Later discussion highlights progress in clarifying the law in this area.

Despite the high cost of antitrust litigation and the uncertainty and consternation generated by antitrust fears, the explosion of antitrust activity in the health care sector should not be a cause for public concern. The process of adapting to a new and fundamentally different system of social control could hardly be painless and cost-free in an industry so large and so complex. There are, however, many reasons to think that the public will enjoy a net gain from making the transition to a competitive regime. Already the application of antitrust principles to the industry has permitted some private reforms that would previously have been frustrated, and further desirable changes can be anticipated as the law clarifies and as emerging cost consciousness is felt.

Perhaps the most important contribution of the antitrust movement to date has been to inform and broaden the policy debate. Application of the antitrust laws to this neglected sector of the economy has illuminated the reasons for the industry's poor past performance, has offered ready-made (and otherwise politically unobtainable) remedies for many institutionalized restraints, and has provided for the first time a realistic basis for anticipating substantial private sector innovation in response to consumer cost concerns. Indeed, the antitrust movement that began in 1975 has supplied a coherent national policy where previously there was nothing worthy of the name, but only an implicit acceptance of existing institutions and practices (including industry-sponsored controls) and an unresolved political struggle over how to make those institutions politically accountable and to improve their performance. Though not itself a complete public policy for the health care industry, the antitrust enforcement effort has taken away policy makers' politically easy option of accepting and perpetuating established institutions without carefully examining them. Even if it does no more, the forcing of fundamental policy choices makes the antitrust movement in the health care industry a constructive development, easily worth its social cost.

Implications of the Law's Strict Insistence on Competition

For the most part, the antitrust principles being invoked in the health care industry are the most basic ones of all—namely, those applicable to competitor collaboration under section 1 of the Sherman Act. Although much antitrust doctrine is currently controversial and is undergoing overdue rethinking both in enforcement agencies and in the courts, the rules applicable to "horizontal" restraints of trade, in addition to being reasonably clear, are generally accepted by antitrust experts.[14] Most of the legal uncertainties in the health care field arise not from controversy over basic antitrust doctrine but from the special forms that competition has taken or might take.

The idea that competition is not compelled by law as rigorously in the health care industry as elsewhere in the economy, though clung to by many lawyers with industry clients, has not been borne out by the courts. Although a few lower court judges have indicated a continuing willingness to defer to physicians and health care institutions and to put favorable constructions on their motives and practices,[15] the trend seems to be running toward the erosion of such interprofessional courtesy. The Supreme Court has stopped short of settling the matter definitively, however, choosing instead to couch each of its decisions involving the professions in guarded language. Nevertheless, while still leaving open the possibility that professionalism might sometime make a difference, the Court's successive statements have progressively narrowed the grounds for possible exceptions.[16] In one of its more recent pronouncements, the Court conceded only the obvious point that, "by their nature, professional services may differ significantly from other business services, and, accordingly, the nature of the competition in such services may vary. Ethical norms may serve to regulate and promote this competition, and thus come within the Rule of Reason."[17] Significantly, the Supreme Court has yet to make professionalism and the fact that a restraint is "premised on public service or ethical norms"[18] the basis for deciding any case in favor of a professional group.[19] Moreover, in its most recent decision in this area, the Court specifically rejected the argument that the usual antitrust rules should be applied more tentatively "because the judiciary has little antitrust experience in the health care industry."[20]

A source of special tension in applying antitrust principles to the health care sector is the perception that, in circumstances frequently encountered in health care, competition can be more harmful than beneficial. Although this perception may sometimes be correct in some sense, the judgment required to verify it can be difficult indeed. In part because arguments of this kind open such complexities, even clearly harmful effects of competition have been made irrelevant to the application of antitrust law. Thus, it has long been held that the Sherman Act requires competition for better or for worse and leaves no room for courts to make the difficult and essentially legislative judgment whether, or how much, competition is desirable in a specific situation.[21] This principle was forcefully reaffirmed in a 1978 case overturning an ethical ban on competitive bidding by professional engineers.[22] In that case, the Supreme Court refused to allow the engineers to defend by showing that price competition would invite unsafe engineering work and specifically rejected the argument that the antitrust rule of reason allows competition to be attenuated where its effects would be contrary to the public interest. Rather, the Court made the effect of the challenged practices on competition the only touchstone. The law is therefore quite clear that only Congress and, to a lesser extent, state legislatures can create exceptions to the basic prohibition against agreements among competitors that impair the competitive process.

The legal principle explained above would also preclude arguing in defense of an agreement among hospitals that, because third-party payment takes the form it does, competition among hospitals will focus on factors other than price and therefore will cause costs to rise rather than to fall. Many thoughtful observers of the hospital industry would find this argument persuasive as a policy proposition, however, and would therefore regard as perverse the legal doctrine that rejects its relevance.

Even antitrust prosecutors, recognizing the peculiar economics of hospital competition, have sometimes seemed reluctant to insist on the letter of the law in the hospital setting. Because of the argument's plausibility, because prosecutorial discretion may legitimately be exercised to avoid compelling results deemed adverse to the public interest, and finally because health care interests have vigorously contended that antitrust is unsuited to the industry's special conditions, it is necessary specifically to consider whether strict insistence by courts and law enforcers on competition in this industry would really be as destructive as many predict.

The crucial premise in the argument advanced against competition in the health care industry is that third-party payment systems remove price considerations as a factor in most consumer decisions. Yet it is not inevitable that payment systems will always be so perverse as to invite undesirable cost escalation. Indeed, in an unrestrained competitive market, both the purchasers of financial protection and the financing plans themselves would have the opportunity as well as the incentive to seek and implement less expensive methods of financing care that do not have this adverse consequence. Furthermore, the effect of tolerating industrywide collaboration as a way of offsetting the worst effects of dysfunctional payment systems would simply be to shelter such systems from the consequences of their own inefficiency, thereby contributing to their perpetuation. Finally, to legitimize such concerted action is to confirm prevalent attitudes toward independent initiatives and to credit industry claims that it is doing all that needs doing about health care costs; if cost increases seem to be the inevitable result of a legitimate collective process, private innovations in health care financing are unlikely to be undertaken.

Nor should enforcement of the antitrust laws be relaxed in order to spare government the higher Medicare and Medicaid costs that might flow from nonprice competition. Enhancing competition that raises these program costs in the short run might well cause Congress finally to break with the cost-reimbursement approach in public programs. (Indeed, this is already occurring.) Moreover, insistence on such competition in the market as a whole might trigger the private development of new financing mechanisms that would benefit government indirectly by stimulating greater efficiency in hospitals and in medical practice. New types of private financing plans might also increase the potential gains to government from shifting to a voucher approach under which federal beneficiaries could opt for private plans giving better protection for the same money. Once again, vigorous insistence on competition without regard to short-run expediency should perform the useful public service of forcing Congress to reexamine its policy choices. Thus, the unsettling effects of firmly applying antitrust doctrine can be seen as an aid to developing not only a more efficient industry but also a better national health policy.

The rigor of the basic antitrust rules for appraising industrywide collaboration by competitors obviously presents severe problems for industry-sponsored reform efforts aimed at cost containment. Because antitrust doctrine focuses on effects on competition and not on motives or on whether prices are raised or lowered or on whether competition has been impaired for a good reason, even the most sincere and well-motivated reformers may find their efforts challenged. In the recent case of *Arizona* v. *Maricopa County Medical Society,* the Supreme Court condemned as price fixing—an automatic (per se) violation—the efforts of two profession-sponsored "foundations for medical care" to place maximum limits on the fees charged by member doctors for services underwritten by insurers who had agreed to adhere to the foundation's fee schedule. Noting some theoretical harms that such fee limits might cause, the Court observed that "[t]he *per se* rule 'is grounded on faith in price competition as a market force [and not] on a policy of low selling prices at the price of eliminating competition.' "[23]

Because the two justices not participating in the four-to-three decision in the *Maricopa County* case might have voted with the dissenters, some observers will continue to harbor hope that the Court will one day bend its rules to accommodate the health care industry's allegedly special problems. Nevertheless, the wisdom of adhering to the requirement of competition and to the firm rule against naked competitor price agreements is so well recognized that the decision is likely to be approved by antitrust experts. Moreover, the case serves as an excellent demonstration of precisely why courts should avoid a complete inquiry into the overall competitive effects of practices that are inherently dangerous to competition. The arguable procompetitive benefits of the foundations' fee-setting would have accrued only in the insurance market and were of minor importance compared with the possible harms in the market for physician services. Nevertheless, a trial court would have found it difficult to balance these alleged benefits against the real but possibly unprovable risk that, by asserting their own responsibility for fee levels, the foundations discouraged insurers from competitively bargaining with individual physicians for lower prices. Similarly, courts would have found it impossible to determine with precision whether the foundations' fees were set at a competitive level or were instead entry-limiting prices discouraging to the creation of independent HMOs and other competitive innovations unwanted by the foundations' physician members. Finally, the dissenting justices seemed to have no appreciation of the value of clear rules in deterring competitors from anticompetitive acts and in relieving the courts from tedious but usually inconclusive inquiries. The majority, on the other hand, observed with approval that, "[f]or the sake of business certainty and litigation efficiency, we have tolerated [in other cases] the invalidation of some agreements that a fullblown inquiry might have proved to be reasonable."[24]

Even if the Supreme Court majority in *Maricopa County* had thought, as the dissenters apparently did, that the foundations had integrated the member physicians into a procompetitive joint venture, the close connection with organized medicine and the large proportion of physicians participating in that venture should still have condemned the plan.[25] The reason for such a result is once again that competition is the preferred vehicle of reform and that collective efforts to improve the industry's overall economic performance proceed from an unacceptable monopolistic premise—namely, the conception of the medical profession, or the health care system, as an economic entity whose performance is to be centrally controlled and judged as a totality. Although it requires sacrificing some seemingly desirable reforms often sponsored by dedicated and well-meaning professionals, the firm antitrust rule makes sense. Experience indicates that the dominant professional interests allow such collective reforms to succeed only when some external threat—either emerging competition or pressures for government regulation—is so palpable that reform appears to be the lesser evil.[26] As a result, the public, though the beneficiary of voluntary reform, is likely to have been denied a greater good. Once again, vigorous antitrust enforcement, by refusing to defer to a claim of collective responsibility by industry interests, leaves issues open for a definitive legislative choice and keeps competition as an available option by not sacrificing it prematurely.

The Antitrust Enforcement Agenda

A brief survey of particular concerted actions in the health care industry that have been or may be attacked under the antitrust laws will illustrate both the depth of the challenge to professional traditions and institutional arrangements and the nature and likelihood of change under an antitrust regime. Although space does not permit a full statement of the law in each area, the discussion identifies particular issues that have been or may be raised. At several points, the availability of certain express or implied exemptions from the antitrust laws is discussed.

Ethical Restrictions on Professional Advertising. An early object of the FTC's interest in the health care industry was the restrictions imposed by professional organizations on their members' advertising. Although the AMA moved to reinterpret its rules on advertising following the *Goldfarb* decision, the FTC insisted on prosecuting and issuing its own order against enforcement of provisions in the AMA's and state societies' codes of ethics.[27] The commission did, however, allow professional organizations to police "false and deceptive" advertising. Such self-regulation could be undertaken only under specific, objective guidelines that the organization adopted in advance to advise professionals of their rights, to minimize the risk of selective enforcement, and to permit the FTC to satisfy itself that there were no abuses.

As a technical legal matter, it is not obvious that professional associations should be allowed to police even deceptive advertising, for an agreement not to compete using deceptive methods is still a naked agreement not to compete. Although Justice Stevens's opinion in the *Professional Engineers* case indicated that "professional deception is a proper subject of an ethical canon,"[28] a substantial question remains whether professional regulation of deceptive advertising would in fact "promote competition" as required by the tests announced by the Court in that case. Although such self-regulation is ostensibly addressed to an aspect of the problem of consumer ignorance, it would be surprising indeed if a professional organization were really committed to increasing consumers' confidence in professional advertising, thereby strengthening competitive forces bearing on its members. In view of the AMA's own overly restrictive policies in the past, the FTC would probably have been justified in refusing to give it a power that might be employed to harass and intimidate professionals whose advertising or other conduct was not to its liking. Although medical societies would theoretically be subject to a treble damage claim if they should abuse this power in disciplining a particular physician, the Supreme Court has indicated in a similar context that a self-regulatory body, if legitimate, is entitled to "breathing space" so that it can function without undue fear of antitrust liability.[29] For this reason and because abuses and actual anticompetitive effects can be quite subtle, self-regulatory powers such as those conceded to medical societies by the FTC carry with them a potential for unchallenged harm.

The FTC's decision against the AMA was affirmed, first (two to one) by the court of appeals and subsequently by an equally divided Supreme Court.[30] The primary issues were whether the Federal Trade Commission Act gives the commission jurisdiction over professional societies and whether the AMA had mended its ways sufficiently and soon enough following *Goldfarb* to render the FTC challenge moot. Because the Supreme Court affirmed without opinion, there is no way of knowing how the justices felt about these issues. Professional organizations have cited the split in the Court as evidence of a need for legislation clarifying—and drastically curbing—the FTC's power over state-regulated professions.[31] Nevertheless, the mootness issue, which

307

occasioned the dissent in the court of appeals, is more likely to have been the question that divided the justices.

Specialty Certification. A program for certifying individual professionals as having special skills is surely a desirable feature of a marketplace in which consumers have difficulty in judging professional qualifications. Even where the certification program is run by a group of competing professionals, it has prima facie validity under Justice Stevens's *Professional Engineers* formula as a collaboration to "promote competition." Antitrust issues would arise only if there were some abuse in the administration of the program so that competitors were unfairly disadvantaged.[32] In order to protect against unfair treatment of potential competitors, such a competitor-controlled certification body would probably be expected to employ fair procedures and to adopt reasonably objective standards. The extent to which antitrust courts will enter into an investigation of the value of the information being conveyed by certification remains an open question, but judges should probably not concern themselves with such technical matters. In the absence of a clear showing of an intent to mislead consumers (which would defeat the claim that competition was being promoted), the marketplace should be allowed to determine what value to attach to certification. First Amendment principles counsel avoidance of any substantial judicial inquiry into the truthfulness or informational value of the claims that certifying groups make for themselves.

The argument that the marketplace can decide what particular certifications are worth suggests that competing certification schemes might usefully coexist. Indeed, both antitrust and First Amendment considerations point toward the desirability of multiple sources of information. As things now stand, however, the American Board of Medical Specialties (ABMS), the profession's overseer of certification programs, strongly discourages any overlap between certification schemes. Because new schemes find it impossible to get established without recognition from the ABMS, that body has been able to foreclose most competition among specialties. Although consumers undoubtedly need to be assured that certification schemes are what they claim to be—that is, there is a need for a body to certify the certifiers—a new certifying body should not have to satisfy the existing bodies before being recognized. The antitrust laws could well be employed to open up the market for the development of new configurations and competing specialties.

Physicians' Hospital Privileges and Exclusive Arrangements. The expanding supply of physicians is increasing the tension between physicians, whose practice requires hospital admitting privileges, and hospitals

308

concerned about the quality of care, efficiency, and interests of their medical staffs. The antitrust issues presented require distinguishing between the concerns of the hospital itself, which is probably free under the antitrust laws to be as selective as it likes, and the possibly self-interested concerns of its medical staff, which is in a position to deny a vital resource to competing physicians.[33] To date, physicians have been generally unsuccessful in winning on their antitrust claims concerning hospital privileges, but it seems clear that hospital medical staffs must maintain fair procedures and must have some reasonably objective grounds for denying staff membership.[34] The hospital should also avoid becoming involved in a conspiracy with the medical staff. Indeed, it must be seen to act as an independent decision maker, taking account only of its own interests. Cases allowing hospitals to make exclusive arrangements with anesthesiologists, pathologists, radiologists, and other hospital-based physicians have been resolved largely on the principle that hospitals' business judgments should be respected.[35]

In general, the antitrust laws, while perhaps yielding few recoveries to disappointed applicants for hospital staff positions, may contribute to the maintenance of fair procedures and discourage abdication by hospital boards of their responsibilities in this area. As the supply of physicians increases and as hospitals become increasingly involved in innovative financing and delivery arrangements, antitrust problems will continue to appear. One area likely to receive attention is the use of limitations on staff privileges as a vehicle for finely dividing the market among competing physicians and surgeons within the hospital.

Nonphysicians' Opportunities. In *Virginia Academy of Clinical Psychologists* v. *Blue Shield,* physician domination of the Blue Shield plans led the court to find that the plans' policy of discriminating against nonphysician providers of psychotherapy violated the Sherman Act.[36] Because professional organizations of physicians can also influence the market opportunities of nonphysician providers in other ways, antitrust claims by disadvantaged providers are increasing. In addition to seeking to have their services covered by prepayment plans, nonphysician practitioners have sued to obtain hospital admitting privileges and access to other doctor-controlled resources.[37]

Again, the issues are difficult.[38] On the one hand, the medical profession is not permitted to act collectively, through boycotts or otherwise, to enforce any particular conclusion about how care should be delivered or by whom. Although physician organizations may engage in legitimate certification and accreditation efforts, competing certification and accreditation schemes must be permitted to coexist. The key issue in a given case is probably whether the physician organization making and enforcing policy with respect to nonphysicians is a broad-based association possessing appreciable market power or is instead an independent delivery organization facing effective competition from similar competing plans. Where such competition exists, the consumer is the ultimate decision maker with respect to the role of nonphysicians, and the market should be deemed to provide all the protection to which nonphysicians are entitled.

Provider Control of Financing Plans. The FTC staff has issued a lengthy report and a statement of enforcement policy challenging the domination of Blue Shield and other medical prepayment plans by state and local medical societies.[39] Whereas the *Virginia Academy* case indicated that profession-controlled plans are subject to special limitations on their power to make decisions disadvantageous to physicians' competitors, the FTC has challenged the control relationship itself, calling attention to the plans' destructive effect on price competition among physicians. Difficulties are presented with respect to what relationships short of outright control might be permissible and what kinds of physician organizations would be denied the right to organize a financing plan. The appropriate test appears to be one that focuses on the percentage of physicians in the market area involved in controlling the particular plan. If the percentage is low enough that competing organizations of physicians can reasonably be expected to coexist, a physician group should be allowed to organize and run an organized health plan without antitrust fears.[40] Indeed, such joint ventures are to be valued for their procompetitive impact.[41]

The FTC's challenge to profession-dominated plans has been quite controversial. In many localities, the medical community has sought to meet the various competitive or regulatory threats it faces by organizing a foundation for medical care or an individual practice association. These profession-sponsored reforms are another example of arguably well-intended reform efforts by professional groups that should not be tolerated because of their incompatibility with competition.[42]

Boycotts and Related Restraints. Professional groups historically employed the classic boycott to achieve many of their objectives. A recent and particularly egregious example involved the Michigan State Medical Society, which solicited powers of attorney authorizing it to withdraw individual physicians as participating providers in an independent Blue Shield plan that had undertaken some unpopular cost-containment measures.[43] Boycotts may also be found where the professional organization simply encourages its members to think (and thus to act) alike on a matter of collective interest. In other words, an explicit call for a boycott may not be necessary if the professional organization has allowed itself to be used to stimulate parallel action by its members.[44] Most professional boycotts need not be unanimous to be effective in warding off perceived threats.

Collective Bargaining. Medical societies and hospital organizations have frequently sought to negotiate with health insurers over reimbursement matters. Because concerted refusals to deal (boycotts) are themselves unlawful, a provider group engaging in such collective bargaining lacks the ultimate sanction needed to ensure its bargaining effectiveness. Even though the group's ability to bargain successfully is therefore in doubt, the law would also independently prohibit the providers' collective negotiation, at least to the extent that it represents a surrender of their competitive independence and precludes insurers from negotiating with them individually.[45] Moreover, an insurer that engages in such negotiations, such as a Blue Cross or Blue Shield plan, might easily be found to be involved in a conspiracy with the provider group if it accepts an anticompetitive arrangement. Litigation is currently in progress in Cleveland over a hospital council's agreement with Blue Cross to use a cost-reimbursement scheme that eliminated the possibility of effective price competition among hospitals.[46]

Preemption by Professional Groups of Decision-Making Authority on Economic Issues. The large number of health insurers does not necessarily mean that they compete by seeking to purchase providers' services on favorable terms. In order to preclude such cost-reducing efforts, which would force physicians into price competition, medical organizations have frequently sought to assume decision-making powers on important economic issues. If third-party payers should instead assume such functions themselves, providers would have to decide individually whether to accept the conditions offered by an insurer as the price of having their services covered on advantageous terms. Thus, both price and willingness to accept administrative requirements aimed at controlling utilization would become the subject of bargaining between health plans and providers. The lack of competitive bargaining explains, more than any other single thing, the industry's high prices and its apparently excessive claims on society's resources.

Professional organizations have moved in several ways to preempt decision making on crucial economic issues. The promulgation of relative value scales by medical organizations has carried with it not only the risk that the value schedules would be employed for price-fixing purposes but also the risk that third parties would generally accept them instead of competing to design better payment systems.[47] More serious,

311

though largely unrecognized, risks are inherent in profession sponsorship of peer-review panels to mediate disputes over fees, utilization, and other economic matters. The existence of such peer-review mechanisms constitutes an invitation to third parties not to compete by bargaining over fees or by establishing their own controls on utilization. Instead, insurers are invited to accept the profession's own controls.

Properly understood, the antitrust movement in the health care industry can be seen as having the primary objective of decentralizing decision making on medical-economic questions. Progress on this front was made in the *Maricopa County* case, which held that foundations for medical care could not set maximum fees on behalf of approved insurers. The Court noted that, "[e]ven if a fee schedule is . . . desirable, it is not necessary that the doctors do the price fixing."[48] It also observed, almost as a matter of judicial notice, that "insurers are capable not only of fixing maximum reimbursable prices but also of obtaining binding agreements with providers guaranteeing the insured full reimbursement of a participating provider's fee."[49] In thus pointing the way toward true competitive bargaining between insurers and physicians, the Court correctly identified why it would be inappropriate to accept profession-sponsored groups as arbiters of economic issues. In another recent case, the Court refused to extend the antitrust exemption enjoyed by the business of insurance under the McCarran-Ferguson Act to cover a chiropractor organization's peer-review program for reviewing the reasonableness of fees.[50] Although the Court did not rule on the merits of the antitrust claim in this case, it would seem that the *Maricopa County* case goes far toward condemning such peer-review programs and forcing insurers to assume responsibility for setting limits and negotiating prices.[51]

Although there has been no challenge as yet to the legality of peer-review programs aimed at controlling utilization, it is logical to expect one. In economics and antitrust theory, agreements to limit output are as troublesome as agreements on price, and thus, despite their arguable benefits, profession-sponsored peer-review programs might fall under a per se rule similar to the one articulated and applied in the *Maricopa County* case. The logic of such a result lies once again in the antitrust policy favoring decentralized decision making. Thus, an HMO or other integrated health plan would be encouraged to maintain internal utilization rules as long as it was not composed of or controlled by a dominant professional group, but a health insurer or employer seeking to control costs would be denied the option of turning to profession-sponsored groups for utilization standards.[52] They would thus be forced to find their own ways of controlling spending through changes in benefits, contractual arrangements with providers, or otherwise.

It is in these areas more than anywhere else that antitrust law penetrates to the heart of the medical monopoly by threatening to deprive the profession of its authority to set standards for the system as a whole.[53] The natural result of foreclosing the profession's decision-making role will be the emergence of competing middlemen, each of them accountable not to the profession as a whole but to the consumers and providers whom they must attract in the marketplace and to any regulators that government sees fit to appoint. There is no denying the seriousness of this challenge to deep-seated professional traditions, which have long maintained that only groups representing professional interests should make medical-economic decisions.

Restraints on the Ways in Which Providers Sell Their Services. Competition can be expected to yield efficient arrangements only if providers are not constrained in accepting new terms of employment or in accommodating their patients' special needs arising from insurers' requirements. In the past, an important barrier to reform of the financing and delivery system has been professional restrictions on the ways in which professionals could market their services. Ethical restrictions on "contract practice" by physicians were found illegal by the FTC in the same case in which it attacked the AMA and its advertising restrictions.[54] An FTC administrative law judge has also condemned a dental organization that encouraged its members to withhold from dental insurers X-rays that were needed for cost-containment purposes.[55] Hospitals have also been penalized for agreeing not to grant price or other concessions to HMOs.[56]

Restraints on HMOs. Had the antitrust laws not been applied to vindicate HMOs in the famous *AMA* case of 1943, it is unlikely that even a vestige of competition would have survived in the medical care industry. HMOs still encounter numerous problems as a result of hostility from local medical groups, however, and it has been hard for antitrust enforcers to intervene effectively on their behalf because intervention can often be self-defeating, causing resistance to the HMO to harden. Although some HMOs have found it helpful to invoke the antitrust laws, much of the resistance they encounter, though concerted, is of such an informal nature that proving the violation and implementing an effective remedy are both problematic.[57]

Partly because group practice HMOs are so readily identified as a threat to professional interests, the appearance of one in a community may have the effect of drawing local professionals together into a more cohesive group. Although the antitrust threat may be useful in curbing egregious conduct, it cannot ensure that entry barriers faced by HMOs will not be artificially high. It is partly because HMOs encounter such problems in getting established that reforms of other kinds, particularly insurer initiatives that would split the fee-for-service community into competing groups, are desirable.

313

Health Planning. Hospital interests have frequently worked with local planning organizations to structure the local market and minimize competition. Despite the argument that hospital competition may sometimes increase costs, interhospital cooperation, even when brought about with the approval and through the good offices of federally sponsored health planning agencies, is probably not exempt from the antitrust laws. The Supreme Court recently held that the National Health Planning and Resources Development Act of 1974 provided no blanket exemption for a private party acting on its own to carry out the will of a federally designated health systems agency (HSA).[58] The Justice Department's Antitrust Division holds the view that there is also no exemption for anticompetitive arrangements negotiated and specifically approved by the health planners themselves. Thus, the department has refused to indicate its approval of an HSA's brokering of market division agreements among hospitals as a way of achieving goals established through federally mandated planning.[59] This view seems supported by careful reading of the planning law and by the many cases holding that antitrust exemptions are not to be "lightly" inferred.

The antitrust challenge to the brokering of anticompetitive agreements by health planning agencies served to highlight the implications of the health planning enterprise and raised sharply the question whether Congress wished to rely on competition or exclusively on planning and regulation to achieve efficiency in health services. In considering amendments to the federal health planning legislation in 1979, Congress was specifically aware of the emerging conflict between the Justice Department and the health planners. Not only did it choose not to resolve the matter in the planners' favor, but it added language to the law placing new emphasis on the desirability of competition, thus further weakening claims that it intended that the antitrust laws not apply.[60] Now that federally sponsored health planning is being phased out (in part because of its anticompetitive character), it should be clear that local hospital councils and other groups, such as purchaser coalitions, are fully subject to the antitrust laws and will not be allowed to take trade-restraining actions. As argued earlier, there are reasons to believe that the long-run benefits of enforcing the law strictly against such industrywide "reform" organizations will more than offset any short-run costs that might be incurred.

Hospital and Other Mergers. Antitrust questions have been increasingly raised with respect to mergers and takeovers in the hospital and nursing home industries. In general, the focus has been exclusively on effects on competition in local markets. The FTC has attacked a series of acquisitions in a small California community, and the Justice Depart-

314

ment has opposed acquisitions by a large nursing home chain.[61] Antitrust questions have also been raised in private litigation about takeover bids involving chains of proprietary hospitals. Among the special problems that have yet to be explicitly addressed is the question whether markets should sometimes be defined more narrowly than hospital services or more broadly than a single community. Another open question is whether proprietary hospitals might be viewed as more effective competitors than some nonprofit and community hospitals, making mergers between them more troublesome than mergers involving voluntary hospitals.

Anticompetitive Use of Antitrust Law: Is It a Two-Edged Sword? Reforms of the type that procompetition theorists wish to see in private financing mechanisms have been retarded somewhat by antitrust litigation initiated by providers against third parties seeking to implement new approaches. The leading case is *Group Life and Health Insurance Co. v. Royal Drug Co.,*[62] in which the Supreme Court held that the McCarran-Ferguson Act did not exempt a Blue Shield plan's prepaid prescription drug program from antitrust attack by aggrieved pharmacies. The theory of the plaintiff pharmacies was that the plan's practice of discriminating against them because they were unwilling to accept the prescribed professional fee as payment in full violated the antitrust laws. Although the Supreme Court had no occasion to consider this substantive question, numerous lawsuits involving similar questions, both in the pharmacy field and in other health professions, sprang up around the country. The first of these cases has recently been decided in favor of the insurers.[63] As a result, many third parties who have been reluctant to challenge providers may now be more aggressive and selective in their dealings with them.

Coverage or benefit limitations that steer consumers away from high-cost providers are a new development and are only beginning to make headway in medical and hospitalization insurance. But such price-conscious selectivity, which can take innumerable forms short of closed-panel prepaid group practice, represents possibly the most promising approach to solving insurers' cost problems. Naturally, fee-for-service providers, unaccustomed to facing such price resistance, feel that they are being victimized by a large insurer with whom they cannot deal on equal terms—partly because of antitrust constraints on their own ability to act in concert. Nevertheless, these provider complaints are almost certainly not meritorious. Insurers are appropriately regarded simply as purchasers of services, and they are entirely within their rights in attempting to limit their costs. Although an insurer acts as its insureds' buying agent and combines their buying power, it does so, not to restrain trade, but as an incident to the pooling of risks that is the basic purpose of insurance.

315

Moreover, because the pooling of risks weakens the insureds' own cost consciousness and gives rise to behavioral distortions that economists call moral hazard, the insurer has a clear business purpose in taking special measures to control its costs. Thus, even a mutual insurer, which is technically a combination of competing buyers, could claim that its efforts to keep providers' prices down are ancillary to the legitimate business objective of efficiently sharing risks. Only if the insurer substantially dominated the market, representing a predominant share of the providers' available business, would there be any issue at all under either section 1 or section 2 of the Sherman Act.

These conclusions, while consistent with basic antitrust analysis, are not easily accepted in the medical and hospital care setting. Observers tend to react against the efficient business arrangements thus fostered because of arguably adverse effects on consumers' freedom of choice, on providers' market opportunities, on clinical independence, and on the quality of care. Analytical clarity has been aided, however, by the surfacing of identical issues in less highly charged arenas. In several cases involving casualty insurers' arrangements with automobile body shops, the courts have had no substantial difficulty in recognizing the legitimacy of, and applauding, individual insurers' aggressive purchasing.[64] The body shop plaintiffs, for whose services the insurers were obligated to pay, have been recognized as sellers whose only grievance sprang from a preference for not selling to cost-conscious buyers. It seems likely that the remaining pharmacy cases, which also present the issue in a fairly straightforward commercial setting, will be decided in the same way. Finally, once the courts have seen the forms that competition can usefully take in markets characterized by extensive insurance coverage, it is unlikely that they will give hospitals, doctors, and other professionals any special protection against competition. A much greater danger to competition is that pharmacists and other professional groups fearful of competition will seek and obtain statutory protection in the states.

Conclusion

Antitrust law now seems rather plainly to command that providers of health services must refrain from collaborating in anticompetitive ways. Whatever the collaborators' professional status, whatever their purposes, and however questionable the value of competition in the particular circumstances, the law insists on competition in health care just as it does in other industries and leaves to the legislative branch any judgments about the wisdom of such a policy in particular circumstances. The application of these tested and time-honored principles to the health care sector has called into fundamental question certain contrary traditions of cooperation and professional self-regulation and has undermined the foundations of providers' market power. With the end of the Supreme Court's 1981–1982 term, a term marked by five significant antitrust decisions involving professional services and health care, the legal revolution appears to be virtually complete.[65] Unless regulation prevents realization of the fruits of that revolution in the marketplace, one can expect to see major competitively inspired changes in the structure and operation of financing and delivery mechanisms. Signs of this anticipated revolution are already appearing.

Notwithstanding recent clarifications of health care providers' obligations under the antitrust laws, some uncertainties remain. Antitrust law does not evolve in complex areas without deviations from the narrow path, and the possibility of future compromises with basic antitrust principles still exists. Indeed, despite the clarity of the Supreme Court's rulings, a majority of the present justices may still be inclined to special tolerance in viewing the trade-restraining activities of professionals. Thus, a new decision reflecting a weak appreciation of the complex nature of competition in insured services or an acceptance of professional claims at face value could reintroduce confusion. Nevertheless, there are no specific cases on the horizon in which the Court will have an opportunity to undercut the principles recently established. The law therefore seems clear enough that professional organizations will no longer be advised to take their chances in the courts, and the lower courts should be able to dispose satisfactorily of the cases that do arise. In general, it appears that an important legal plateau has been reached and that there are few chances of losing the ground gained. Even though the medical profession is currently leading a legislative campaign to limit the antitrust jurisdiction of the FTC over professional organizations, adoption of that proposal would have no effect on substantive antitrust doctrine applicable to the health care industry. The most substantial dangers to competition in the health care field at the moment lie not in the area of antitrust law but in the field of state regulation.

In addition to clearing the way for the private sector to pursue efficiency in the financing and delivery of health services, antitrust law has contributed importantly to competition's emergence in the national political arena. Even as political observers speculated over whether or not the Reagan administration would propose and Congress would adopt a procompetitive health policy, the courts were gradually clarifying antitrust doctrine to a point where the federal government's policy toward the health care industry can now be declared firmly procompetitive in fact. Federal policy is after all a matter of law, and the courts, finding no sweeping antitrust exemptions in federal health legislation or elsewhere, have now concluded that competition in health care is the law of the land. Significantly, this crucial determination of policy was reached outside the political process and therefore did not require the formation of a solid political consensus in support of either the general concept or its complex and unpopular implications. Because competition has had few political supporters and has been opposed, openly or covertly, by nearly all of the important industry interest groups, the political process alone could never have yielded a procompetitive policy as coherent and as stable as the current one seems to be.

The recent crystallization of federal health policy around the idea of competition obviously owes a great deal not only to antitrust law but also to recent changes in political attitudes about the proper role of government in the private economy. Even though political processes may yet undo the current commitment to competition, this is an appropriate time to recognize and cautiously applaud the success of the antitrust movement in giving the nation at least the rudiments of its first conceptually sound health policy. Much more needs to be done, of course, to adapt existing laws, regulations, and public financing programs to fit the new policy framework. Nevertheless, one should be impressed by what the nation's institutions, by adhering to sound principles in the face of spurious arguments and serious temptations and pressures, have so far been able to accomplish.

Notes

1. United States v. Oregon State Medical Soc'y, 343 U.S. 326 (1952).

2. Ibid., p. 336.

3. 130 F.2d 233 (D.C. Cir. 1942), aff'd, 317 U.S. 519 (1943).

4. 130 F.2d at 249.

5. American Column & Lumber Co. v. United States, 257 U.S. 377, 411 (1921).

6. United States v. National Ass'n of Real Estate Boards, 339 U.S. 485, 489 (1950).

7. In re Community Blood Bank, Inc., 70 F.T.C. 728 (1966), rev'd on other grounds, 405 F.2d 1011 (8th Cir. 1969).

8. See generally "The American Medical Association: Power, Purpose, and Politics in Organized Medicine," *Yale Law Journal*, vol. 63 (May 1954), pp. 976–96; Clark C. Havighurst, "Professional Restraints on Innovation in Health Care Financing," *Duke Law Journal*, vol. 1978 (May 1978), pp. 303–87.

9. United States v. Oregon State Medical Soc'y, 343 U.S. 326 (1952).

10. See Lawrence G. Goldberg and Warren Greenberg, "The Effect of Physician-Controlled Health Insurance: U.S. v. Oregon State Medical Society," *Journal of Health Politics, Policy and Law*, vol. 2 (Spring 1977), pp. 48–78.

11. For the relevant principles, see California Retail Liquor Dealers Ass'n v. Medcal Aluminum, Inc., 445 U.S. 97 (1980). For a constructive application of them in a professional field, see United States v. Texas State Bd. of Public Accountancy, 464 F. Supp. 400 (W.D. Tex. 1978), modified and aff'd, 592 F.2d 919 (5th Cir. 1979) (per curiam).

12. 421 U.S. 773 (1975).

13. See, for example, McLain v. Real Estate Bd., 444 U.S. 232 (1980) (fixing of commission and brokerage fees by members of the real estate board); Hospital Bldg. Co. v. Trustees of Rex Hosp., 425 U.S. 738 (1976) (alleged conspiracy to block the relocation and expansion of a private hospital); McDonald v. Saint Joseph's Hosp., 524 F. Supp. 122 (N.D. Ga. 1981) (alleged antitrust violation arising out of denial of physicians' applications for staff privileges at two hospitals).

14. See, for example, Michael Wines, "Reagan's Antitrust Line—Common Sense or an Invitation to Corporate Abuse?" *National Journal,* vol. 14 (July 10, 1982), pp. 1204–9.

15. See, for example, Arizona v. Maricopa County Medical Soc'y, 643 F.2d 553 (9th Cir. 1980), rev'd, 102 S.Ct. 2466 (1982); United States v. American Soc'y of Anesthesiologists, 473 F. Supp. 147 (S.D.N.Y. 1979).

16. See Arizona v. Maricopa County Medical Soc'y, 102 S.Ct. 2466, 2475–76 (1982); National Soc'y of Professional Eng'rs v. United States, 435 U.S. 679, 696 (1978); Bates v. State Bar, 433 U.S. 350, 368–72 (1977); Goldfarb v. Virginia State Bar, 421 U.S. 773, 788 n. 17 (1975); United States v. Oregon State Medical Soc'y, 343 U.S. 326, 336 (1952).

17. National Soc'y of Professional Eng'rs v. United States, 435 U.S. 679, 696 (1978).

18. Arizona v. Maricopa County Medical Soc'y, 102 S.Ct. 2466, 2475 (1982).

19. The nearest thing to a victory for a professional organization was American Medical Ass'n v. FTC, 452 U.S. 960 (1982) (per curiam), affirming, by an equally divided Court, 638 F.2d 443 (2d Cir. 1980). See also Arizona v. Maricopa County Medical Soc'y, 102 S.Ct. 2466 (1982). This 4–3 decision is discussed below in this chapter.

20. 102 S.Ct. 2466 (1982) at 2476.

21. See United States v. Addyston Pipe & Steel Co., 85 F. 271 (6th Cir. 1898), aff'd, 175 U.S. 211 (1899).

22. National Soc'y of Professional Eng'rs v. United States, 435 U.S. 679, 688 (1978).

23. 102 S.Ct. 2466, 2475 (1982), quoting James A. Rahl, "Price Competition and the Price Fixing Rule—Preface and Perspective," *Northwestern University Law Review,* vol. 57 (May–June 1962), p. 142.

24. Ibid., p. 2473.

25. See section below on "Provider Control of Financing Plans."

26. See Clark C. Havighurst and Glenn M. Hackbarth, "Enforcing the Rules of Free Enterprise in an Imperfect Market: The Case of Individual Practice Association," in Mancur Olson, ed., *A New Approach to the*

Economics of Health Care (Washington, D.C.: American Enterprise Institute, 1981), pp. 396–401.

27. In re American Medical Ass'n, 94 FTC 701 (1979), modified and enforced 638 F.2d 443 (2d Cir. 1980), affirmed by an equally divided Court, 452 U.S. 960 (1982) (per curiam).

28. 435 U.S. 679, 696 (1978).

29. Silver v. New York Stock Exchange, 373 U.S. 341, 360 (1963).

30. American Medical Ass'n v. FTC, 638 F.2d 443 (2d Cir. 1980), affirmed by an equally divided Court, 452 U.S. 960 (1982) (per curiam).

31. At this writing, a bill to deny the FTC jurisdiction over professional organizations was pending before Congress and was reported to have a good chance of passing. S. 2499, 97th Congress, 2d session (1982); Judy Sarasohn, "Panel's Vote Squeezing FTC May Threaten Authorization," *CQ Weekly Report,* vol. 40 (May 15, 1982), pp. 1131–32.

32. See Philip C. Kissam, "Applying Antitrust Law to Medical Credentialing," *American Journal of Law & Medicine,* vol. 7 (Spring 1981), pp. 1–31; Lewin and Associates, Inc., *Competition among Health Practitioners: The Influence of the Medical Profession on the Health Manpower Market* (Washington, D.C.: Federal Trade Commission, 1982), ch. 3.

33. Philip C. Kissam, William L. Webber, Lawrence W. Bigus, and John R. Holzgraefe, "Antitrust and Hospital Privileges: Testing the Conventional Wisdom," *California Law Review,* vol. 70 (May 1982), pp. 595–685; Andrew K. Dolan and Richard S. Ralston, "Hospital Admitting Privileges and the Sherman Act," *Houston Law Review,* vol. 18 (May 1981), pp. 707–78; Lewin and Associates, Inc., *Competition among Health Practitioners,* ch. 4.

34. See, for example, Robinson v. Magovern, 521 F. Supp. 842 (W.D. Pa. 1981).

35. See, for example, Dos Santos v. Columbus-Cunes-Cabrini Medical Center, 1982–2 Trade Cases (CCH) ¶64,887 (7th Cir. 1982) (anesthesiologists); Dattilo v. Tucson Gen. Hosp., 23 Ariz. App. 392, 533 P.2d 700 (1975) (nuclear medicine services); Centeno v. Roseville Community Hosp., 107 Cal. App. 3d Supp. 62, 167 Cal. Rptr. 183 (1979) (radiologists). But see Hyde v. Jefferson Parish Hosp., 1982–2 Trade Cases (CCH) ¶64,945 (5th Cir. 1982) (using tying theory to overturn exclusive contract with anesthesiologist group).

36. 624 F.2d 476 (4th Cir. 1980), cert. denied, 450 U.S. 916 (1982).

37. See, for example, Shaw v. Hospital Auth., 507 F.2d 625 (5th Cir. 1975) (podiatrist); Touchton v. River Dist. Community Hosp., 76 Mich. App. 251, 256 N.W.2d 455 (1977) (podiatrist); Stribling v. Jolley, 241 Mo. App. 1123, 253 W.2d 519 (1953) (osteopath); Greisman v. Newcomb Hosp., 40 N.J. 389, 192 A.2d 817 (1913) (osteopath seeking privileges at private hospital). See also "Antitrust Suit Claims JCAH Bars Psychologist," *Medical World News,* vol. 21 (February 4, 1980), pp. 26–27.

38. See Lewin and Associates, Inc., *Competition among Health Practitioners.*

39. Federal Trade Commission, Bureau of Competition, *Staff Report on Medical Participation in Control of Blue Shield and Certain Other Open-Panel Medical Prepayment Plans,* April 1979; 46 Fed. Reg. 48982 (1981).

40. For a discussion of percentage tests, see 46 Fed. Reg. 48982 (1981).

41. On the distinction between naked restraints and restraints occurring in the context of a joint venture, see Arizona v. Maricopa County Medical Soc'y, 102 S.Ct. 2466, 2479–80 (1982).

42. See discussion of the *Maricopa County* case above in the section on the "Implications of the Law's Strict Insistence on Competition"; also see Havighurst and Hackbarth, "Enforcing the Rules of Free Enterprise in an Imperfect Market."

43. In re Michigan State Medical Soc'y, 3 Trade Reg. Rep. (CCH) ¶21,836 (FTC Dkt. No. 9129, June 30, 1981).

44. See Havighurst, "Professional Restraints on Innovation in Health Care Financing," pp. 343–68.

45. Columbia River Co. v. Hinton, 315 U.S. 143 (1942); United States Steel Corp. v. Fraternal Ass'n of Steelhaulers, 1970 Trade Cases (CCH) ¶73,187 (W.D. Pa. 1970), aff'd, 431 F.2d 1046 (3d Cir. 1970).

46. Ohio v. Greater Cleveland Hosp. Ass'n, No. C80-1305 (W.D. Ohio, filed July 25, 1980).

47. But see United States v. American Soc'y of Anesthesiologists, 473 F. Supp. 147 (S.D.N.Y. 1979). Compare Clark C. Havighurst and Philip C. Kissam, "The Antitrust Implications of Relative Value Studies in Medicine," *Journal of Health Politics, Policy and Law,* vol. 4 (Winter 1979), pp. 48–86, with Rickard F. Pfizenmayer, "Antitrust Law and Collective Physician Negotiation with Third Parties: The Relative Value Guide Object Lesson," *Journal of Health Politics, Policy and Law,* vol. 7 (Spring 1982), pp. 128–62. Many of the arguments in the latter critique would seem to be refuted by the Supreme Court's decision in the *Maricopa County* case.

48. 102 S.Ct. 2466, 2477 (1982).

49. Ibid. The Court relied primarily on the practice of using pharmacy agreements documented in *Group Life & Health Ins. Co. v. Royal Drug Co.,* 440 U.S. 205 (1979). Physicians have seldom been employed on a similar contract basis.

50. Union Labor Life Ins. Co. v. Pireno, 102 S.Ct. 3002 (1982).

51. The FTC has indicated a willingness to allow peer review of professional fees for insurers if the program is kept purely voluntary. Iowa Dental Association, 3 Trade Reg. Rep. (CCH) ¶21,918 (FTC Advisory Opinion, April 9, 1982).

52. Recent amendments to the federal legislation on peer review, which repealed earlier provisions creating Professional Standards Review Organizations, require the successors of these peer-review organizations to make their "facilities and resources" available to private financing plans. Though helpful in giving insurers a new means of implementing their contractual limitations on coverage at the local level, this legislation does not appear to change the antitrust status of such an organization's acceptance of delegated

responsibility for generally defining what services should and should not be paid for.

53. On the importance of breaking down professional authority, see Clark C. Havighurst, "Decentralizing Decision Making: Private Contract versus Professional Norms," chapter 2 in this volume.

54. American Medical Ass'n v. FTC, 638 F.2d at 443, aff'd by an equally divided Court, 452 U.S. 960 (1982) (per curiam).

55. "FTC Judge Orders Indiana Dentist Group to Dissolve, End Boycott of Insurance Companies," *Antitrust & Trade Regulation Report,* No. 958 (April 3, 1980), pp. A-13 and A-14.

56. See, for example, Ohio ex. rel. Brown v. Mahoning County Medical Soc'y, 5 Trade Reg. Rep. (CCH) (1982-1 Trade Cases) ¶64,557 (Jan. 22, 1982) (consent decree); United States v. Halifax Hosp. Medical Center, 1981-1 Trade Cases (CCH) ¶64,151 (June 24, 1981) (consent decree); In re Forbes Health Sys. Medical Staff, 3 Trade Reg. Rep. (CCH) ¶21,656 (FTC Dkt. No. C-2994, Oct. 15, 1979) (consent decree).

57. Ibid.

58. See National Gerimedical Hosp. & Gerontology Center v. Blue Cross, 452 U.S. 378 (1981).

59. Letter from Sanford M. Litvack, assistant attorney general, Antitrust Division, U.S. Department of Justice, in the matter of Central Virginia Health Systems Agency, May 6, 1980.

60. See Clark C. Havighurst, *Deregulating the Health Care Industry* (Cambridge, Mass.: Ballinger Publishing Company, 1982), pp. 159–76.

61. In re American Medical International, Inc., 3 Trade Reg. Rep. (CCH) ¶21,851 (July 30, 1981) (complaint); "Justice Opposes Merger in Nursing Home Industry," *Antitrust & Trade Regulation Report,* vol. 42 (April 22, 1982), p. 823.

62. 440 U.S. 205 (1979).

63. See, for example, Sausalito Pharmacy v. Blue Shield, 1981-1 Trade Cases (CCH) ¶63,885 (N.D. Cal. 1981), aff'd per curiam, 677 F.2d 47 (9th Cir. 1982); Medical Arts Pharmacy v. Blue Cross and Blue Shield, 518 F. Supp. 1100 (D. Conn. 1981), aff'd per curiam, 675 F.2d 502 (2d Cir. 1982).

64. See Quality Auto Body, Inc. v. Allstate Ins. Co., 1981–2 Trade Cases (CCH) ¶64,303 (7th Cir. 1981); Chick's Auto Body v. State Farm Mut. Auto Ins. Co., 168 N.J. Super. 68, 401 A.2d 722 (1979), aff'd per curiam, 176 N.J. Super. 320, 423 A.2d 311 (1980).

65. In addition to the cases already discussed, two other cases increased the exposure to private treble-damage remedies of defendants in cases involving professional restraints of trade. Blue Shield of Virginia v. McCready, 102 S.Ct. 2540 (1982) (recovery allowed for cost of patronizing nonphysician providers illegally excluded from insurance coverage); American Soc'y of Mechanical Eng'rs, Inc. v. Hydrolevel Corp., 102 S.Ct. 1935 (1982) (recovery allowed against organization sponsoring industrial standard-setting programs for anticompetitive abuses by some professional participants).

16

Health and Antitrust:
The Case for Legislative Relief

William G. Kopit

Although the Sherman Act—the first federal antitrust statute—was enacted in 1890, the wholesale application of antitrust laws and policies to the health care field only began in the mid-1970s. Before then, the conventional wisdom held that health care was exempt from the application of the antitrust laws.[1] Perhaps the most famous judicial expression of the exemption was contained in the 1952 case of *United States* v. *Oregon State Medical Society,* in which the Supreme Court stated:

> Since no concerted refusal to deal with private health associations has been proved, we need not decide whether it would violate the antitrust laws. We might observe in passing, however, that there are ethical considerations where the historic direct relationship between patient and physician is involved which are quite different from the usual considerations prevailing in ordinary commercial matters. This court has recognized that forms of competition usual in the business world may be demoralizing to the ethical standards of a profession.[2]

While the above statement was dictum, it was nonetheless dictum that was widely accepted as an accurate statement of the law of the land. As one prominent commentator on the subject put it, the medical profession, like the other learned professions, enjoyed a "virtual exception from the antitrust laws" from the enactment of the Sherman Act in 1890 until the mid-1970s.[3]

This widespread assumption of immunity was, however, dramatically and abruptly brought to an end in 1975 by the case of *Goldfarb* v.

NOTE: Prepared for the American Enterprise Institute's Task Force on Legal Issues relating to the competition proposals. Several of the ideas regarding practices requiring legislative clarification were taken from a list submitted to the task force by John Hoff, one of its other members. The complete list appears in the appendix to this chapter.

Virginia State Bar.[4] In that case, the Supreme Court unanimously rejected any claim to a "professional" exemption. As stated by the Court:

> The nature of an occupation, standing alone, does not provide sanctuary from the Sherman Act . . . nor is the public service aspect of professional practice controlling in determining whether section 1 [of the Sherman Act] includes professions.[5]

If *Goldfarb* left any lingering doubt regarding the vitality of a professional exemption, that doubt was laid to rest by the Supreme Court's 1978 decision in the case of *National Society of the Professional Engineers* v. *United States.*[6] This case involved the canons of ethics of the National Society of Professional Engineers, which included a prohibition against competitive bidding for engineering services. The defendants' rationale for the prohibition involved a claim that competition could adversely affect the quality of service provided and thus create danger to the public health and safety. The Supreme Court refused to accept this claim, stating that the proper role of the courts in applying the Sherman Act to professional conduct was to "form a judgment about the competitive significance of the restraint . . . not to decide whether public policy favoring competition is in the public interest or in the interest of the members of an industry."[7]

Thus, there can no longer be any doubt that a professional exemption providing broad protection for the actions of physicians or others involved in the health care field is dead. It is far less clear, however, whether there are, nonetheless, circumstances that can be used to distinguish restraints in the health field from those accomplished in a purely commercial area. In footnote 17 of the *Goldfarb* case itself, for example, the Supreme Court explicitly mentioned the existence of possible differences between the professions and purely commercial activities. As stated by the Court:

> The fact that a restraint operates upon a profession as distinguished from a business is, of course, relevant in determining whether that particular restraint violates the Sherman Act. It would be unrealistic to view the practice of professions as interchangeable with other business activities, and automatically to apply to the profession's antitrust concepts which originated in other areas. The public service aspect, and other features of the professions, may require that a particular practice, which could properly be viewed as a violation of the Sherman Act in another context, be treated differently. We intimate no view on any other situation than the one with which we are confronted.[8]

In *Professional Engineers,* that view was subsequently reiterated, if somewhat narrowed. There the Court again acknowledged that "by their nature, professional services may differ significantly from other business services, and accordingly, the nature of the competition in such services may vary."[9]

Significantly, the Court's emphasis shifted from differences imposed by public policy to competitive differences imposed by the nature of the market. Still, just what those differences might be, and how they might affect the outcome of litigation, was not discussed in either case.

The Supreme Court's emphasis again appears to have shifted in the more recent case of Arizona and Maricopa County Medical Society (June 18, 1982).[10] In that case a Medical Care Foundation established maximum allowable fees for participating physicians in foundation-sponsored insurance programs. In a decision the Supreme Court held that the arrangement was price fixing, a per se violation of the antitrust laws. The Court said, "the respondents' claim for relief for the per se rule is simply that the doctors' agreement not to charge certain insurers more than a fixed price facilitates the successful marketing of an attractive insurance plan. But the claim that the price restraint will make it easier for customers to pay does not distinguish the medical profession from any other provider of goods or services."

The Court then went on to reiterate that "the public service aspect and other features of the profession may require that a particular practice, which could properly be viewed as a violation of the Sherman Act in another context, be treated differently." However, the Court concluded that in *Maricopa* the arrangement was not premised on public service, ethical norms, or quality of care consideration.

Thus, it is still fair to say that ninety years after the enactment of the Sherman Act, we have no clear idea of exactly how the antitrust laws apply in the health field. As stated by one proponent of antitrust enforcement in health care, the "application of antitrust laws to the professions . . . is, in some respects, still in its infancy."[11] A less polite way of characterizing the situation is that it involves both substantial confusion and uncertainty.

Imprecision of Antitrust Principles

Before discussing the effects of this uncertainty, it may be useful to make a general point about antitrust principles: For the most part, they are imprecise. As stated by the Federal Trade Commission in a recent publication:

> As with most other facets of antitrust law, very few precise or hard and fast rules can be given in this area, because such rules

usually cannot take into account the many variables that may affect a practice's competitive impact.[12]

Perhaps the most imprecise standard of all is the so-called rule of reason.

In order to simplify and clarify the rules regarding the antitrust laws, one thing the courts have attempted to do is to carve out from the rule of reason certain practices that are so completely without justification that they can be termed per se illegal. Those practices are treated as illegal, without regard to their purpose and effect.[13] However, the "courts have been reluctant to adopt wholesale characterizations developed in other commercial contexts" in determining whether a per se approach should be used in the health care field.[14]

Therefore, health care issues, for the most part, will continue to be guided only by the dim light of the rule of reason. Under this rule,

> There must be an examination of the purpose for which the parties have entered into the agreement or course of conduct and of the effects that have resulted or are likely to result from their concerted activity. Any pro-competitive effects are weighed against anti-competitive effects in determining whether the restraint, on balance, is unreasonable. This standard permits consideration of factors which are unique to a particular industry or profession, and it permits justification that relates not merely to price competition, but also to competition based on quality and convenience.[15]

Effects of Uncertainty

Unfortunately, the use of this amorphous standard, though perhaps necessary given the circumstances surrounding the health industry, merely serves to intensify the already high level of uncertainty that permeates the area because of the lack of judicial guidance and the differences in the health care market. As a result, the spectrum of possible antitrust enforcement is likely to have a chilling effect on a number of activities that most people would classify as laudatory or, at worst, benign.[16]

That this should be so is not surprising. Antitrust litigation can be long and costly—particularly under the rule-of-reason standard. Moreover, prevailing parties may receive attorneys' fees and the actual extent of any damages is multiplied by three under the treble damages provision—a point not lost on individuals making decisions, particularly as personal liability sometimes also may be assessed.[17] To make matters worse, any one of a group of defendants can be sued for all the alleged damages, not simply their respective share.[18]

To understand how this works in practice, it is helpful to describe some situations that highlight the problems. First, one should examine voluntary agreements by hospitals and/or other health providers to limit specified services. It is widely conceded that the rapid increases in the costs of health care have been created, in part, by unnecessary duplication of services. Thus, in many areas—particularly urban areas—there are far too many acute care hospital beds, as well as certain kinds of specialty beds such as those reserved for obstetrics/gynecology. Moreover, certain high-priced, high-technology equipment like computerized axial-tomographic (CAT) scanners have proliferated unnecessarily. Nevertheless, hospitals and other providers have no confidence that they can voluntarily agree to limit their services in conjunction with any kind of a mutually acceptable plan, even though they involve the state or local health planning agency.[19] The problem with such agreements restricting or limiting services is that in a purely commercial area they would be viewed as a "division of markets"—a per se offense. Although it could be argued that because health is different the activity should be judged under the rule of reason, this provides little security for those contemplating the conduct, particularly after *Maricopa County*. As a result, most health care providers simply eschew all opportunities for this type of voluntary concerted activity.

Hospital staff privileges provide another good example. Most people would agree that patients benefit if hospitals, in conjunction with their medical staffs, act to supervise the quality of care provided by those with staff privileges. The problem is that any exclusion or expulsion can be viewed as a group boycott—often treated as a per se offense, as well as an attempt to monopolize in areas where there are no other hospitals. Again, any possible assurance that the conduct probably would be evaluated under the rule of reason rather than the per se rule because of the unique characteristics of the health care market is unlikely to provide much comfort. The result is that hospitals and medical staffs are less willing to enforce quality standards rigorously, and the level of patient care suffers.

Individual voluntary not-for-profit hospitals are increasingly contemplating joint arrangements regarding shared services or purchasing as a means of competing more effectively with the proliferating large investor-owned hospital chains. These arrangements are obviously more effective if the participants can be selective—indeed, it is important that entry can be denied to competitors. Yet, this kind of conduct could be considered an illegal group boycott.

Business groups in about 100 cities are now organizing into health care coalitions in conjunction with labor, insurers, and providers. These groups are designed to reduce health care costs through the sharing of information and joint bargaining. Any such conduct, however, creates the danger of price-fixing and boycott charges.

327

Similar problems occur with health maintenance organizations (HMOs). Most health care observers, including those committed to the introduction of increased competition in health care, support the HMO concept. Indeed, perhaps more than any single element, HMOs have been responsible for injecting increased competition into the health care field over the last five years. To compete effectively, as well as to maintain standards of patient care, HMOs must be able to restrict participation by health professionals. However, attempts to exclude or expel a health care practitioner from participation are subject to the same claims that could be levied against hospitals with regard to staff privileges. The result has been a reluctance to act, with a concomitant diminution of effectiveness.

One final illustration regarding health maintenance organizations is perhaps in order. The Federal Health Maintenance Organization Act of 1973 specifically recognizes HMOs of the individual practice association (IPA) type. Moreover, the HMO census compiled by the federal office of HMOs demonstrates that, on the average, IPA-type HMOs perform almost as well as group-model HMOs, and twice as well as the non-HMO sector of the health care market with regard to hospitalization. IPA-type HMOs must establish a schedule of maximum physician fees for each type of procedure undertaken by physicians in order to establish the premium they will charge consumers. The problem is that the maximum payment schedule can be characterized as price fixing, a per se offense. Assurance of the possible application of joint venture analysis, as suggested by the Supreme Court in *Maricopa County,* does little to change the level of concern of participating IPA physicians. The full extent to which this fact has limited the growth and development of IPA-type HMOs is unclear, but it cannot have helped.

Need for Legislative Relief

The above examples provide evidence of the potentially deleterious effects of applying the antitrust laws to the health care field. Yet these examples are meant to be merely illustrative, not exhaustive. Indeed, many of the potential conflicts between sound public policy and antitrust enforcement in the health care area may not even be known at this time.[20]

Indeed, this very impossibility of defining standards that will deal adequately with all situations is perhaps the best argument against any broad-scale revision of the antitrust laws in the health care field.[21] It is not, however, a justification for inaction. There are activities—such as those listed above—that most people would agree should be permissible. Many of these can be identified. They should, therefore, be protected—by legislation. Because their underlying purpose is the encouragement of competition, the consumer choice proposals would be an ideal vehicle for such legislative relief of some kind.

The problems regarding the application of antitrust law to the health care industry would not, of course, be created by the "consumer choice" proposals. The problems exist now. Nevertheless, if these problems are not solved, they will create a potential incompatibility between the consumer choice proposals and antitrust that could serve to reduce substantially any beneficial competitive impacts such proposals could have if enacted.

Given the skeletal nature of most of the consumer choice proposals and the uncertain probabilities of their passage, it is impossible to provide a complete blueprint to ensure compatibility between the workings of these programs and the operation of the antitrust laws at this time. It is possible, however, to identify at least some of the critical activities that should be accorded antitrust protection.

All of the consumer choice proposals at least encourage a broad choice of insurers to the employed population. To make these choices meaningful to a purchasing employer or to the ultimate consumer, however, insuring entities must have the right to enter into agreements, including exclusive agreements, with groups of practitioners and providers. They must have the right to enter into preferential arrangements with hospitals and other providers. Such agreements should be accorded antitrust protection. Moreover, groups of practitioners should be permitted to exclude physicians—at least as long as the group does not have monopoly power.[22] Finally, employers must be free to get together—through business coalitions or otherwise—and share information and bargain collectively with insurers.[23]

Finally, other actions could be taken to encourage competition between competing plans, but these involve reducing restrictive state regulatory requirements—for example, capital and reserve requirements.[24] However, these probably require preemption of state laws—as well as the possible substitution of federal standards. In the present political climate, both are extremely unlikely, regardless of their desirability.

Appendix: Antitrust Issues in Health Care
John Hoff

At the AEI Legal Task Force meeting on September 28, I agreed to identify antitrust issues that, while already relevant under the present system, are likely to be more important under competition. I submit the following list for consideration. (The hypotheticals assume, where relevant, that all the hospitals in a community are involved in the conduct.)

1. May the hospitals agree on which one will perform what services to avoid duplication?

2. May they make joint purchases of equipment to be shared by them?

3. May they sell/lease excess capacity to each other?

4. May a hospital impose a condition upon membership on the medical staff that a member may not be a member of the staff of a competing hospital?

5. May health plans maintain lists of participating (nonemployed) providers and limit reimbursement to those providers?

6. May competing hospitals engage in joint efforts to recruit nurses or to operate nursing schools?

Notes

1. It is true that in 1943 the Supreme Court held that the American Medical Association and the District of Columbia Medical Society had violated the Sherman Act by conspiring against a prepaid health plan. American Medical Association v. United States, 317 U.S. 519 (1943). Nonetheless, this case appeared to be aberrational for the next thirty years.

2. 343 U.S. 326, 336 (1952).

3. Clark C. Havighurst, "The Antitrust Challenge to Professionalism," University of Maryland Law Review, vol. 41 (1981), p. 30.

4. 421 U.S. 773 (1975).

5. Ibid., p. 787.

6. 435 U.S. 679 (1978).

7. Ibid., p. 692.

8. 421 U.S. 773, 778 n. 17 (1975).

9. 435 U.S. 679, 696 (1978).

10. 102 S.Ct. 2466 (1982).

11. Pollard and Leibenluft, "Antitrust in the Health Professions," Policy Planning Issues Paper (Washington, D.C.: Federal Trade Commission, Office of Policy Planning, July 1981), p. 24.

12. Federal Trade Commission, "Enforcement Policy with Respect to Physician Agreements to Control Medical Prepayment Plans" (September 25, 1981), p. 5.

13. Assessing the general utility of the per se doctrine is obviously beyond the scope of this paper.

14. Pollard and Leibenluft, "Antitrust in the Health Professions," p. 32. This reluctance is entirely understandable. As previously mentioned, there is little court experience with health, and the workings of the health care marketplace are not fully understood. It has been widely recognized, moreover, that there are substantial differences between the health care industry and other areas. These differences include the fact that reimbursement for services is, for the most part, made on a "cost" basis, and that payment is

made by third-party payers rather than consumers of health care. Equally important, the field remains dominated by nonprofit institutions and professionals and, as a result, decisions typically are not made on a purely commercial basis.

15. Federal Trade Commission, "Enforcement Policy with Respect to Physician Agreements," p. 8.

16. The fact that the health care market remains dominated by small entities and people who perceive themselves as volunteers and/or professionals rather than businessmen probably means that the lack of certainty is more inhibitory than it would be in a commercial setting.

17. There is also a possibility of criminal enforcement, although this is less likely to inhibit those with any degree of sophistication undertaking reasonable ventures.

18. Those who undertake the activities without regard to the dangers may find that even a potentially successful antitrust defense is too costly.

19. In the recent case of National Gerimedical Hospital v. Blue Cross, 101 S.Ct. 2415 (1981), the Supreme Court rejected the claim that the Federal Health Planning Law created any broad-scale repeal of the antitrust laws. Although in footnote 18 of that decision the Court did hold out the hope that in certain cases a more limited immunity might be found, it provided no meaningful guidance on this subject.

20. This discussion is not meant to suggest either that the health care industry should be immune from the antitrust laws or that the application of the antitrust laws to the health field is always unclear. Certainly, there are many situations, such as medical society and hospital staff boycotts of physicians participating in HMOs, where antitrust principles clearly should be applied. Moreover, that can be done with certainty and substantial precision. Nevertheless, it remains true that the areas of antitrust uncertainty regarding health care are far larger and of far greater consequence than in commercial areas.

21. It is also argued that health care should not be singled out, because other areas need legislative relief as well. Although this may be true, it is not convincing. It amounts to saying that, if all problems cannot be solved, it is better to solve none.

22. In the absence of such protection, the legitimacy of such restraints could depend on whether the plan, the hospital, or the physician group was considered the relevant market. To date, no judicial guidance has been given on this important point.

23. Interestingly, insurers would be able to agree among themselves regarding the development of their premiums under existing law. See, for example, Proctor v. State Farm Mutual (Cir. Ct. D.C. March 16, 1982) (Civ. Action No. 249-72), CCH Trade Case # 64606.

24. These are unnecessary where there are contractual commitments to provide services.

A NOTE ON THE BOOK

This book was edited by Robert Faherty
and by Claire Theune of the
Publications Staff of the American Enterprise Institute.
The staff also designed the cover and format, with Pat Taylor.
The figures were drawn by Hördur Karlsson.
The text was set in Times Roman, a typeface designed by Stanley Morison.
Hendricks-Miller Typographic Company, of Washington, D.C.,
set the type, and R. R. Donnelley & Sons Company,
of Harrisonburg, Virginia, printed and bound the book,
using paper made by the S. D. Warren Company.

SELECTED AEI PUBLICATIONS

Meeting Human Needs: Toward a New Public Philosophy, Jack A. Meyer, ed. (469 pp., cloth $34.95, paper $13.95)

Medicaid Reimbursement of Nursing-Home Care, Paul L. Grimaldi (194 pp., cloth $15.95, paper $7.95)

A New Approach to the Economics of Health Care, Mancur Olson, ed. (502 pp., cloth $18.25, paper $10.25)

Drugs and Health: Economic Issues and Policy Objectives, Robert B. Helms, ed. (344 pp., cloth $16.25, paper $8.25)

International Supply of Medicines: Implications of U.S. Regulatory Reform, Robert B. Helms, ed. (156 pp., cloth $14.25, paper $6.25)

Tropical Diseases: Responses of Pharmaceutical Companies, Jack N. Behrman (80 pp., $4.25)

National Health Insurance: What Now, What Later, What Never? Mark V. Pauly, ed. (381 pp., cloth $16.25, paper $8.25)

National Health Insurance in Ontario: The Effects of a Policy of Cost Control, William S. Comanor (57 pp., $4.25)

National Health Insurance: Now, Later, Never? John Charles Daly, mod. (25 pp., $3.75)

Prices subject to change without notice.